Language Across the Curriculum

When Students Are Deaf or Hard of Hearing

B. Luetke-Stahlman, Ph.D.

Butte Publications, Inc.
Hillsboro, Oregon, USA

Language Across the Curriculum
When Students Are Deaf or Hard of Hearing
by B. Luetke-Stahlman, Ph.D.

Acknowledgments:
Editor: Jane Van Dusen
Design and Layout: Anita Jones

Butte Publications, Inc.
P.O. Box 1328
Hillsboro, OR 97123-1328
U.S.A.

ISBN: 1-884362-27-3

Dedication

This book is dedicated to

Deborah Sue Stryker
Nancy Sue Montgomery
Lisle Kauffman

my first doctoral students, without whom references and
publishers' permissions would never have been completed,

and to Kent Douglas, Breeze Elizabeth, Hannah Schell, Mary Pat,
and Marcy Anasova Luetke-Stahlman,
with love and gratitude.

Foreword

Readers who are familiar with Barbara Luetke-Stahlman's work will expect to find a nice blend of theory, research, and practice in her latest book, *Language Across the Curriculum*. This book will meet their expectations and more. In fact, Luetke-Stahlman makes it look easy to proceed from theoretical concepts to practical applications; however, this is a skill that cannot readily be accomplished without a great deal of effort.

The first line in Chapter 1 is a question, which actually sets the tone for the rest of the text: "What can team members do when students who are deaf or hard of hearing are not benefiting from general instruction?" Citing the theoretical concepts of Vygotsky (mediated learning), Cummins (communicative and academic proficiency), and others, Luetke-Stahlman provides interpretive perspectives on developing appropriate supports and services for these students. No stone appears to be left unturned; her ideas cover aspects of instruction, curriculum, assessment, and the physical learning environment. One of the most important recurring themes is the notion of accessibility, which from Luetke-Stahlman's perspective depends on prudent and critical modifications in language, mode of instruction, and other instructional factors.

The use of the words "across the curriculum" in the title is apt and descriptive, since instructional strategies for major areas of the curriculum are included. Chapters 2 and 3 focus on assessing and facilitating oral communication skills such as audition (hearing), speech, and speechreading; Chapter 4 addresses social interaction; Chapters 5 and 6 deal with reading; Chapter 7 covers writing; Chapter 8 focuses on spelling; Chapter 9 applies to mathematics; and Chapter 10 is centered on other school subjects including science, social studies, and current health issues. In every chapter, Luetke-Stahlman reminds us of the pervasive influence of the receptive and expressive power of language, especially for students who are deaf or hard of hearing.

Because of my deep fascination with literacy and deafness, I had a strong, biased interest in the contents of Chapters 5 through 8. Not only are these chapters well-written, comprehensive, and balanced, but they also enabled me to improve in my use of story mapping, networking, dialoguing, and mediating—all high-level skills that are necessary and important for developing proficient literacy skills in deaf and hard of hearing students and, indeed, in all students. Readers of this text will be amazed, as I was, with the devotion of a whole chapter to one of the most neglected areas in the field of deafness: spelling. Educators may have forgotten or may simply be unaware of the close connections among spelling (via writing), phonemic awareness, and proficient literacy ability. Even the simple process of copying words seems to strengthen children's memory and recognition skills. More important, as Luetke-Stahlman demonstrates nicely, the strong connection between knowledge of spelling patterns and sound patterns enhances the ability to remember or figure out how a "new" word is spelled.

Readers with strong biases and interests in the other areas (oral communication, social interaction, mathematics, and other school subjects) will not be disappointed with the comprehensive treatment by Luetke-Stahlman. In addition, it will become clear that this text is user friendly as well as extremely informative. In every chapter, the author provides a list of topics that will be discussed, references for further study, appendices and activities that clarify and enhance the contents of the chapter, and study guide questions that are strategically placed to facilitate the application and understanding of major chapter concepts.

There is no question that this text is accessible, informative, and a valuable contribution to the field of deafness. Readers will want to grab a second cup of coffee and proceed through this book again and again and again. But, as Luetke-Stahlman points out, rereading is a good way for any learner to approach a subject.

Peter V. Paul, Ph.D.
Professor of Education
School of Teaching and Learning
College of Education
The Ohio State University

Acknowledgments

This text could not have been written without the work of other researchers and professionals in the field of education and, more specifically, deaf education. I am very grateful for the research they have conducted, the strategies they have developed, and the practical materials they have provided to teachers.

I would especially like to thank the founder of Butte Publications, Matt Brink, who encouraged me to write this textbook series and who listened thoughtfully to my concerns throughout the entire process. He does every aspect of his job extremely well.

To my colleagues—Ruth Fletcher-Carter of New Mexico State University, Jess Freeman King of Utah State University, and Connie Mayer of the Metropolitan Toronto School for the Deaf—who reviewed an early draft of the text and made helpful comments, I am indebted. Ruth and Connie in particular provided me with the encouragement needed to complete a difficult project. In addition, my heart skipped a beat when I first read the introduction to this text written by Peter Paul. His comments continuously lifted my spirits.

I would also like to thank Lynn Hayes, Director of the Hartley Family Center, for her interest and support of my work and family. A big round of applause is also due Judy Conley, Secretary of the University of Kansas Medical Center, who was responsible for typing and formatting many drafts of each chapter. Judy was assisted by Nancy Montgomery and Deb Stryker, who will always have a warm place in my heart for all the hard work they did as my first doctoral students.

Thank you to my editors, Jane Van Dusen, Susan Blackaby, Ellen Todras, and Patricia Beis, as well as to Anita Jones, the designer of the text and of the cover.

My deep appreciation to Rebecca Villarreal, Instructional Supervisor for the Deaf in the Regional Day School for the Deaf, McAllen, Texas, for a friendship that I especially value. Many, many thanks to the principals, teachers, and support staff employed by the Olathe School District in Kansas, and others in the Kansas City area schools—they allowed me to visit their programs and watch them facilitate learning, and discussed with me many of the practices and materials suggested in this text.

A special thank you to those professionals and staff at Scarborough Elementary School in Olathe, Kansas—especially Cindy Griffiths, Nettie Johnson, Norina Meyers, Jo Taylor, and Beth Owens—who have taught my own daughters with such expertise for some eight years now. Many teachers, interpreters, and students at Scarborough served graciously as subjects for the pictures used in the learning modules that are now available on the world wide web site accompanying this text. Scarborough teachers of the deaf and students were also the subjects of countless videotapes I filmed and use for demonstration purposes during consultation and inservice workshops.

A kiss and a hug to Breeze (now 20), Hannah (15), Mary Pat (13), and Marcy (11), my children, for their understanding when I wasn't there mentally to give them the attention they deserved. I feel so lucky to be their mother, sharing their lives and watching them grow into independent thinkers.

And finally, a thank you "as big as the world wide web" to my husband and best friend, Kent. There aren't even words in the English language adequate to describe his support during the three years that I have been researching, writing, and revising these books. He held me in my darkest hours; hundreds of times he cooked dinner, cleaned house, and carted our children around town; and, all the while, he proclaimed his pride in my professional mission! I love you, Honey.

Contents

Introduction xiii

Chapter 1: Program, Curricular, and Instructional
Modifications..1

Appropriate Supports and Services...2
Mediated Instruction 13
Mediation and the Cummins Model 18
Mediation Strategies..19
Summary 34
Activities 34
Appendix 1–A: Programmatic and Curricular
    Modifications Checklist..35
Appendix 1–B: Examples of Using Programmatic and
    Curricular Modifications..43
Appendix 1–C: Incorporating Principles of Effective
    Instruction into Lessons 52
References 54

Chapter 2: Assessing and Facilitating Audition 59

Motivating Students to Listen to Speech 61
Assessment of Audition Abilities...62
Detection Assessment 66
Discrimination Assessment...71
Identification Assessment 75
Comprehension Assessment 77
Audition Curricula 79
Audition Facilitation 80
Summary 92
Activities 93
Appendix 2–A: Meaningful Auditory Integration Scale 94
References 102

Chapter 3: Assessing and Facilitating Speechreading
and Speech..105

Speechreading Assessment 106

Speechreading and the Cummins Model 107
Speechreading Facilitation 110
Speech Assessment 112
Speech Facilitation 118
Summary 140
Activities 140
Resources 141
Appendix 3–A. Meaningful Use of Speech Scale (MUSS)....142
References 149

Chapter 4: Social Interaction and Language 153

The Need for Attention to Social Interaction 154
Social Interaction Assessment.......................................155
Available Curricula..160
Social Integration Facilitation Strategies.........................162
The Adult's Role in Students' Social Interactions 168
Evaluation 171
Signing in Schools...173
Summary 177
Activities 177
Resources 178
Appendix 4–A: Formal Social Assessment Tools 179
Appendix 4–B: Children's Books about Deafness 182
References 183

Chapter 5: Reading to Students 187

Language and Reading 189
Reading Assessment..191
Facilitation of Text Reading and Comprehension 193
Adults Get Ready to Read..197
The Essential Practices 199
Examples of the Adult Reading Practices.........................222
Summary 229
Activities 229
Appendix 5–A: Making the Most of an Adult-Read Session:
     How Do You Rate?..230
Appendix 5–B: Examples of Text Structure Graphic
     Organizers 234
References 238

Chapter 6: Students Reading to Adults and Reading Independently 251

Day One: Rereading, New Read, and Analyzing 253
Day Two: Decoding Strategies and Facilitating Meaning 255
Day Three: Reinforcing Through Word Work and Writing 258
Day Four: Rereading and Response Activities 265
Independent Reading 269
Summary 271
Activities 271
Resources 272
Appendix 6–A: Making the Most of a Student Reading
    Session: How Do You Rate? 274
Appendix 6–B: Narrative Lesson Report 280
Appendix 6–C: Sight Word Learning: An Orthographic
    Strategy 284
Appendix 6–D: Activities to Extend Reading at School or
    at Home 285
Appendix 6–E: Literature to Hook Reluctant Readers 288
References 292

Chapter 7: Assessing and Facilitating Writing 295

Writing Assessment 296
Beginning Writers 301
Process Writing 303
Reading about Writing 315
Using Computers 316
Summary 318
Activities 318
Resources 319
Appendix 7–A: Six Trait Rubric 320
References 326

Chapter 8: Assessing and Facilitating Spelling 329

Spelling Assessment 330
Three Spelling Approaches 331
Phonological Awareness and Students Who Are D/HH 333
Spelling Facilitation 334
Summary 345

Activities 345
Appendix 8–A: Basic Sight Vocabulary List: The 200 Most
    Frequently Used Words..346
Appendix 8–B: Spelling and Phonics Monitoring Form 348
References 354

Chapter 9: Math and Language 357

Math Assessment 358
Cognition and Math 360
Semantics and Math..361
Syntax and Math..363
Teaching about Time and Money....................................364
Word Problems 365
Math Facilitation Tips 370
Summary 375
Activities 375
Resources 376
Appendix 9–A: Ten-Step Word Problem Worksheet 378
References 379

Chapter 10: Other School Subjects and Language 383

School Subject Assessment 384
Linguistic Demands of School Subjects............................385
Facilitating English Needed for School Subjects 390
Choosing Curricula 395
School Subject Facilitation..396
Using an Interpreter 401
Using Computers 403
Teaching about HIV/AIDS and Sexually Transmitted
    Disease 406
Summary 412
Activities 412
Resources 413
Appendix 10–A: Lesson Plan for Science............................423
Appendix 10–B: Recommended Computer Programs..........425
Appendix 10–C: Graphics Supporting the HIV/AIDS
    and STI Curriculum 429
References 432

Index 435

Introduction

In this text, I present models and techniques for assessment and facilitation of subject area skills when students are deaf or hard of hearing. This is the second of two texts: The companion is *Language Issues in Deaf Education* (Butte Publications, 1998) in which I discuss theories, issues, and procedures for language assessment and facilitation with these students. This second text focuses on how language needs affect speech, auditory training, socialization, reading, writing, math, and other school subjects. I present and explain numerous specific strategies for facilitating language development in the context of learning across the curriculum.

In writing this text, I have focused on procedures
- that are of benefit to students primarily ages 5 to 18
- that are applicable to students who use a variety of communication methods (oral English only, SEE, ASL, and so forth)
- that are useful across school subjects
- that encourage collaboration and collective problem solving

Both texts are replete with examples and graphics. I have included graphic organizers not only to highlight key points in the text but also to demonstrate the kinds of visualizations that can be useful to learners—be they students or educational team members!

Because terminology can be complex in deaf education, I want to clarify my use of some important terms. I have used
- the word "language" to mean "any language"
- the words "English" and "ASL" only when the intent was to specifically delineate one of these languages
- the word "system" primarily to mean English-with-the-hands, believing that grammatically-correct English can be made accessible in this way
- the terms "general education" or "general instruction" to apply to both public and residential school settings

In addition, I have used the term "team members" throughout the text to refer to those professionals who are involved with the education of a particular student as well as the student's parents or guardians. Traditionally, an administrator, the school psychologist, general and special education teachers, an educational interpreter, a speech-language pathologist, an audiologist, and the student's parents work together on this team. If the student receives other special services, representatives of these disciplines might also be team members.

Exciting adjuncts to this text are the Internet web sites containing units that parallel text chapters, including condensed versions of parts of the text, graphics, and photographs. We now teach two deaf education courses primarily using these world wide web sites. A set of interactive modules has also been developed that parallels text chapters and provides discussion topics, submission activities, and contact with others in the field of deaf education.

Join us on the web! For information, or to provide feedback on the text, e-mail Barbara Luetke-Stahlman: bluetke@kumc.edu

Chapter 1

Program, Curricular, and Instructional Modifications

Appropriate Supports and Services

Mediated Instruction

Mediation and the Cummins Model

Mediation Strategies

Appendix 1-A: Programmatic and Curricular Modifications Checklist

Appendix 1-B: Examples of Using Programmatic and Curricular Modifications

Appendix 1-C: Incorporating Principles of Effective Instruction into Lessons

What can team members do when students who are deaf or hard of hearing (D/HH) are not benefiting from general instruction? These students, as well as students who are language challenged in other ways (have learning disorders, mild mental retardation, are multi-lingual, and so forth), may require modifications in the learning environment, instruction, or activities. Specific adaptations in supports and services and a teaching strategy known as mediated instruction are described in this chapter.

Appropriate Supports and Services

Learning cannot occur if students who are deaf or hard of hearing do not have access to it. Providing access may involve modifying the languages or modes of instruction used along with numerous environmental and monitoring modifications. Team members should remember that the supports and services that provide access to learning for one student may differ from the supports and services required by another.

A review of adaptations that can be made in the school program and in the curriculum (Luetke-Stahlman, 1996) is presented in the checklists in Appendix 1–A and 1–B. Appendix 1–A is a more general form for listing activities or classes in which adaptations will be made, tracking who will ensure that adaptations are made and continued, and noting any comments made by team members. Appendix 1–B provides examples in a format that may be helpful when team members discuss specific school subjects. This appendix also includes a blank form which can be copied and adapted for trial use. These lists are not all-inclusive but will be of assistance to team members in discussing what is needed to enable individual students to achieve their academic and social potential (Luetke-Stahlman, 1996).

To facilitate learning for students who are D/HH, team members need to divide up responsibilities for (a) providing inservice sessions to determine the need for modifications and how they can be implemented, (b) planning monitoring procedures, and (c) collecting data to evaluate the effectiveness of adaptations. Team meetings concerning a student should be called whenever any team member is concerned about that student's needs. Such discussions provide opportunities to brainstorm strategies for adapting instruction or changing placement as required. An overview of the major categories of modifications follows.

Communication

The most common resource provided to students who are D/HH in inclusive settings is interpreter services (Egelston-Dodd, 1995). Students who are D/HH typically use some form of oral English or English sign at school (Woodward, Allen, & Schildroth, 1985). All students, however, should have access to the language of instruction as well as that of social interaction and be able to use their dominant language/system when involved in analytical conversations (Luetke-Stahlman, 1997). This means that hearing adults and students will need to make one or both of these accommodations:

- change their mode of communication to match that of the student who is D/HH
- enlist the skills of another person (an interpreter, teacher) to assist during instructional and social interactions

Federal laws in the United States mandate that all school-sponsored activities (instruction, recess, lunch, sports, holiday events) be accessible to all students. To comply with these laws, public school programs have modified the communicative environment for students who are D/HH in a variety of ways:

- offering sign instruction throughout the school day (see, for example, the ideas about social interaction in Chapter 4)
- hiring interpreters based on student need, not on availability or financial constraints
- training educational interpreters to conform to certain attitudes toward signing and signing skill
- monitoring those hired to ensure they follow the school's sign policy
- labeling objects and activities in the school with single signs, signed phrases, and English print

Linguistic Level

Team members may need to discuss the adaptation of the syntactic or semantic level of a particular language or system used with a particular student. To do so, they will need to
- collect current information about the use, meaning, and form abilities of the student
- involve the educational interpreter if one is employed
- monitor changes so that the language modeled for the student is at a developmentally appropriate level as much of the time as possible

It would be inappropriate for an educational interpreter to change the level of instructional language without first consulting with or being asked to do so by team members. If a student is not comprehending grammatical complexity, use of figurative English, or vocabulary used by the general education teacher, the interpreter should inform the teacher so that concerns can be addressed at the student's team meeting.

The Listening Environment

An ideal acoustic environment is critical to success for many students participating in an inclusive setting. "The combined effects of noise, reverberation, and distance can be devastating to the communication reception of a student who is [deaf or hard of hearing]" (Berry, 1988, p. 335).

Proper use of curtains, rugs, and acoustical tiles can benefit many students who are D/HH. Advocating for quieter alarms to inform hearing students that classes are beginning, changing, or ending and asking that peers make less noise during informal times at school may also be warranted. Students who can benefit from FM systems should be afforded this technology, and team members should know how to keep this equipment in proper working order. Captioning is a must have! There are over 60 libraries that produce closed captioned (CC) films and videotapes; the inclusion of captions or subtitles is indicated by the "CC" logo (Conway, 1990).

The Physical Environment

Teachers should seat students who are D/HH in locations where they can see adults and student speakers, yet be distanced from sounds such as hallway noise, air conditioners, pencil sharpeners, and so on. These students should not be seated in "special" locations that result in their being isolated or singled out (Berry, 1988). Two suggested placements are shown in Figure 1–1.

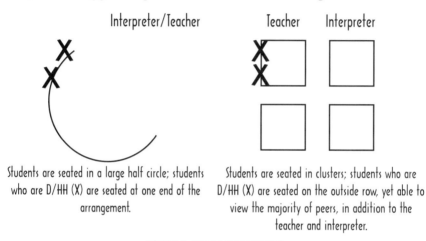

Interpreter/Teacher

Teacher   Interpreter

Students are seated in a large half circle; students who are D/HH (X) are seated at one end of the arrangement.

Students are seated in clusters; students who are D/HH (X) are seated on the outside row, yet able to view the majority of peers, in addition to the teacher and interpreter.

FIGURE 1–1: SEATING ARRANGEMENTS

Tests and Grading

Team members might work together to write school policy regarding the adaptation of student tests and grading schemes. Possibilities include providing test study guides that feature a variety of answer forms (essay, multiple choice, fill in the blank); giving frequent mini-tests; and using alternative response forms when existing formats appear to be a barrier to comprehension (Mercer & Mercer, 1989). Teachers might also give practice tests and have students test each other (Mercer & Mercer). Ample white space left between test questions, key words underlined in the directions and test items, use of simplified grammar whenever possible, and additional time may also be required. Students who have questions during a quiz or test should ask the teacher rather than the interpreter; the interpreter should interpret teacher responses only and should not respond to questions from students directly.

In adapting grading schemes, team members might consider criterion-referenced grading, curriculum-based measurement (CBM), self-referenced grading, norm-referenced criterion, and portfolio analysis. Any changes in grading schemes should be communicated to parents in writing prior to sending report cards home. Parents often miss or do not comprehend symbols used to indicate adaptations on report cards. Lack of this realization can cause confusion later when additional program, curricular, or placement modifications are discussed. Pass/fail grades should be avoided since they do not provide specific feedback (Mercer & Mercer, 1989).

Organizational Structure

The structure of the classroom can be discussed in the context of the following questions: Will personal assistance (a paraprofessional or student buddy) be needed to ensure appropriate participation for learning and socializing in the classroom? Would peer-mediated instruction be beneficial? Would it be helpful if an older or same-aged (hearing or deaf) peer tutored or coached the student? Is a notetaker needed? Students who are D/HH can also benefit from study skills training (for example, use of an assignment notebook), time management training, and clear expectations with regard to organization (Conway, 1990).

Rapport and Affect

All students should feel that they are equal members of the group. General education teachers may need to schedule a specific time to chat with the students who are D/HH. If teachers find they are not interacting with these students as often or as spontaneously as they do with others in the group, the teachers may need to learn how to use the interpreter. They may also need to be reminded to call on the student with at least the same frequency as they call on hearing peers and to monitor the frustration of students who are D/HH and academically or socially challenged. Conway (1990) reminded staff that inattention or negative behavior, especially in the later part of the day, may be a result of fatigue from watching either spoken or signed communication. Finally, all students need to cultivate peer friendships that are genuine and comfortable.

Instructional Format

Often students who are D/HH do not know as much about topics being discussed as do their hearing peers. As a result, content may need to be modified so that the key ideas, facts, and concepts can be understood. Procedures for adapting the instructional format are explained later in this chapter.

"The visualization of instruction is relevant to any population and especially so for deaf students" (Egelston-Dodd, 1995, p. 27). Teachers might reformat text to provide pictorial or graphic cues. They might supply wide margins so that students can add their own context to what is being read or studied. Context can be added in many different ways. Numerous ideas provided by teachers for adding context to English are presented below; additional adaptations are used daily by creative adults who work with students who are D/HH.

Ways to Supply Context to Help Students Comprehend Instruction

1. Clarify directions.
2. Define key vocabulary.
3. Encourage text-to-life, life-to-text connections.
4. Repeat what has been said more slowly.
5. Provide English or ASL sentence starters to help the students express their ideas.
6. Provide direct feedback about the appropriateness of students' ideas, comments, etc.
7. Use self talk, parallel talk, inform talk (see Luetke-Stahlman, 1998).
8. Use graphic organizers (Venn diagrams, word webs, etc.).
9. Use real objects.
10. Fingerspell signed words to build specific/technical vocabulary.
11. Role play.
12. Give multiple-choice options.
13. Pair English with ASL.
14. Use space, directionality, eye-gaze, etc.

15. Facilitate peer communication.
16. Practice/review related or prerequisite skills.
17. Use dash lines to cue spelling.
18. Use manipulatives to clarify math computation.
19. Use story frames or sentence starters to facilitate written responses to a story.
20. Use a book with a lower reading level for the same subject content.
21. Pair figures of speech with more literal translations.
22. Use or draw pictures.
23. Use captioned filmstrips and movies.
24. Provide oral interpreting.
25. Use colored pictures.
26. Use a computerized encyclopedia program.
27. Provide a notetaker.
28. Monitor seating arrangements.
29. Hire only certified, skilled educational interpreters.
30. Attend to the room acoustics.
31. Ensure that assistive listening devices are working.
32. Require the completion of fewer problems than peers are doing.
33. Provide linguistic access to all school events.
34. Chunk phrases when using complex sentences.
35. Use specific teaching strategies.
36. Implement efficient (assessment-based) lessons.
37. Teach spelling rules and word patterns.
38. Teach learning strategies.
39. Provide synonyms and definitions to new vocabulary.
40. Teach and require the six trait writing components (Chapter 7).
41. Demonstrate science experiments.
42. Use maps, globes, relief maps, topography maps, etc.
43. Use the format of student's learning style (visual, auditory, global learner).
44. Use videos.
45. Take field trips.
46. Make models.
47. Use visual phonics.

The use of learning centers is another way to adapt the instructional format. As suggested by Gearheart and Weishahn (1984), there are some advantages to using learning centers:

Study Guide Question
Review the list of ways to supply context when working with students who are D/HH. What would you add to this list?

- They provide an alternative to pencil and paper seatwork.
- They allow students to work at their own rate.
- They provide an opportunity to learn through various modes.
- They allow the teacher time to work with individuals or smaller groups.
- They help develop responsibility and foster self-discipline through accomplishment and success.
- They provide immediate self-evaluation.

Learning center content might parallel classroom instruction, provide review, or provide enrichment experiences and activities. Basic skill review centers, discovery or enrichment centers, and creativity centers are three types to consider using, always being sure to require use of key vocabulary and high-level thinking skills (Luetke-Stahlman & Luckner, 1991).

Instructional Language

In addition to the obvious techniques that teachers can employ to assist students who are D/HH (reducing their rate of communication, repeating themselves, avoiding meaningless hand movements), there are several specific strategies that can be used so that instructional and social language is comprehensible. Primary among these is being conscious of the student's English language level, as well as ASL language level when appropriate (for an assessment and tracking system, see Luetke-Stahlman, 1997). Conway (1990) suggested that the language level used by adults should be slightly above the student's currently assessed abilities in the areas of use, meaning, and form.

Berry (1988) stated that a difficult task for a student who is D/HH is to determine when the topic of conversation has shifted. Teachers should develop a signal and alert a student of such shifts

("*We were talking about urban or city areas, and Rieka said she has a grandmother who lives on a farm in a rural area*"). To help students who are attempting to speechread, adults should keep their voices at an appropriate volume, keep hands away from their faces, and remain facing the student (many teachers of the deaf have learned to write on the board while facing the class!).

To reduce the complexity of the language, a teacher might state a thought in a typical way and then proceed with the following strategies:

- Repeat the thought.
- Substitute familiar words for difficult ones ("*The peacock— that bird with the beautiful tail feathers—lives in this habitat— place*").
- Change word order (change "*Go outside after lunch*" to "*After lunch go outside*").
- Reduce complexity ("*Eat lunch. Go outside.*").
- Chunk clauses (follow "*The littlest goat went across the bridge*" with clauses separated by a pause: "*The littlest goat . . . went across the bridge*").
- Translate figurative expressions ("*The wind rolled—blew— across the plain*").

To increase the redundancy of the message, adults can employ natural mime, gesture, and pointing; use facial expressions; and add synonyms, definitions, and critical features to explain important terms. Figure 1–8, provided later in this chapter, is an example of a worksheet used to assist with such adaptations. Berry (1988) suggested including repeating and rephrasing (paraphrasing) in instructional language for students who are D/HH.

Lesson Format

Often the pacing of new information needs to be slowed for students who are D/HH to allow time for comprehending teacher comments and questions, as well as student comments and questions. If information is provided too quickly and lag time is not provided by interpreters in public schools, these students cannot participate and do not have an equal opportunity to learn. Using effective principles of instruction and question prompts (explained later in this chapter) along with learning strategies may be required to help students who are D/HH access learning.

Materials

When a student who is D/HH is not successful in the general educational classroom, your team might focus on the desired outcomes of the lesson: What is to be learned that is important in life? In addition, Gallagher (1988) provided examples of alterations that can be made to existing materials to enhance students' chances for success. These examples include clarifying directions; covering the same material at a lower reading level; and reading (and signing) to the student with materials that use simpler sentences, less figurative English, and easier vocabulary words. She also suggested highlighting essential information and providing a set of books for home.

Comprehension Checking

Teachers may need to adapt the curriculum by asking students who are D/HH to respond frequently to comprehension questions— perhaps more frequently than their hearing peers. When students who are D/HH are asked to repeat what others have said, adults might request that they use new key vocabulary and phrases to provide more practice.

Activities

Team members may need to provide alternate activities for students who are D/HH in lieu of classroom assignments that are too difficult. If such an adaptation is made often, team members would need to discuss the value of the placement in the general classroom. This placement should be based on student need and not on economic considerations. It may be that a student can learn more efficiently if seen by a teacher of the deaf in a contained classroom setting. In public schools, hearing students might be asked to join such students in the resource or speech room for some activities as well.

Assignment Completion

Teachers should be mindful that time away from class for tutoring or other special needs makes it difficult for students who are D/HH to complete as much work as their hearing peers. Therefore, teachers should consider presenting work to be completed by these students in small amounts or prioritizing assignments and grading accordingly. Discussion about information provided or missed can be a learning experience in itself. Adults should provide parallel examples and allow a student to rethink questions or comments. Specific feedback without giving the answers away will be more useful to the student than general comments (see Table 1–1).

TABLE 1–1: EXAMPLES OF FEEDBACK WHEN DISCUSSING ASSIGNMENTS

General Comments	Specific Feedback
Oh, you did some nice work here.	You listed a screw, a wedge, and an incline plane as simple machines. You needed one more. Can you think of another one now?
Oops, you were confused here.	You wrote down these bodies of water from smallest to largest—puddle, stream, river, ocean—but you missed a few. If I add lines where you needed other bodies of water, can you fill them in?

Monitoring

Conway (1990) noted that students who are D/HH may be unaware of their comprehension difficulties and may lack the strategies necessary to request clarification or additional information. Therefore, consistent monitoring is absolutely necessary (Berry, 1988). Students may require daily or weekly monitoring of assignments turned in, projects in process, books being read, and so forth. Most families appreciate a home/school communication form, and these need not be time consuming to complete.

Placement

A full range of placement options should be discussed at least annually in team meetings. The placement options listed in Section XIV of Appendix 1–A are only examples. To ensure an *appropriate* education, a wide variety of options could be created for meeting the academic and social needs of students who are D/HH.

Mediated Instruction

Many of the curricular modifications discussed above could be labeled "mediated instruction." Mediated instruction is known by a number of different terms including "mediated learning strategies," "instructional conversation," "the mediated learning experience," "constructivist instruction," and "scaffolding" (Figure 1–2). The terms refer to particular ways in which students are guided by more mature learners (adults) until independent comprehension is possible (Winne & Marx, 1983; Wittrock, 1983). Such instruction has been recommended when students do not demonstrate an age-appropriate English language base (Echevarria & McDonough, 1995; Pressley, Harris, & Marks, 1992).

Study Guide Questions

1. Show the blank form provided in Appendix 1–B to a teacher. How would she or he complete it for a student who is D/HH?

2. Can you and a peer select three placements from the options provided in Section XIV of Appendix 1–A that might be appropriate for a student you work with or know about?

3. What information would you include in an inservice session about supports and services that are appropriate for compliance with federal law?

Facilitation
Co-construction
Mediated Learning
Instructional Conversation
Mediated Learning Experience
Constructivist Instruction
Scaffolding
Guided Learning

FIGURE 1–2: TERMS FOR MEDIATED INSTRUCTION

The concept of mediated instruction emerged from work by Vygotsky and his notion of a "zone of proximal development" (Vygotsky, 1962, 1978). However, earlier theorists—including Binet (1909), Dewey (1916), and Piaget (1967)—emphasized guided learning in academic contexts in which adults acted as catalysts for students' comprehension. The zone of proximal development has been described as the distance between thinking about something independently and thinking about it when assisted or mediated by a more competent person (Figure 1–3).

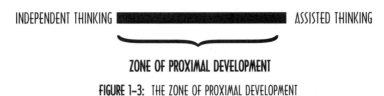

INDEPENDENT THINKING ▰▰▰▰▰▰▰▰▰▰▰▰ ASSISTED THINKING

ZONE OF PROXIMAL DEVELOPMENT

FIGURE 1–3: THE ZONE OF PROXIMAL DEVELOPMENT

The role of adults in mediated instruction is one of facilitation, co-construction, or scaffolding (Bruner, 1968), helping each student to understand academic material that could not otherwise be comprehended independently (Echevarria & McDonough, 1995). Providing students who are D/HH with mediated instruction will surely result in the positive learning effects that hearing monolingual and bilingual students have experienced (Brown & Palincsar, 1982; Chamot, 1985; Cummins, 1984; Durkin, 1995; Echevarria & McDonough, 1995; Feuerstein & Jensen, 1980; O'Malley & Chamot, 1986; Ortiz, 1986; Poplin & Stone, 1992; Palincsar & Brown, 1984).

 ## Scaffold = Help to understand what can't be comprehended independently

Nelson (1995) provided a useful table of the philosophy and tools of mediated instruction (scaffolding). It is adapted in Table 1–2 to serve as a checklist for team members as this important concept is discussed and integrated across the curriculum.

TABLE 1–2: THE PHILOSOPHY AND TOOLS OF MEDIATED INSTRUCTION

Base actions on beliefs about relevant learning.

____ ▸ Believe that change is possible.

____ ▸ Keep sense-making, active learning, and constructivist thinking as the goal.

____ ▸ Appreciate the instructional value of transactional conversations and value divergent questions and answers as much as convergent ones.

____ ▸ Keep the general education curriculum and real-life communication demands in focus.

____ ▸ Collaborate with parents, teachers, and the student to identify zones of significance based on the needs of the learner.

____ ▸ Remember that definitions of *sense* vary for members of different cultures.

Use contextually based assessment strategies.

____ ▸ Design assessment tools to match curriculum concepts.

____ ▸ Use participant observation to look at the experience through the lens of the learner.

____ ▸ Consider the communication demands of the context.

____ ▸ Consider both what a learner say/signs and what a learner does as evidence of internalized processing.

____ ▸ Compare observed responses with expected responses.

____ ▸ Identify new knowledge, skills, grammar, and strategies the learner would need to function more successfully in similar contexts.

Select facilitation contexts in consultation with others.

____ ▸ Select facilitation targets on the basis of the learner's needs and priorities.

____ ▸ Decide where to facilitate learning.

____ ▸ Involve the student's whole team in the change process.

____ ▸ Convey the attitude that professionals should collaborate.

Use mediation techniques to build independence.

____ ▸ Segment the experience into manageable chunks without violating its wholeness.

____ ▸ Keep in mind the knowledge, skills, grammar, and strategies identified through assessment.

____ ▸ Foster a better match between sense-making justified by the information and its processing by the student.

____ ▸ Use questioning strategies to assist more than to assess.

____ ▸ Provide feedback that focuses the learner's attention on mismatches between observed response and expected response.

cont.

From "Scaffolding in the Secondary School: A Tool for Curriculum-Based Intervention," by N. Nelson, 1995, in D. Tibbits (Ed.), *Language Intervention*, pp. 375-419. Austin, TX: Pro-Ed. Copyright 1995 by Pro-Ed. Adapted with permission.

TABLE 1–2, CONT.

___ ‣ Encourage the learner to verbalize observations about points of mismatch and to paraphrase where appropriate.
___ ‣ Frame significant features that support sense-making.
___ ‣ Point out regularities and patterns that have meaning across contexts.
___ ‣ Look for opportunities to review and reinforce newly acquired knowledge, skills, grammar, and strategies.
___ ‣ Encourage the learner to take risks, not to be afraid to make mistakes, and to identify mistakes independently.
___ ‣ Provide brief instruction whenever teachable moments present themselves.
___ ‣ Coach or tutor before, during, and after lessons, as appropriate.
___ ‣ Keep the process moving forward.
___ ‣ Encourage completion of products and a sense of competence.

Help the learner acquire metacognitive tools.
___ ‣ Use questions to guide actions, organize concepts, and support retrieval from memory.
___ ‣ Transplant questions from the mind of the facilitator to the mind of the learner.
___ ‣ Help the learner acquire organizing cognitive structures for evaluating, grouping, and sequencing perceptions, memories, and actions.
___ ‣ Help the learner acquire mnemonic strategies.
___ ‣ Encourage reflection and recognition of learning opportunities associated with mistakes.
___ ‣ Encourage reflection and self-appreciation associated with successes.

Be accountable for relevant and lasting change.
___ ‣ Provide no more scaffolding support than necessary.
___ ‣ Keep checking on independent competence in real contexts.
___ ‣ Systematically "up the ante" and challenge the student.
___ ‣ Document success in terms of functional outcomes.
___ ‣ Periodically stand back and survey collaboratively for new concepts that are challenging.

Norris and Hoffman (1993) noted that language is both enhanced and serves as a tool for learning when team members use mediation strategies (Figure 1–4). Mediated instruction strategies (rather than incidental learning, lectures by teachers, or worksheets done with teacher supervision) are advocated in this textbook as the preferred method for students who are D/HH.

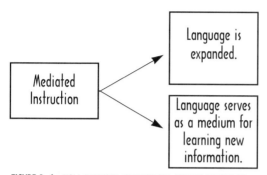

FIGURE 1–4: HOW MEDIATED INSTRUCTION AFFECTS LANGUAGE

Mediated instruction enables a high degree of student participation, regardless of the student's language abilities (Echevarria & McDonough, 1995). Three suggested reading methods (discussed in Chapters 5 and 6) that exemplify this principle are read alouds, shared reading, and adult-guided reading (also referred to as directed reading). In these active reading situations, as well as those involving instructional conversation and process writing in other subject areas, the teacher's role is neither to lecture nor control, but rather to "decenter" (Webster, Beveridge, & Reed, 1996) and create a nonthreatening atmosphere in which all students' contributions are accepted. Figure 1–5 presents some examples of mediated experiences.

Study Guide Questions

1. One college professor lectures for two hours of a weekly, evening course. Another professor lectures for 15–20 minutes, breaks into discussion groups, lectures for another 15–20 minutes, shows a demonstration video, lectures for another 15–20 minutes, and then has students role play in pairs. How are each of these professors demonstrating or not demonstrating mediated instruction?

2. How might study guide questions, graphics, and applied activities such as those supplied throughout this text be examples of devices that mediate learning?

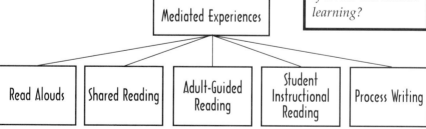

FIGURE 1–5: EXAMPLES OF MEDIATED EXPERIENCES

Mediation and the Cummins Model

Cummins (1981), a Canadian researcher working in the field of hearing bilingual education, found that academic learning is influenced both by the amount of context provided and the degree of cognitive demand in the language used in the classroom (Figure 1–6). The language used in academics, for instance, is sometimes referred to as "decontextualized" because it is abstract and removed from the immediate setting (Durkin, 1995).

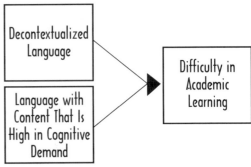

FIGURE 1–6: LANGUAGE CHARACTERISTICS INFLUENCE ACADEMIC LEARNING

Team members can use many strategies (appropriate supports and services, analytical conversations, effective instruction, mediated learning) to make academic language comprehensible. The Cummins model, shown in Figure 1–7 (and discussed more extensively by Luetke-Stahlman, 1998), provides a means of discussing which strategies can be used to assist a student who is D/HH participate with peers in acquiring age-appropriate subject matter (science, social studies, math, and so forth). Demonstrating the use of this model, some of the key strategies discussed in this chapter are plotted in the upper left quadrant of the model, on the side characterized by the inclusion of context.

Cognitively Demanding

■ use graphic organizers
■ teach learning strategies
■ shape independence
■ collaborate   C   D

Context   Context
Embedded   Reduced

                 A   B

Cognitively Undemanding

FIGURE 1–7: THE CUMMINS MODEL AND MEDIATION STRATEGIES

Mediation Strategies

Mediation strategies include a wide range of techniques varying from adapting conversational content to using learning centers and graphic organizers. General strategies for facilitating school subject learning in students who are D/HH are presented in this section. Strategies specific to particular subject areas are presented in later chapters. When students are provided these strategies they may be better able to comprehend subject content *without a need to lower typical (age-appropriate) academic expectations.*

Use Analytical Conversation

As illustrated in Figure 1–7, team members can assist students to understand cognitively demanding content. Dickinson and Smith (1994) suggested that the type of conversation used in this assistance is as important as the cognitive concepts presented.

   The type of conversation is as important as the subject content.

Goldenberg (1991) encouraged teachers to "weave participants comments into a larger tapestry of meaning" during mediated instruction to the cognitive benefit of all learners (p. 3). Students who are D/HH should be placed with general or special education teachers who are committed to dialogue, engaging them in conversations about what they are learning in school. These conversations are cognitively challenging in that students are asked to reflect on what they have learned, compare new concepts to acquired ones, make inferences and judgments, and so forth.

Many researchers and educators have suggested that for students to comprehend the cognitive and linguistic operations of school, they must be involved in interactions that are cognitively challenging, that is, requiring the understanding and use of extended discourse (de Villiers, 1995; Dickinson & Smith, 1994; Idol & Jones, 1991; Snow, Cancino, Gonzales, & Shribert, 1989). Cognitively challenging conversations (or analytical conversations) have been

defined by Dickinson and Smith (1994) as those involving
- the meaning of English vocabulary and grammar
- the perspective of others
- nonpresent events and prediction
- character, element, or event analysis
- summaries of extended discourse or text
- evaluation of new information
- explicit discussion of emotional states

 Challenging conversational interactions ⟶ **Improved academic comprehension**

Watson (1989) found that parents' use of cognitive verbs (thinking, considering) and superordinate terms (categories of objects such as furniture, vehicles, continents) had positive influences on students' cognitive and metalinguistic abilities at school. Teachers should also expand on students' linguistic learning and on the meaning of student comments by
- using semantically related utterances (recasting the meaning of information students are attempting to express)
- paraphrasing verbal (sign or voice) or written information
- adding distinguishing information to define how vocabulary or concepts are alike and unlike
- using antonyms and synonyms to expand comprehension of key vocabulary and figures of speech
- supporting novel or rare vocabulary and concepts with context (graphic organizers, real objects)
- requiring students to define words using categorical terms (Dickinson, Cote, & Smith, 1993)
- asking students to think beyond the information provided (for instance, analyzing a character's personality or motivation; Dickinson et al., 1993)

Analytical conversation has been found to be of critical importance as a mediation strategy (Dickinson et al., 1993). "Exchanges in which teachers and students were actively engaged with each other in *intellectually challenging* discussions are those that foster the greatest language and academic growth" (p. 75).

Activate Learning

Students who are D/HH should be placed with teachers who require them to be active learners and are constantly monitoring their engagement (Norris & Hoffman, 1993; Rosenshine, 1986). Teachers should frequently ask for comments and observations from these students to help evaluate cognitive and linguistic involvement. Activating these students' learning can be accomplished by

> **Study Guide Question**
> *How would you construct a web for the concept of analytical conversation? Work with a peer and construct this web.*

- using verbal focusing cues (*"Look at the first paragraph on page 45."*)
- using nonverbal focusing cues (flashing the classroom lights, pointing)
- calling on students frequently
- incorporating these students' comments in the discussion
- creating a classroom in which students feel comfortable taking risks

> **Study Guide Question**
> *What other strategies could you use to activate learning?*

Relate New Information to Old Information

Students who are D/HH should be placed with teachers who link "text-to-life" and "life-to-text" (Cochran-Smith, 1984; Heath, 1982) or "discussion-to-life" and "life-to-discussion." The term "life" in this context refers to past home, community, and school experiences. Linking new and old information can be accomplished by

- using familiar, concrete objects or events to demonstrate abstract principles
- using graphic organizers to depict relationships between new and old information
- providing feedback to students when they have expressed appropriate or inappropriate linkages

> **Study Guide Question**
> *How would you relate old and new information when teaching a science unit on consumers and producers? Explain your strategy to a peer.*

Use the Principles of Effective Instruction

The principles of effective instruction (Rosenshine, 1986) are beneficial for all students and should be practiced by all teachers. When working with students who are D/HH, it is essential that adults

- secure attention
- review prerequisite learning
- state objectives
- introduce new material in small steps
- give clear directions and explanations
- provide guided practice
- ask questions and obtain responses from all students
- provide systematic feedback and correction
- monitor learning to ensure confidence with independent practice

Further explanations of these practices were provided by Luetke-Stahlman and Luckner (1991). A lesson planning sheet incorporating the principles of effective instruction is provided in Appendix 1–C.

Facilitate the Retention of Concepts

Many times adults worry that students who are D/HH are not retaining information covered in class or explained during a tutorial session. Difficulty in retention most often occurs because adults lecture or talk at students rather than engaging them in dialogue. A sample of a worksheet found to be useful in assisting students to retain conceptual information, define words, and compare and contrast examples is provided in Figure 1–8. This form is of

> **Study Guide Question**
> *How might you use the principles of effective instruction in the lesson plan guide provided in Appendix 1–C to teach a peer a familiar task?*

particular benefit because it provides for an interactive, analytical dialogue; requires a superordinate term when giving a definition (denoted by the term written in the box); provides a syntax sentence frame which should be faded when students no longer require it; provides space to compare correct and incorrect examples that are highly similar; and provides space to indicate the student's success in defining the target term in his or her own words.

| A _____ is a [   ] that |
| Key Vocabulary |

A characteristic of a _____ is

An example of a _____ is

| Examples | Non-Examples |

(Turn this sheet over so it can't be seen. Indicate the student's success in defining the target word in his or her own terms.)

FIGURE 1-8: CONCEPT WORKSHEET

An Example Using the Concept Worksheet

Marcy is a nine-year-old deaf third grader who participates in the general education classroom for science despite an assessed two-year English language delay and a one-year reading delay. Recently, her class studied a unit including the words *prey* and *predator*. The teacher of the deaf, Mrs. Owens, assisted Marcy in formulating a definition for the word *predator* using the Concept Worksheet

(Figure 1–8). Mrs. Owens didn't tell Marcy the definition or have her copy it from the glossary of her science textbook; they worked together to decide on a definition: "a predator is an animal that catches and eats other animals." To reach this definition, Mrs. Owens used question prompts (explained later in this chapter) as well as the pictures in Marcy's science textbook.

Using the Concept Worksheet, Marcy's attention was directed to the superordinate category, *animal*, which assisted her both with organizing information and formulating the definition. Providing syntax (*A _____ is a _____ that . . .*) allowed her to focus on the content of the discussion rather than the grammar. (This syntactic phrase for definitions had been used for a year to help Marcy with definitions because of the difficulties she has had expressing English grammar.)

After completing their preliminary definition, Marcy and Mrs. Owens decided to check the glossary at the back of the text. In that definition, the words *organism* and *living thing* were substituted for their choice, *animal*. Mrs. Owens wrote these terms above the boxed superordinate term and draw a circle around all three of them, indicating that they were synonyms. This simple type of graphic display has helped many students to attach the meaning of new words to known ones.

As they discussed examples of predators, Mrs. Owens tried to incorporate critical features to contrast *prey* and *predator*. For instance, in the Examples column they wrote:
> *Daddy hunting pheasants*
> *tigers, lions, bears*

Mrs. Owens used synonyms of the superordinate term to create more examples:
> *an animal that kills*
> *an organism that eats other organisms*

Marcy read to Mrs. Owens from her science book and discovered that predators kill prey, so she recorded that as a characteristic of a predator. She told Mrs. Owens about her cat catching a mouse, and they added *cat* as an example of a predator.

To complete the Non-Examples column, Marcy and her teacher discussed the items and phrases they had written as examples, considering whether pheasants, bears, and cats are predators. Eventually, Marcy listed *mouse* and *deer* as non-examples since they do not hunt live prey.

When this work was finished, Mrs. Owens flipped the worksheet paper over and asked Marcy to define *predator*. Marcy independently said/signed, *"A predator is an animal that catches and eats other animals."* A week later she correctly identified definitions of *prey* and *predator* on her science test.

Use Reciprocity

Reciprocal teaching is a component of analytical conversation. It can be defined in its broadest sense as a dialogue in which students and teachers take turns facilitating discussion about a topic or text. Palincsar, Ranson, and Derber (1989) described a more structured instructional practice that included four specific elements (generating questions, summarizing, clarifying, and predicting), but the term is used here to refer to their more global definition: "conversation with a purpose" (p. 37). The term is conceptually similar to instructional conversation or mediated learning. Students who are D/HH should be placed with teachers who use this method to facilitate or lead dialogue; verbally model construction of meaning (*"Oh, I see now that the properties here are similar . . . and these here are dissimilar"*); monitor self-comprehension (*"Oh, I can use a map to find it"*); expect everyone to participate; and gradually transfer leadership to the students.

> **Study Guide Question**
> *How would you compare some of the ideas to activate learning provided in this chapter with the ideas about using reciprocity?*

Use Question Prompts

Students who are D/HH need multiple opportunities to indicate their comprehension of concepts and vocabulary. They may need to be given question prompts and asked analytical questions (Dickinson, Temple, Hirchler, & Smith, 1992). For example, students may not realize that a question has been asked for which an answer is expected or they may provide an answer that does not match the question. When this happens, teachers can simply preface a repetition of the question with an attention-getting phrase (*"Judy, listen to my question now . . ."*) or ask the student to pay attention while a peer answers. The teacher should then re-ask the initial student the same question or a similar one. These strategies are called "question prompts" (ten of them are described and exemplified by Luetke-Stahlman and Luckner, 1991, and several are used where appropriate in this text).

When teachers ask analytical questions (calling for comparisons, judgments, analysis, synthesis), it may be that a student is capable of supplying the content to a question but is unsure of the syntax to use in the response. Teachers can give sequence or listing prompts (*"First you line the two numbers up under each other, right; and then you subtract this one from this one . . . and then what do you do?"*). They can also provide a multiple choice question (of at least three choices) or ask another student to model the response to the same or a highly similar question.

It is always helpful if adults use context when asking questions (graphic illustrations, real objects) so that the language they are using is supported by visualizations. Signing in a manner that forms a visual picture of how some things are related to other things in space also provides context. When asking questions themselves, students may need adults to supply the first few words (*"In this story, who is . . . you say it with me . . . Who is . . . "*).

Question prompts, in summary, include
- repeating questions, beginning with an attention-getting phrase
- supplying sequence or listing prompts
- providing multiple choice questions
- asking another student to model the response
- adding context

Using a variety of these question prompts will help facilitate comprehension both of concepts and vocabulary for students who are D/HH.

Encourage Peer Teaching and Cooperative Learning

Study Guide Questions

1. *Can you design a question prompt for each of five higher-level thinking skills (evaluate, judge, compare and contrast, and so forth)?*

2. *How would you teach others about question prompts? Make a grid that includes the name of the question prompt, a description of it, and an example from a relevant content area (free play, art, reading, civics) for each prompt described in this section.*

Students who are D/HH should be placed with teachers who maximize active participation by all students by using peer tutoring, cooperative learning, students working as partners, and collaboration at learning centers. Students are apt to converse more and have more opportunities to use novel vocabulary to express their thoughts and ideas in smaller groups when the affective filter is low (Krashen, 1982; see also Luetke-Stahlman, 1998). In addition, students may be better able to hear and read speech when they are sitting closer to peers in small groups. Monitor equal participation by all students working together and group students with complementary abilities. One example of an organizational plan that might work when students who are D/HH participate in learning groups is called "The Jigsaw" (Aronson, Blaney, Stephan, Sikes, & Snapp, 1978). The steps of the plan are as follows:

1. Academic material is divided into segments and students are divided into groups.
2. Each group member is assigned one segment and given a specific task.
3. All the students in the room who have been assigned the same segment come together in new groups and discuss their role jointly.
4. Students then return to their original groups and teach each other their material.

Roles usually change in cooperative learning groups and adults should always clarify each student's role and monitor each group to ensure students are actively completing their assigned task. The following is an example of assigned roles for cooperative learning when students are practicing reading:

1. One student reads to a peer.
2. The peer paraphrases the main idea and one to three details without looking at the text.
3. The first student expands or corrects the peer's summary as needed.
4. The pair refers back to the text to check the accuracy of each contribution.
5. The students reverse roles and continue reading.

Engage Students in Active Problem Solving

Students who are D/HH should be placed with teachers who assist them in active problem solving (Schoenfeld, 1985) by giving them choices (*"Do you think that word is* black *or* block?*"*), presenting real needs (*"Could you write those instructions down for me so that I can use them again next time we play this game?"*), and acting like learners themselves (*"I'm not sure about that. Let's look in the dictionary"*). Teachers should also "think aloud" to express their thoughts, feelings, and attitudes as they figure something out—modeling puzzlements, revisions, and "on-line processing" of thinking as it occurs in reality (Palincsar & Brown, 1988). Palincsar and Brown (1984) stressed that modeling also demonstrates variety among people in how they construct meaning due to different perspectives about a similar topic.

> **Study Guide Question**
> *How have teachers met the challenge of using cooperative learning groups with students who are D/HH? Interview teachers and ask them what some of the challenges have been and how they met them. Share your findings with a peer.*

Provide Elaboration Strategies

To elaborate is to add a symbolic construction to what is learned. This makes learning more personally meaningful (Weinstein, Ridley, Dahl, & Weber, 1989). Students who are D/HH should be placed with teachers who assign them elaboration activities to apply and remember new knowledge. These strategies include

> **Study Guide Question**
> *Reflect on your own learning. What strategies are helpful when you are actively problem solving?*

- providing analogies and coaching students in creating analogies

- paraphrasing concepts and asking students to repeat the essence of the paraphrase
- identifying main points, explaining the reasoning for the selection, and asking students to critique the selection
- summarizing information in their own words (perhaps using the text structure as a guide) and asking students to state reasons why they agree or disagree
- transferring new ideas into charts, graphs, and other visual organizers

Elaboration also includes asking students to go beyond the facts and discuss other possible endings, make inferences, or offer conditional conclusions (*"What would happen if . . . ?"*). Asking students to apply or compare what they have learned to other situations (*"How was the problem in this story similar to the one faced by the characters in the story we read last week?"*) is another elaboration strategy.

> **Study Guide Question**
>
> *What is elaboration? Perhaps the concept is new to you. Read the description of it again, put the material out of view, and provide a definition and several examples for a peer. Ask that peer to evaluate your response.*

Use Graphic Organizers

Graphic organizers are used to illustrate information visually. Students who are D/HH should be placed with teachers who constantly sketch flow charts, pie charts, family trees, networks, word webs, Venn diagrams, matrices, and so forth, during reading, writing, or discussions of otherwise abstract material. Graphic organizers allow students a means of tangibly displaying relationships among pieces of information as well as serving as support for verbal (signed or spoken) explanations (Jones, Pierce, & Hunter, 1989).

Durkin (1979) found that students' ability to recognize patterns (text structures) in both narrative and expository material affected comprehension. Because students who are D/HH often lack background knowledge, are unfamiliar with text structures, and find complex grammatical forms difficult, de Villiers (1995) recommended that they be helped to construct graphic organizers. He documented improved English writing abilities when compare-and-contrast tables, cause-and-effect diagrams, and so forth, were used and English transition words (*because, but*) directly taught.

Darnell (1998) has provided the following summary defining graphic organizers and explaining their uses. Examples of graphic organizers appear as figures throughout this text.

Graphic Organizers

What are graphic organizers?
Graphic organizers are visual representations of ideas and details and their relationships to each other.

Why use graphic organizers?
- They support visual learners by providing a vehicle for analyzing and constructing meaning.
- They illustrate relationships among ideas.
- They can efficiently show an entire process.
- They can help students represent their thinking.
- They permit, and often encourage, nonlinear thinking.
- They can encourage teachers to focus on essential grouped information versus fragmented parts.
- They support instructional design based on conceptual learning.

When do you use graphic organizers?
Use graphic organizers if students
- have an underdeveloped language base
- are stronger visual than auditory learners
- need support in seeing structure in complex information and the relationships among parts
- need assistance in representing ideas in written or expressive English
- need assistance in recalling information from previous instruction or reading
- need support in comprehending, analyzing, applying, synthesizing, or evaluating complex information that they have heard, read, or observed
- require assistance in preparing for tests and other types of assessments

How do you create a graphic organizer?

■ Review examples (sample graphic organizers were provided by Luetke-Stahlman, 1998, and appear in many other texts and articles; examples are also provided throughout this text).

■ List the critical ideas and details from what was heard, signed, read, or observed.

■ Group related ideas and details, and display them by using or adapting one of the sample graphics (or creating your own).

■ Create labels that describe the grouped information.

From *Graphic Organizer* handout, by R. Darnell, 1998, Township High School, District 214, Arlington Heights, IL. Adapted with author's permission.

Teach Learning Strategies

"Learning strategies" have been defined by Derry (1989) as cognitive processes that involve tactics (planning, rehearsal, imaging, outlining, comprehension monitoring) to execute a plan for accomplishing a learning goal. The term is not used in this text to mean program or curricular modification such as those discussed at the beginning of this chapter.

Students who are D/HH should be placed with teachers who do not tell them the answers but teach them systematic learning strategies for decoding and spelling new words, figuring out problems, taking risks in giving responses, and so forth. Many of the learning strategies available have not been tried on students who are D/HH and will require thoughtful adaptation. Teachers may need to encourage the use of such strategies over long periods of time but may eventually be rewarded by student demonstrations of independence. The chapters following this one present descriptions and examples of learning strategies that may be appropriate for school subjects. Additional information can be found in texts that focus on learning disabilities.

One example of a learning strategy is the technique designed by Ogle (1989) that is commonly used in elementary schools in the United States. It is called the "K-W-L" and is useful when students are reading expository text. The *K* in the model stands for "What I already know about this topic." The *W* stands for "What I want to learn about this topic," and the *L* stands for "What I learned" after reading and discussing the material. These three components are presented as three columns to be completed. Typically the first two columns are completed as a group activity prior to asking the students to read a section of a textbook. Later in the unit, perhaps when the students are preparing to take a test on the material, the last column is also completed as a group activity.

> ## Texts That Focus on Instruction of Students with Learning Disabilities
>
> *Effective Instruction of Students with Learning Difficulties* (1995). P. Cegelka & W. Berdine; Allyn & Bacon.
>
> *Language Instruction for Students with Disabilities* (1992). E. Polloway & T. Smith; Love.
>
> *Teaching Secondary Students with Mild Learning and Behavior Problems: Methods, Materials, and Strategies* (1994). L. Masters, B. Mori, & A. Mori; Pro-Ed.
>
> *Teaching Special Learners in the General Classroom: Methods and Techniques* (1995). K. McCoy; Love.

Shape Independence

Fading, or gradually removing adult support, is essential for independent learning (Idol & Jones, 1991). DeFord, Lyons, and Pinnell (1991) noted that students need to be helped to be aware of why they are learning and be guided eventually to monitor their own acquisition of information.

Students who are D/HH need to be placed with teachers who are aware of the skills the students have acquired and who challenge

> ### Study Guide Question
>
> *What is your success with using learning strategies? Select one strategy and use it with a student who is D/HH. Evaluate the success of this strategy.*

them to use their new linguistic and cognitive abilities independently as content becomes more complex and diverse. Wong-Fillmore (1995) found in a study of hearing second-language learners of English that students were successful when individual work was assigned after formal lessons (in which adults used effective teaching principles) and completion was monitored.

Archer, Gleason, Englert, and Isaacson (1995) suggested guide-lines for independent work assignments. Their guidelines include having students demonstrate a specified level of ability (supervised by a teacher) *before* work is sent home and expecting parents to provide only minimal additional instruction.

Teach Collaboratively and Secure Organizational Support

Students who are D/HH need to be placed with general educa-tion teachers who are willing to collaborate with specially trained teachers. In addition, these students need to be placed in programs where administrators provide the time team members require to assess student needs, review curricular goals for all students and decide which are obtainable for students who are D/HH, supply required mediated learning, and support students in learning envi-ronments that promote constant linguistic and cognitive growth. Dickinson et al. (1992) also suggested that teachers of language-challenged students should work with smaller groups, minimize background noise, and display enthusiasm for facilitating learning. These kinds of behaviors require active administrators who are understanding and supportive.

In addition, for team members to supply mediated learning experiences and engage in analytical conversations to the extent required by some students who are D/HH, they obviously need to be able to communicate in the language or system that is most beneficial for each student's learning of new and cognitively difficult concepts. This could be Spanish, American Sign Language, Cued Speech, Signing Exact English, or any other language or system. School staff unable to communicate proficiently in a student's dom-inant language should employ the services of someone who can (such as a teacher of the deaf, interpreter, or transliterator) and team teach.

Summary

A variety of modifications can be made in supports and services to facilitate learning by students who are D/HH. In addition, the use of mediated instruction is essential in providing an effective education for these students. Mediated instruction is a process of facilitation that is designed to move students away from dependence in learning and toward independence. Scaffolding, or mediated instruction, by more mature learners can bring about positive change in the cognitive and linguistic abilities of students, as well as promote academic skill development. Students who are D/HH must be placed with teachers who have adopted this methodology or are willing to learn it.

Activities

1. Videotape yourself working with a student who is D/HH and mediating learning. Critique your effectiveness.

2. Make a modification sheet for a different subject area modeled after those provided in Appendix 1–B.

3. Videotape examples of using the principles of effective teaching both well and poorly.

4. Interview an administrator of a program that enrolls both hearing students and those who are deaf or hard of hearing. Ask how teachers are provided adequate planning time to apply the strategies suggested in this chapter and to team teach. Is this time allotment different from what is afforded teachers who are not working in teams? Discuss your findings with several of your peers.

Appendix 1-A

Programmatic and Curricular Modifications Checklist

PROGRAM MODIFICATION	ACTIVITY	ACCOUNTABILITY	COMMENTS
I. Mode/Flow of Communication __ Access to all activities __ Adequate interpreting (oral, Cued Speech, manual) __ Assessed dominant language/system (L/S) __ Match between adult and student L/S __ Decisions made about English language level __ Decisions made about writing level __ Decisions made about reading level __ Other appropriate assessment conducted __ Decisions made about ASL language level __ Interpreter(s) informed __ Other:			

II. School/Class Environment
__ No changes
__ Captioning/real time
__ Listening environment
__ FM equipment
    __ quiet rooms
    __ carpet
    __ acoustic tiles
    __ window treatments
__ Visible alarms
			cont.

PROGRAM MODIFICATION	ACTIVITY	ACCOUNTABILITY	COMMENTS

__ Visual strain
    __ allow for physical movement into sightline
    __ provide visual breaks
    __ wear plain clothing
__ Seating environments
    __ preferential seating (horseshoe)
    __ able to see peers
    __ eliminate visual distractions
__ Other:			

III. Testing/Grading
__ No changes
__ Provide test study guides
__ More frequent mini-tests
__ Alternative response mode
__ Video signed tests
__ Additional time
__ Alternative grading
    __ curriculum-based tests
    __ criteria-referenced tests
    __ self-referenced tests
    __ daily/weekly grade report
__ Other:
			cont.

CURRICULUM MODIFICATION	ACTIVITY	ACCOUNTABILITY	COMMENTS
IV. Organizational Structure __ No change __ Buddy; peer tutor; peer mediated instruction __ Notetaker __ Use assignment sheets, notebook, monthly calendars __ Write down assignments; have student check them off __ Give interim due dates on longer assignments __ Teach time management skills for daily work __ Initial/intermittent assistance in organizing self as appropriate __ Additional personnel/ paraprofessional __ Other:			
V. Rapport/Affect __ Schedule regular times to chat __ Increase honest praise __ Treat the student as a member of the class (called on as others, expectations as appropriate) __ Reinforce appropriate participation regularly __ Monitor frustrating situations and fatigue __ Discuss rejection or superficial peer encounters __ Be aware of what embarrasses students __ Other:			

cont.

CURRICULUM MODIFICATION	ACTIVITY	ACCOUNTABILITY	COMMENTS
VI. Instructional Format __ No change __ Small group interaction; activities __ Add context (graphic organizers)/overhead projector __ Relevant and real information __ Learning style match (global, analytical) __ Use of games, simulations, role plays, presentations (activity-based), etc. __ Thematic, integrated instruction __ Learning centers/computers __ Other:			
VII. Instructional Language __ Reduce volume __ Don't block mouth __ Don't turn away __ Reduce rate __ Present instruction two, three, four times __ Avoid meaningless hand movements __ Modify syntax/grammar __ Use more common words/phrases __ Simplify word order __ Reduce complexity __ Chunk clauses in message __ Translate figurative English			*cont.*

CURRICULUM MODIFICATION	ACTIVITY	ACCOUNTABILITY	COMMENTS
VII. Instructional Language, cont. __ Increase message redundancy __ Employ natural gestures/mime/pointing __ Use meaningful facial expressions __ Use synonyms for perceived difficult words, definitions, critical features __ Other:			
VIII. Lesson Format __ Slow pace of instruction __ Task analyze to determine level __ Make certain directions are understood __ Use effective instruction principles (increased guided practice, multisensory approach, summarize, etc.) __ Use a variety of question types and prompts __ Use cues __ Provide study notes/outline __ Help student acquire a study buddy __ Use/teach strategies for acquiring/remembering __ Other:			
IX. Materials __ No change __ Clarify instructions			*cont.*

CURRICULUM MODIFICATION	ACTIVITY	ACCOUNTABILITY	COMMENTS
IX. Materials, cont. __ Same material/lower reading level __ Read (sign) to the students rather than having them read themselves __ Rewrite materials to simplify grammar __ Highlight essential information __ Change response mode __ Provide second set of books to be used at home __ Other:			
X. Comprehension Checking __ Ask questions more frequently than to peers __ Ask student to repeat an explanation/answer __ Other:			
XI. Activity __ No change __ Parallel activity of simpler nature __ Other:			
XII. Assignment Completion __ Provide examples of what's expected __ Give specific comments to correct responses __ Provide individual assistance time __ Encourage quality __ Reduce quantity required __ Other:			*cont.*

CURRICULUM MODIFICATION	ACTIVITY	ACCOUNTABILITY	COMMENTS
XIII. Monitoring __ Daily/weekly monitoring report __ Chart continuous progress (or lack of) __ Develop/maintain home/ school communication plan __ Other:			
XIV. Placement __ Full day special classes at a residential school __ 1/2 day special classes and 1/2 day general classes at a residential school __ Full day general classes at a residential school __ Full day placement in a cooperative school program __ Full day resource in a public magnet school __ 1/2 day resource with TOD* and 1/2 day with TOD in general education classes __ 1/2 day resource with TOD and 1/2 day with an interpreter in general education classes __ 1/4 day resource with TOD and 3/4 day with an interpreter in general education classes __ Almost full day general education classes with an interpreter and tutoring with TOD			*cont.*

*TOD = teacher of the deaf

CURRICULUM MODIFICATION	ACTIVITY	ACCOUNTABILITY	COMMENTS
XIV. Placement, cont. __ Full day general education classes with consultation provided by TOD __ Full day in the student's home school with or without an interpreter __ Other:			

Appendix 1-B

Examples of Using Programmatic and Curricular Modifications*
Example #1

Target Goal: THE STUDENT WILL READ GRADE-LEVEL NARRATIVE OR EXPOSITORY MATERIAL TO AN ADULT

Possible Objectives	Modifications	Testing/Grading

The student will
__ use dominant language to clarify material
__ participate in an interactive dialogue about what is read
__ state purpose for reading
__ demonstrate enjoyment throughout session
__ explain appropriate concepts of print
__ make text-to-life connections
__ decode all words (word recognition)
__ explain the meaning of words, phrases, or text structures
__ explain written syntactic structures relevant to the meaning of text
__ engage in one or more response activities that require high-level thinking skills and use of targeted grammar and vocabulary
 	
Modifications to Objective Given:
__ a reduced length of material to read
__ a story/text frame to organize the material
	Communication
	__ Access to all activities
	__ Adequate interpreting (oral, Cued Speech, manual)
	__ Assessed dominant language/system (L/S)
	__ Match between adult and student L/S
	__ Decisions made about English language level
	__ Decisions made about writing level
	__ Decisions made about reading level
	__ Other appropriate assessment conducted
	__ Decisions made about ASL language level
	__ Interpreter(s) informed
	
	Learning Environment
	__ Listening
	__ FM system
	__ Captioning
	__ Quiet rooms
	__ Carpet, acoustic tiles, window treatments
	__ Visible alarms
	
	Seating Arrangement
	__ Visual strain
	   __ allow for physical movement into sightline
		Testing and Grading
		__ Provide test study guides
		__ More frequent mini-tests
		__ Alternative response mode
		__ Video signed tests
		__ Additional time
		__ Alternative grading
		   __ curriculum-based tests
		   __ criteria-referenced tests
		   __ self-referenced tests
		   __ daily/weekly grade report
		
		cont.

*From B. Luetke-Stahlman and N. Montgomery, 1997

Target Goal: THE STUDENT WILL READ GRADE-LEVEL NARRATIVE OR EXPOSITORY MATERIAL TO AN ADULT		
Possible Objectives, cont.	**Modifications, cont.**	**Testing/Grading**

__ a signed summary prior to reading
__ highlighting of the main ideas prior to the reading
__ choral reading with others
__ opportunities to reread the text to or with others
__ multiple comprehension activities
	__ provide visual breaks
	__ wear plain clothing
	__ Seating environments
	  __ preferential seating (e.g., horseshoe)
	  __ able to see peers
	  __ eliminate visual distractions
	
	Organizational Structure
	__ Work with a buddy/peer tutor
	__ Use a notetaker
	__ Use assignment sheets, notebook, monthly calendars
	__ Write down assignments; have student check them off
	__ Give interim due dates on longer assignments
	__ Teach time management skills for daily work
	__ Initial/intermittent assistance in organizing self as is appropriate
	
	Rapport/Affect
	__ Use honest praise
	__ Reinforce appropriately & regularly
	__ Monitor frustration & fatigue
	
	Instructional Format
	__ Wear plain clothing
	__ Use cooperative learning
	__ Provide visual breaks (graphics, overheads)
	__ Add context	

		cont.

Target Goal: THE STUDENT WILL READ GRADE-LEVEL NARRATIVE OR EXPOSITORY MATERIAL TO AN ADULT		
Possible Objectives, cont.	Modifications, cont.	Testing/Grading
	__ Make material relevant & real __ Match learning styles (visual, auditory, tactile) __ Use games or simulations __ Thematic instruction (spelling words from the reading) **Mediated Instruction** __ Relate new information to known __ Use reciprocal teaching __ Use a variety of question types __ Engage active problem solving __ Provide elaboration strategies (students create analogies, paraphrase) __ Provide progressively less assistance	

Other Modifications

General Education Communication
Know ASL and/or English language level
Reduce rate; don't block mouth; don't turn away
Present instruction numerous times
Avoid meaningless hand movements
Modify syntax/grammar
Increase message redundancy

Lesson Format
Slow the pace of instruction
Task analyze to determine level
Make certain the student understands directions
Use effective instruction principles (increase active learning, use guided practice) *cont.*

Other Modifications, cont.

Clarify importance (*this point is important*)
Provide study notes/outline
Help student acquire a study buddy
Use/teach strategies for acquiring/remembering

Materials
Same material/lower reading level
Read/sign to the students rather than having them read
Rewrite materials to simplify grammar
Highlight essential information
Change response mode
Provide second set of books to be used at home

Comprehension Checking
Ask questions more frequently than to hearing peers
Ask student to repeat an explanation/answer

Assignment Completion
Provide examples of what is expected
Give specific comments to correct responses
Provide individual assistance time
Encourage quality (spellcheck, proofreading, rewrites)
Reduce quantity required

Activity
Parallel activity of simpler nature

Monitoring
Daily/weekly monitoring report
Chart progress (or lack of)
Develop and maintain home/school communication plan

Placement
Full day special classes at a residential school
1/2 day special classes and 1/2 day general classes at a residential school
Full day general classes at a residential school
Full day placement in a cooperative school program
Full day resource in a public magnet school
1/2 day resource with TOD* and 1/2 day with TOD in general education classes
1/2 day resource with TOD and 1/2 day with an interpreter in general education classes
1/4 day resource with TOD and 3/4 day with an interpreter in general education classes
Almost full day general education classes with an interpreter and tutoring with TOD
Full day general education classes with consultation provided by TOD
Full day in the student's home school with or without an interpreter
Other:

*TOD = teacher of the deaf

Example #2

Target Goal: THE STUDENT WILL USE CORRECT SPELLING DURING CREATIVE, RESPONSE, AND JOURNAL WRITING		
Possible Objectives	**Modifications**	**Testing/Grading**

The student will
__ apply relevant phonics rules/spelling rules
__ apply word pattern knowledge
__ spell most frequently misspelled words correctly
 	
Modifications to Objective
__ Decrease/increase number of words
__ Use spellcheck
__ Allow use of a personal dictionary
__ Use a lower grade level spelling list
__ Monitor correct spelling of known words
	Communication
	__ Access to all activities
	__ Adequate interpreting (oral, Cued Speech, manual)
	__ Assessed dominant language/system (L/S)
	__ Match between adult and student L/S
	__ Decisions made about English language level
	__ Decisions made about writing level
	__ Decisions made about reading level
	__ Other appropriate assessment conducted
	__ Decisions made about ASL language level
	__ Interpreter(s) informed
	
	Learning Environment
	__ FM system
	__ Captioning
	__ Window treatments
	__ Quiet rooms
	__ Carpet, acoustic tiles
	__ Visible alarms
	
	Seating Arrangement
	__ Visual strain
	   __ allow for physical movement into sightline
	   __ provide visual breaks
		Testing and Grading
		__ Provide test study guides
		__ More frequent mini-tests
		__ Alternative response mode
		__ Video signed tests
		__ Additional time
		__ Alternative grading
		   __ curriculum-based tests
		   __ criteria-referenced tests
		   __ self-referenced tests
		   __ daily/weekly grade report

cont.

Target Goal: THE STUDENT WILL USE CORRECT SPELLING DURING CREATIVE, RESPONSE, AND JOURNAL WRITING		
Possible Objectives, cont.	Modifications, cont.	Testing/Grading

	__ wear plain clothing
	__ Seating environments
	   __ preferential seating (e.g., horseshoe)
	   __ able to see peers
	   __ eliminate visual distractions
	
	Organizational Structure
	__ Work with buddy/peer tutor
	__ Use a notetaker
	__ Use assignment sheets, notebook, monthly calendars
	__ Write down assignments; have student check them off
	__ Give interim due dates on longer assignments
	__ Teach time management skills for daily work
	__ Initial/intermittent assistance in organizing self as is appropriate
	
	Rapport/Affect
	__ Use honest praise
	__ Reinforce appropriately & regularly
	__ Monitor frustration & fatigue
	
	Instructional Format
	__ Small group and cooperative learning activities
	__ Add context
	__ Use games or simulations
		cont.

| **Target Goal:** THE STUDENT WILL USE CORRECT SPELLING DURING CREATIVE, RESPONSE, AND JOURNAL WRITING |||
Possible Objectives, cont.	Modifications, cont	Testing/Grading
	__ Make material relevant & real __ Match learning style (visual, auditory, tactile) __ Thematic instruction (spelling words from the reading) **Mediated Instruction** __ Relate new material to known __ Use reciprocal teaching __ Use a variety of question types __ Engage active problem solving __ Provide elaboration strategies (students create analogies, paraphrase) __ Provide progressively less assistance	

Blank Form for Trial Use

Target Goal: THE STUDENT WILL		
Possible Objectives	Modifications	Testing/Grading
The student will **Modifications to Objective**	**Learning Environment** __ FM system __ Quiet rooms __ Carpet, acoustic tiles __ Window treatments **Seating Arrangement** __ Preferential seating __ Able to see peers __ Eliminate visual distractions **Organizational Structure** __ Work with buddy/peer tutor **Rapport/Affect** __ Use honest praise __ Reinforce appropriately & regularly __ Monitor frustration & fatigue **Instructional Format** __ Small group and cooperative learning activities __ Add context __ Make material relevant & real __ Match learning style (visual, auditory, tactile) __ Use games or simulations __ Thematic instruction (spelling words from the reading)	 *cont.*

Target Goal: THE STUDENT WILL		
Possible Objectives, cont.	Modifications, cont.	Testing/Grading
	Mediated Instruction __ Relate new information to known __ Use reciprocal teaching __ Use a variety of question types __ Engage active problem solving __ Provide elaboration strategies (students create analogies, paraphrase)	

Appendix 1-C

Incorporating Principles of Effective Instruction into Lessons

___ 1. Use the language/system that is most beneficial to the student(s) in learning new and difficult information (age-appropriate)

___ 2. Secure the student's attention and state the purpose of the lesson (or ask the student to do so)

___ 3. Ascertain what the student knows about the material/concept you are about to teach; praise anything known and move to new material; repeat prerequisite material if unknown

___ 4. State the objective(s) of the lesson

___ 5. Introduce new material in small steps

___ a. Name the concept, using a subordinate term if possible

___ b. Provide synonyms for words or phrases

___ c. Define key words providing distinguishing details and have student repeat

___ d. Identify essential characteristics and also give non-examples

___ e. Ask for examples of the concept or provide them; also provide non-examples

___ f. Ask comprehension questions using partial information, analogy, or multiple choice question prompts if necessary; require higher-level thinking (summarize, compare and contrast, judge, evaluate, infer, etc.)

___ g. Use one or more graphic organizers to display new information

___ h. Ensure that anything needing to be read is at the student's instructional reading level

___ i. Plan anything written with a graphic organizer before beginning

cont.

___ 6. Give clear and detailed instructions for active practice with a partner

    ___ a. Repeat the directions or highlight them

    ___ b. Ask the student to repeat the directions

    ___ c. If working in cooperative groups, make sure the student is working with partners of similar ability and has an assigned job

    ___ d. Design active learning sessions that involve role play, hands-on demonstration, experimenting, arts, etc.

___ 7. Provide systematic feedback and correction

___ 8. Provide clear explanations of seat work (sequenced in the order of the task, repeated by others, etc.) and monitor the student's progress; rote or copied answers are unacceptable

___ 9. Continue practice sessions until the student demonstrates 80% or higher comprehension of the material

___ 10. Do not send work home for which the student has not demonstrated #9; ask parents to report on abilities at home

References

Andrews, J., & Mason, J. (1986). Strategy use among deaf and hearing readers. *Exceptional Children, 57,* 536-545.

Archer, A., Gleason, M., Englert, D., & Isaacson, S. (1995). Meeting individual instructional needs. In P. Cegelka & W. Berdine (Eds.), *Effective instruction of students with learning difficulties* (pp. 195-226). Boston: Allyn & Bacon.

Aronson, E., Blaney, N., Stephan, C., Sikes, J., & Snapp, M. (1978). *The jigsaw classroom.* Beverly Hills, CA: Sage.

Berry, V. (1988). Classroom intervention strategies and resource materials for the auditory handicapped child. In R. Roeser & M. Downs (Eds.), *Auditory disorders in school children* (2nd ed.) (pp. 325-349). New York: Thieme Medical.

Binet, A. (1909). *Les idees modernes sur les enfants.* Paris: Ernest Flammarion.

Brown, A., & Palincsar, A. (1982). Inducing strategic learning from text by means of informed, self-control training. *Topics in Learning and Learning Disabilities, 2*(1), 1-17.

Bruner, J. (1968). *Towards a theory of instruction.* New York: Norton.

Chamot, A. (1985). *English language development through a content-based approach.* (ERIC Document Reproduction Service No. ED 273 150)

Cochran-Smith, M. (1984). *The making of a reader.* Norwood, NJ: Ablex.

Conway, L. (1990). Issues related to classroom management. In M. Ross (Ed.), *Hearing-impaired children in the mainstream* (pp. 131-158). Parkton, MD: York Press.

Cummins, J. (1981). The role of primary language development in promoting educational success for language minority students. In *Schooling and language minority students: A theoretical framework.* Los Angeles: California State University Evaluation, Dissemination, and Assessment Center.

Cummins, J. (1984). *Bilingualism and special education: Issues in assessment and pedagogy.* San Diego, CA: College-Hill Press.

Darnell, R. (1998). *Graphic organizers.* (Available from Township High School, District 214, 2121 S. Goebbert Rd., Arlington Heights, IL 60005)

Deford, D., Lyons, C., & Pinnell, G. (1991). *Bridges to literacy: Learning from reading recovery.* Portsmouth, NH: Heinemann.

Derry, S. (1989). Putting learning strategies to work. *Educational Leadership, 46*(4), 4-10.

de Villiers, P. (1995, October). *Expository writing, extended discourse, and science: Towards an integrated curriculum for deaf students.* Paper presented at the 10th Annual Issues in Language and Deafness Conference, Nebraska City, NE.

Dewey, J. (1916). *Democracy and education.* New York: Free Press.

Dickinson, D., Cote, L., & Smith, M. (1993). Learning vocabulary in preschool: Social and discourse contexts affecting vocabulary growth. *New Directions for Child Development, 61,* 67-78.

Dickinson, D., & Smith, M. (1994). Long-term effects of preschool teachers' book readings on low-income children's vocabulary and story comprehension. *Reading Research Quarterly, 29*(2), 104-122.

Dickinson, D., Temple, J., Hirchler, J., & Smith, M. (1992). Book reading with preschoolers: Construction of text at home and school. *Early Childhood Research Quarterly, 7,* 104-122.

Durkin, D. (1979). What classroom observations reveal about reading comprehension instruction. *Reading Research Quarterly, 14*(4), 481-533.

Durkin, D. (1995). *Language issues: Readings for teachers.* New York: Longman.

Echevarria, J., & McDonough, R. (1995). An alternative reading approach: Instructional conversations in a bilingual special education setting. *Learning Disabilities Research and Practice, 10*(2), 108-119.

Egelston-Dodd, J. (1995). Inclusion in higher education. In R. Rittenhouse & J. Dancer (Eds.), *The full inclusion of persons with disabilities in American society* (pp. 23-34). Levin, New Zealand: National Training Resource Centre.

Feuerstein, R., & Jensen, M. (1980). Instructional enrichment: Theoretical basis, goals, and instruments. *The Educational Forum, 46,* 401-423.

Gallagher, P. (1988). *Teaching students with behavior disorders: Techniques and activities for classroom instruction.* Denver: Love.

Gearheart, B., & Weishahn, M. (1984). *The exceptional student in the regular classroom* (3rd ed.). St. Louis: Times Mirror/Mosby.

Goldenberg, C. (1991). *Instructional conversations and their classroom applications* (Educational Practice Report No. 2). Santa Cruz, CA: National Center for Research on Cultural Diversity and Second Language Learning.

Heath, D. (1982). What no bedtime story means: Narrative skills at home and school. *Language in Society, 11*, 49-76.

Idol, L., & Jones, B. (1991). *Educational values and cognitive instruction: Implications for reform.* Hillsdale, NJ: Lawrence Erlbaum.

Jones, B., Pierce, J., & Hunter, B. (1989). Teaching students to construct graphic representations. *Educational Leadership, 46*(4), 20-25.

Krashen, S. (1982). Accounting for child-adult differences in second language rate and attainment. In S. Krashen (Ed.). *Child-adult differences in second language acquisition,* (pp. 202-226). Cambridge, MA: Newbury House.

Luetke-Stahlman, B. (1996). A helpful checklist for schools and students. *Perspectives in Education and Deafness, 15*(1), p. 16-17.

Luetke-Stahlman, B. (1998). *Language issues in deaf education.* Hillsboro, OR: Butte Publications.

Luetke-Stahlman, B., & Luckner, J. (1991). *Effectively teaching students with hearing impairment.* New York: Longman.

Luetke-Stahlman, B., & Montgomery, N. (1997). *Programmatic and curricular modification form.* Unpublished form, University of Kansas Medical Center, Kansas City.

Mercer, C., & Mercer, A. (1989). *Teaching students with learning problems.* New York: Merrill.

Nelson, N. (1995). Scaffolding in the secondary school: A tool for curriculum-based intervention. In D. Tibbits (Ed.), *Language intervention: Beyond the primary grades* (pp. 375-419). Austin, TX: Pro-Ed.

Norris, J., & Hoffman, P. (1993). *Whole language intervention for school-age children.* San Diego, CA: Singular.

Ogle, D. (1989). The know, what to know, learn strategy. In K. D. Muty (Ed.), *Children's comprehension of text: Research into practice.* Newark, DE: International Reading Association.

O'Malley, J., & Chamot, A. (1986). What will happen to Tran and other LEP children? *PTA–Today*, 11, 6-10.

Ortiz, A. (1986). Characteristics of limited English proficient Hispanicstudents served in programs for the learning disabled: Implications for policy and practice (Part II). *Bilingual Special Education Newsletter, 4*, 1-5.

Palincsar, A., & Brown, A. (1984). Reciprocal teaching: A means to a meaningful end. In J. Osborn, P. Wilson, & R. Anderson (Eds.), *Reading education: Foundation for a literate America* (pp. 299-309). Lexington, MA: D. C. Heath.

Palincsar, A., & Brown, A. (1988). Teaching and practicing thinking skills to promote comprehension in the context of group problem solving. *Remedial and Special Education, 9*(1), 53-59.

Palincsar, A., Ranson, K., & Derber, S. (1989). Collaborative research and development for reciprocal teaching. *Educational Leadership, 46*(4), 37-40.

Piaget, J. (1967). *Biologie et connaissance.* Paris: Gallimard.

Poplin, M., & Stone, S. (1992). Paradigm shifts in instructional strategies: From reductionism to holistic/constructivism. In W. Stainback & S. Stainback (Eds.), *Controversial issues confronting special education: Divergent Perspectives* (pp. 156-179). Boston: Allyn & Bacon.

Pressley, M., Harris, K., & Marks, M. (1992). But good strategy instructors are constructivists! *Educational Psychology Review, 4*, 3-31.

Rosenshine, B. (1986). Synthesis of research on explicit teaching. *Educational Leadership, 43*(7), 60-69.

Schoenfeld, A. (1985). *Mathematical problem-solving.* New York: Academic Press.

Snow, C., Cancino, H., Gonzales, P., & Shribert, E. (1989). Giving formal definitions: An oral language correlate of school literacy. In D. Bloome (Ed.), *Classrooms and literacy.* Norwood, NJ: Ablex.

Vygotsky, L. (1962). *Thought and language* (E. Hanfonann & G. Vakar, Trans.). Cambridge, MA: MIT Press.

Vygotsky, L. (1978). *Mind and society: The development of higher psychological processes* (M. Cole, V. John-Steiner, S. Scribner, & E. Souberman, Eds. and Trans.). Cambridge, MA: Harvard University Press.

Watson, R. (1989). Literate discourse and cognitive organization: Some relations between parents' talk and 3-year-old's thought. *Applied Psycholinguistics, 10,* 221-236.

Webster, A., Beveridge, M., & Reed, M. (1996). *Managing the literacy curriculum: How schools can become communities of readers and writers.* Florence, KY: Routledge.

Weinstein, C., Ridley, D., Dahl, T., & Weber, S. (1989). Helping students develop strategies for effective learning. *Educational Leadership, 46* (4), 17-19.

Winne, P., & Marx, R. (1983). *Students cognitive processes while learning from teaching.* (Vols. 1 & 2). Instructional Psychology Research Group, (NIE Final Report, Grant No. NIE-G-79-0098). Burnaby, British Columbia: Simon Fraser University.

Wittrock, M. (1983). *Generative reading comprehension.* Boston: Ginn.

Wong-Fillmore, L. (1995). When does teacher talk work as input. In S. Gass & C. Madden (Eds.), *Input in second language acquisition: Series on issues in second language research* (pp. 17-50). New York: Academic Press.

Woodward, J., Allen, T., & Schildroth, A. (1985). Teachers and deaf students: An ethnography of classroom communication. In S. DeLancy & R. Tomling (Eds.), *Proceedings of the First Annual Meeting of the Pacific Linguistics Conference* (pp. 479-493). Eugene, OR: University of Oregon.

Chapter 2

Assessing and Facilitating Audition

Motivating Students to Listen to Speech

Assessment of Audition Abilities

Detection Assessment

Discrimination Assessment

Identification Assessment

Comprehension Assessment

Audition Curricula

Audition Facilitation

Appendix: Meaningful Auditory Integration Scale

"In the last ten years, a major change has occurred in the way that speech-language pathologists (SLPs) deliver services in school settings" (Beck & Dennis, 1997, p. 146). Although it is typically the responsibility of SLPs or teachers of the deaf to assess the audition, speechreading, and speech abilities of students who are D/HH, they are now often assisted by other team members in facilitating skills in these areas. The interrelated outcomes of such collaboration can include students' improvements in speech perception, speech reception, voice quality, and English language abilities (Luetke-Stahlman & Luckner, 1991).

Research reported by Novelli-Olmstead and Lind (1984) indicated that *it is more beneficial across the skills areas to integrate training in audition, speechreading, speech articulation, and language with play or academics than to address each behavior separately.* Team members should focus on facilitating the development of these skills across the curriculum and outside of school, enabling the student to function more independently and acquire a more natural ability to respond to and monitor communication in various settings (Luetke-Stahlman & Luckner, 1991).

Moeller, Osberger, and Morford (1987) noted that the integration of communicative abilities is critical. They proposed a broad-based approach that requires integration on several levels:
- in theoretical and practical terms
- among all team members throughout the day
- with regard to English use, meaning, and form, as well as underlying social, cognitive, and perceptual dimensions
- in auditory training and speechreading training aligned with English language goals
- in English language instruction combined with the facilitation of thinking skills

In this chapter, several frameworks are used to assist in organizing auditory assessment and facilitation ideas. These include work by Norm Erber, Jim Cummins, Daniel Ling, and Amy Robbins. Material within each framework is updated through the experiences of SLPs currently working in academic contexts. The assessment and facilitation of speechreading and speech which should occur simultaneously with the assessment and facilitation of audition, are discussed in Chapter 3.

Motivating Students to Listen to Speech

Auditory assessment and facilitation is a waste of time if students cannot hear sound when wearing assistive listening devices, are not motivated to wear such equipment, or are not willing to try to use the sound they hear. Therefore, it is essential that students be fitted with appropriate amplification devices and that they wear them consistently throughout the day (Luetke-Stahlman & Luckner, 1991). It is vital to combine *consistent* use of an amplification device *with* auditory training to enable a student to interpret sound.

Attention to sound should be made meaningful; behavior management techniques should be used; and environments in which the ability to hear is valued should be created and maintained throughout the day. Simply calling a student's name for no reason other than to see his or her head turn is *not* a good motivation strategy. A positive indicator of motivation and determination is demonstrated when a student who is D/HH spontaneously shows concern that equipment is not working. Students will begin intrinsically over time to recognize the benefits of amplification if given meaningful opportunities to value hearing.

Some professionals suggest that adults assessing and facilitating students' listening skills situate themselves in such a way as to prevent speechreading. For instance, an adult might stand behind or sit beside the student, or might look down naturally while engaged in activities. Others suggest using a puppet to simulate talking so that young children are distracted from watching the adult's mouth.

> **Study Guide Question**
> *Observe a group of young students who are D/HH. How do they demonstrate a motivation to listen to speech?*

Listening screens are useful for blocking all speechreading cues when adults need to be seated across from students. Screens are preferable to using a hand or paper to block speech, methods that can distort the auditory signal and allow the possible interpretation of facial cues from cheek muscle movement. A screen can be made from fabric stretched across an embroidery hoop. It is best to use two thicknesses of the fabric used on stereo speakers, but holiday prints are occasionally an acceptable substitution. Firszt and Reeder (1996) suggested making several screens and placing them in different areas for easy access.

> **Study Guide Question**
> *Visit a program in which listening activities are integrated into other areas of the curriculum. How is speechreading naturally discouraged or blocked?*

Assessment of Audition Abilities

The assessment of student audition (and speech) abilities demands that time be taken to evaluate the school acoustical environment. Completion of the modification checklist in Chapter 1 (Appendix 1–A) is helpful in this process. Needs such as carpeting in all noisy areas, wall and ceiling treatments, and newer FM systems should be included in a five-year administrative plan for implementation over time.

In preparation for the assessment of audition abilities, Luetke-Stahlman and Luckner (1991) suggested that team members plot each student's aided and unaided audiological results on an audiogram, such as the one that appears in Figure 2–1. In this figure, sounds with more than one major format appear in more than one location. The values given are based on data reported by Ling and Ling (1978). They should be considered only as approximations. Cochlear implant detection thresholds might be plotted as well (possibly using the letter C).

It has also been suggested that an auditory test battery contain both informal and formal measures (Moeller et al., 1987) that are question driven. The audiologist may have administered several tests to obtain the detection and speech reception abilities of a particular student. When there is a concern that young students might fatigue, the audiologist should be asked to conduct aided testing prior to unaided thresholds. The audiologist can explain the audiological report to

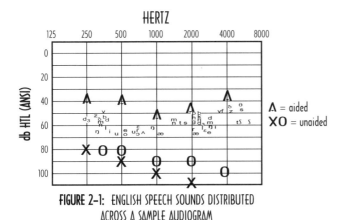

FIGURE 2-1: ENGLISH SPEECH SOUNDS DISTRIBUTED
ACROSS A SAMPLE AUDIOGRAM

Adapted from *Introduction to Aural Rehabilitation* (p. 83) by R. Schow and M. Nerbonne, 1989, Baltimore, MD: University Park Press. Copyright 1989. All rights reserved. Reprinted with permission of Allyn & Bacon.

team members, who will need this information if their desire is to facilitate the audition abilities of each student who is D/HH in academic and/or home settings.

One of the most useful auditory assessment taxonomies was developed by Erber (1982). It is a matrix that can be used to guide the evaluation and facilitation of auditory training. Using the matrix, informal but realistic tasks can be organized by team members to determine whether a student can respond auditorially to spoken stimuli as they become phonemically, syllabically, and linguistically more complex (see Figure 2–2).

Study Guide Question
Review several audiograms. Are aided thresholds charted? Practice explaining the information on each audiogram to a peer.

SPEECH STIMULUS

RESPONSE TASK		Speech Elements	Syllables	Words	Phrases	Sentences	Connected Discourse
	Detection						
	Discrimination						
	Identification						
	Comprehension						

FIGURE 2–2: GUIDELINES FOR EVALUATING AND FACILITATING AUDITORY TRAINING (ERBER MATRIX)

From *Auditory Training* (p. 38), by N. Erber, 1982, Washington, DC: Alexander Graham Bell Association for the Deaf. Copyright 1982 by Alexander Graham Bell Association for the Deaf. Reprinted with permission.

Speech stimuli are listed across the top of the matrix. Along the left-hand side of the matrix are the four basic auditory levels:

- *Detection* refers to the process of determining whether sound is present or absent.

- *Discrimination* is the ability to perceive similarities and differences between two or more speech stimuli. To distinguish sound in a discriminating manner, the student is required to understand the concepts of "same" and "different." For example, a teacher might ask (with his or her face not in view), *"Are these words the same or different: Kansas, Ohio."* A student who responds that they are different can discriminate between two-syllable and three-syllable words.

- *Identification* refers to the process of demonstrating recognition of what has been said. The student could demonstrate this skill by pointing to a picture, reading a specific word, or retrieving a specific object, as requested.

- *Comprehension* of speech is the most difficult auditory skill to master. It requires that the student understand an acoustic message and react appropriately. When students who can not see the speaker's face follow oral-only directions, participate in oral-only conversations, or answer oral-only questions, they are demonstrating their ability to comprehend spoken language.

The following examples of objectives written for auditory training for one student who is D/HH are based on Erber's work:

1. The student will daily demonstrate an ability to detect sounds with 90% accuracy, using the Six Sound Hearing Test administered by an adult at various distances under quiet and noisy classroom conditions.

2. The student will demonstrate an ability to detect (discriminate, identify, or comprehend) single words (common phrases, commands) with 90% accuracy, while engaged in typical school activities.

3. The student will identify common nouns, using classroom materials, with 90% accuracy, using audition only.

4. The student will follow simple, routine directions from the classroom teacher in school contexts with 90% accuracy, using audition only.

> **Study Guide Question**
> *Review the auditory training objectives for student who is D/HH. Which of Erber's four basic auditory levels are targeted?*

In Erber's work, the four levels of auditory assessment are tested in "closed set" situations: The student is aware that the acoustic signal will be one of two or more choices. If each of the auditory levels is graphed on the Cummins model (Cummins, 1984), "open set" or real-life stimuli can be assessed and facilitated (see Figure 2–3). Team members can use the Cummins model both to assess and to task-analyze the audition abilities of a particular student. (See Chapter 1 and Luetke-Stahlman, 1998, for explanations of the Cummins model.)

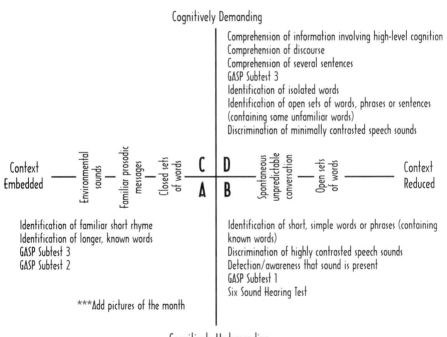

FIGURE 2–3: THE CUMMINS MODEL ADAPTED FOR AUDITION

Detection Assessment

Detection is the ability to perceive whether sound is or is not present. Following are descriptions of some recommended detection assessment tools: the Six Sound Hearing test, the GASP Subtest 1, and the MAIS.

Students who are D/HH should be given the opportunity to demonstrate detection skills. However, if after a period of time and after working with the audiologist to make modifications to amplification, a student is unable to demonstrate an ability to detect the sounds of the Six Sound Hearing Test or any vowels and phonemes of the GASP Subtest 1, then no objective for audition would be necessary. If the student is able to hear one or more of these sounds, then an IFSP/IEP objective for this skill would be written.

The Six Sound Hearing Test

The Six Sound Hearing Test (Ling, 1983) is a detection assessment procedure that can easily be taught to team members and used intermittently to assess closed set detection abilities in many different settings during the day. Its purpose is to determine whether a student who is D/HH notices when sound (provided at various frequencies) is or is not present. The evaluator thus receives information about which speech sounds a student is able to hear. For example, an adult might suspect that a student is not hearing his or her voice and might ask, *"Can you hear me?"* To confirm the student's response, the adult might use the Six Sound Hearing Test. This test can help determine

- whether the student has his or her assistive listening device on
- whether the equipment is working
- whether the battery is dead
- whether the student can hear in a noisy environment (such as in a cooperative learning group)
- whether the student can hear in an acoustically poor environment (such as the restroom or sink area)
- whether the student can hear from where he or she is seated

- a baseline for comparison to future improvement or decline in auditory ability

---

Six Sound Hearing Test (Ling, 1983)

---

1. Detection of six sounds
   a. The student is requested to clap his or her hands when first hearing one of the six sounds (/m/, /a/, /ee/, /oo/, /sh/, /s/) presented in random order and with different amounts of spacing between the sounds.
   b. The teacher turns the volume of the assistive listening device to a low position and stands behind or to the side of the student.
   c. The teacher says the six sounds and gradually increases the volume (older students may adjust the volume themselves).
   d. The detection level has been reached when the student indicates that all of the sounds capable of being heard have been heard. The volume on the assistive listening device should never be below this point.
   e. The teacher moves slowly away from the student, each time saying the sound with the same intensity but from a greater distance. This will demonstrate the maximum distance from the sound source at which the student may function auditorially. The teacher needs to maintain consistent volume while moving away from the student.

2. Discrimination of six sounds
   a. The student is requested to listen carefully with eyes closed for any one of the six sounds and is asked to repeat the sound that is heard.
   b. One sound at a time is presented from normal teaching/therapy distance.

3. Comparison of audiogram with formats

Comparison of the student's audiogram with the English speech sounds chart in Figure 2–1 will determine those sounds in the Six Sound Hearing Test that the student is capable of hearing with a properly fitted assistive listening device set at the proper volume.

From *Speech and the Hearing-Impaired Child,* by D. Ling, 1983, Washington, DC: Alexander Graham Bell Association for the Deaf. Copyright 1983 by Alexander Graham Bell Association for the Deaf. Adapted with permission.

Sometimes a change in response on the Six Sound Hearing Test may indicate audiological concerns. If problems continue, it is vital for team members to work closely with the audiologist to rule out the following:

- middle ear dysfunction and the associated decrease in hearing levels
- changes in acoustic properties of the ear mold
- permanent changes in hearing levels due to progressive hearing loss

When assessing a student's ability to detect the presence of sound, age-appropriate signals should be used as reinforcements. For example, reinforcement for a toddler might be a ring from a colorful stack; for a third grader it might be a thumbs-up signal; for a teenager it might be eye contact. Successful student responses assure the adult that the student realizes a sound has occurred. Conversely, if a student cannot detect sound—either routinely or just for the day (because of faulty equipment or middle ear infection)—team members will need to change their behavior, utilizing visual communication strategies.

> **Study Guide Question**
> *Give the Six Sound Hearing Test to a student from several locations. What were you able to determine from the results?*

The GASP Subtest 1

The detection segment of the Glendonald School for the Deaf Auditory Screening Procedure or GASP (Erber, 1982) can provide team members with more specific information about a student's sound detection abilities than can be derived from the Six Sound

Hearing Test. Vowels and phonemes screened are displayed on the data collection sheet for Subtest 1 in Figure 2–4.

Student:_____ Date:_____

PHONEME DETECTION - Place dot(s) in the yes/no box(es) to indicate student's response(s).

	seat	sit	set	sat	hot	sought	hook	hoot	hut	heard	no sound	nasals		laterals		voiced fricative				unvoiced fricatives			
												ma	no	rat	late	zoo	Measure	vet	the	Sam	shh	fan	thin
	i	I	ɛ	æ	ɑ	ɔ	ʊ	u	ʌ	3^		m	n	r	l	z	3	v	ð	s	ʃ	f	θ
yes	○	●	●	●	●	●	●	●	○	●		●	●	●	●	○	○	●			○		
no	●										●●●●●							●	●	●	●	●	●

● = normal intensity   ○ = increased intensity

FIGURE 2–4: GASP SUBTEST 1 RESPONSE FORM (PHONEME DETENTION)]

From *Auditory Training* (p. 56), by N. Erber, 1982, Washington, DC: Alexander Graham Bell Association for the Deaf. Copyright 1982 by Alexander Graham Bell Association for the Deaf. Adapted with permission.

To give the test, an adult produces the sounds specified, using a speech screen (or standing behind the student) and varying the order of the stimuli as well as the duration between stimuli. After each trial, the student indicates whether the sound was present. Sometimes the adult may only mouth a sound without voicing it. This foil is used to ensure that the student is really responding to sound and not to facial movements.

Students can be asked in this test to repeat the sound they hear, or sometimes they will do so automatically. However, a student can be credited for detecting sound by responding nonverbally (for instance, dropping blocks in a can), and oral repetition of the sound is not required. The response form for the test provides a symbol system to indicate whether it was helpful to the student's detection ability if (a) the sound was produced with more intensity, either by increasing the volume or by moving closer, or if (b) it was repeated.

Study Guide Question

What would you include in an IFSP/IEP objective that would be appropriate for a student who consistently missed two sounds of the Six Sound Hearing Test and could not hear the voiced and unvoiced fricatives tested by the GASP Subtest 1?

The MAIS

Robbins, Svirsky, Osberger, and Pisoni (1996) suggested assessing detection abilities by using the Meaningful Auditory Integration Scale (MAIS), which consists of ten probes asked of parents during an interview. The MAIS is provided in Appendix 2–A. Areas assessed include bonding to the equipment, spontaneously alerting to sound, and deriving meaning from sound.

The MAIS technique does not cue parents as to the desired answers, nor does it use yes/no questions. Information collected via the MAIS is considered by some practitioners to be more accurate than standard survey questioning (Robbins et al., 1996).

MAIS Technique	**Non-MAIS Questioning**
Tell me about Campbell's routine for wearing his assistive listening device (aids, FM system, cochlear implant, etc.).	*Does Clay wear his hearing aids all the time at home?*

Closed and Open Detection Assessment

Detection assessment in both closed-set situations where a context is available as well as open-set situations where context is reduced

Study Guide Question
Where would you add the MAIS on a Cummins model form such as the one in Figure 2–3?

may be useful for discussion during team meetings. Adults may find "charting" a helpful way to take systematic data (see Table 2–1).

TABLE 2–1: COLLECTING DETECTION DATA

Date	Stimuli	Context/Closed-Set Observance (Contrived)	Reduced Context/Open-Set Observance (Real Life)
	vowels		
	phonemes		
	environmental sounds		
	other		

Discrimination Assessment

Study Guide Question
How could you use Table 2–1 for collecting data in either a closed- or open-set situation?

The task of discrimination differs from that of simply detecting sound. Attaching meaning to sound can occur when students are cognitively aware of the acoustic events that surround them (Luetke-Stahlman & Luckner, 1991). For example, a student may hear enough of the characteristics of sound to realize that her father is angry (discrimination) but not enough to understand the content of her father's message (comprehension).

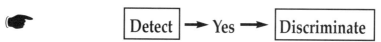

"The primary purpose of assessing auditory discrimination is to determine objectives for the student who can detect sound but who is having difficulty discriminating between two or more stimuli" (Luetke-Stahlman & Luckner, 1991, p. 206). Discrimination tasks require students who are D/HH to do one of two things:

- listen to whether *sounds*, not necessarily *speech*, are the same or different
- listen for a particular stimulus and ignore all others

Examples

Ms. Fletcher: Can you tell me whether you hear one or three sounds, Mary Pat? (beats a drum out of view of the student)

Mary Pat: Three!

Mr. Luckner: You can talk to your friends for a while when you hear the word *talk* (a one-syllable word). Ignore all other sounds or words, OK?

Sue: OK. (motivated to listen because she's excited to get a break from schoolwork and talk with her peers)

Mr. Luckner: (covers his mouth or walks behind her) Sooooo, hi, hi, hi, talk.

The GASP Subtest 2

The GASP Subtest 2 (Erber, 1982) is designed to assess both discrimination and identification ability. The stimulus items for the subtest should only include vocabulary words known to the student. Erber provided the example (shown in Figure 2–5) of words and pictures representing four different stress pattern categories used to elicit a student's response.

1	1—2	1—2	1 2—2
Picture of a shoe	Picture of a pencil	Picture of an airplane	Picture of an elephant
Picture of a ball	Picture of water	Picture of a toothbrush	Picture of a butterfly
Picture of a fish	Picture of a table	Picture of popcorn	Picture of a valentine

FIGURE 2–5: DISCRIMINATION AND IDENTIFICATION USING GASP SUBTEST 2

From *Auditory Training* (p. 59), by N. Erber, 1982, Washington, DC: Alexander Graham Bell Association for the Deaf. Copyright 1982 by Alexander Graham Bell Association for the Deaf. Adapted with permission.

The GASP Subtest 2 should be administered in the following manner:

1. A team member ensures that a student can label each picture correctly (typed words could be used instead of pictures for students who can definitely read them). To check that the stimuli are known to the student, the adult might sign or allow the student to speechread the question *"Where is the _____?"*

2. The adult presents the words to be used in random order enough times to ensure that the student understands the task.

3. After training, the adult stands behind the student or covers the face with a listening screen and randomly asks for an indication of each word identified by "audition only."

4. The student points to the picture or says the word that was heard.

5. The adult makes a dot on the appropriate place on the scoring guide after the student's response.

An example of a GASP Subtest 2 word identification response form is shown in Figure 2–6. Because of the test design, team members can record and analyze the GASP Subtest 2 data in two ways:

- Categorization—the student is able to discriminate the number of syllables in a word (dots marked in the squares of the scoring guide)
- Identification—the student can actually identify specific words (dots marked on the diagonal line of the scoring guide)

In the example in Figure 2–6, the data indicate that the student was able to discriminate words with the four stress patterns. This finding is illustrated by the examiner's markings (dots) that appear

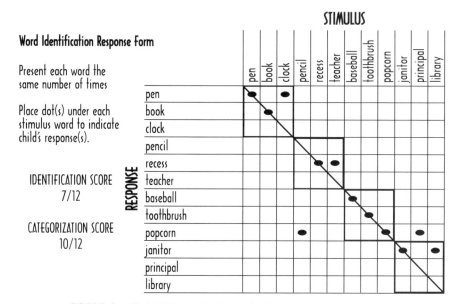

FIGURE 2–6: GASP SUBTEST 2 RESPONSE FORM (DISCRIMINATION AND IDENTIFICATION)

From *Auditory Training* (p. 62), by N. Erber, 1982, Washington, DC: Alexander Graham Bell Association for the Deaf. Copyright 1982 by Alexander Graham Bell Association for the Deaf. Adapted with permission.

in the categories (boxes) of one-, two-, and three-syllable words. Markings in the boxes (but not on the line) indicate that the student could usually recognize the number of syllables and the syllable stressed but could not identify exactly which word was being said. Results when given three-syllable words indicated that the student had difficulty identifying words in this category. The number of examiner's markings that do not appear on the diagonal line of the scoring guide indicates that the student could identify the exact word at only a 58% accuracy level (7 out of 12 on the line). This identification assessment is discussed later in this chapter.

Objectives

The results for the hypothetical student assessed using the GASP Subtest 2 (Figure 2–6) warrant that objectives be written to clarify that stimuli of various syllable constructions need to be manipulated—one syllable, two syllable, spondees, and stressed-unstressed syllables. (A spondee is a word with equal stress on each syllable, such as *toothbrush*). The condition segment of the objective is where this information is most likely to be incorporated. For example:

Once a week Lyle will discriminate social studies and science words that differ in number of syllables with 80% accuracy.

The following examples adapted from a hierarchy by Patterson (1992) could be used in the writing of discrimination objectives:

- single word as contrasted with short phrases (*boat* vs. *the boat is in the water*)
- words that vary in acoustic properties and syllable length (*boat, airplane, sheep, banana*)
- pairs of words that are acoustically similar (*father/brother, producer/consumer*)
- initial consonants that are similar; vowels and final consonants that are different (*down, dime, dance, door; Wisconsin/West Virginia*
- initial consonants that differ with the rest of the word rhyming or acoustically similar (*bean, team, dream, mean*)
- initial sounds that are the same while the ends of the word are different (*kick, kill, kiss, king*)

Identification Assessment

Study Guide Question
What would you include in an objective for discrimination written for a student who is D/HH with whom you work?

The purpose of auditory identification assessment is to determine whether a student who can discriminate the number and stress of syllables can recognize a spoken word or phrase and match it, point to it, or retrieve it when asked to do so in spoken English.

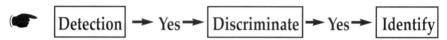

Robbins and Kirk (1996) suggested a list of formal speech perception measures that require students to identify speech stimuli accurately. The measures suggested are listed along a continuum from closed-set tools of pattern perception to open-set tools using sentences and single words (Table 2–2).

TABLE 2–2: FORMAL IDENTIFICATION MEASURES

Test	Material	Mode	Response Format
1. GASP Subtest 2 (Erber, 1982)	12 nouns (as shown in Figure 2–5)	live voice: auditory	closed-set picture pointing (12 choices)
2. Hoosier Auditory-Visual Enhancement Test (HAVE) (Renshaw, Robbins, Miyamoto, Osberger, & Pope, 1988)	40 items of primarily one-syllable word triplets	live voice	closed-set picture pointing (3 choices)
3. Minimal Pairs Test (Robbins, Renshaw, Miyamoto, Osberger, & Pope, 1988)	Word pairs differing by one feature; four pairs per feature	live voice: auditory	closed-set picture pointing (2 choices)
4. Pediatric Speech Intelligibility Test (PSI) (Jerger, Lewis, Hawkins, & Jerger, 1980)	Single words and sentences	live voice: auditory only, visual only, and combined	closed-set picture pointing (6 choices) *cont.*

From "Speech Perception Assessment and Performance in Pediatric Cochlear Implant Users," by A. Robbins and K. Kirk, 1996, *Seminars in Hearing, 17*(4), p. 355. Copyright 1996 by Thieme Medical Publishers, Inc. Adapted with permission.

TABLE 2–2:, CONT.

Test	Material	Mode	Response Format
5. Phonetically Balanced–Kindergarten (PB-K) (Haskins, 1949)	Four lists of 50 mono syllabic words	live voice: auditory	open-set word recognition
6. Lexical Neighborhood Test (LNT) (Kirk, Pisoni, & Osberger, 1995)	List of easy and hard monosyllabic words	live voice: auditory	open-set word repetition
7. Multisyllabic Lexical Neighborhood Test (MLNT) (Kirk et al., 1995)	List of easy and hard multisyllabic words	live voice: auditory	open-set word repetition
8. Common Phrases (Robbins, Renshaw, & Osberger, 1988)	2–6 command or question word phrases and combined	live voice: auditory only, visual only,	open-set phrase repetition

To assess identification using the GASP Subtest 2 (Erber, 1982) with a closed set of items, the following procedure is typically used:

> **Study Guide Question**
> *Assemble several of the tools listed in Table 2–2. How do they compare and contrast?*

1. The adult gathers stimulus items or uses those that are in view (choosing words that are in the student's receptive vocabulary and that require responses the student is capable of making).

2. The adult holds up or points to the stimulus items and says and/or signs the names of each of the items, allowing the student full access to all auditory and visual cues.

3. The adult says the names of each of the items (without holding up or pointing to the stimulus items), allowing the student to use both auditory and speechreading cues to make an auditory and visual match for each item.

4. The adult covers his or her mouth and cheek area and says the names of the items, asking the student for the identification of each item at random.

Team members should remember to choose words for the GASP Subtest 2 that are familiar to the student. If a high percentage (50% or above) of the student's responses are scored on the diagonal line of the scoring grid (see Figure 2–6), more challenging auditory identification abilities should be assessed. After assessment, the Cummins model adapted for audition (Figure 2–3) would be useful in deciding how to increase the challenge systematically to facilitate a student's identification abilities.

Comprehension Assessment

Comprehension of acoustic signals is the most difficult auditory skill to acquire. It is the ability not only to understand what is heard but also to respond in a fitting manner. Both home and academic settings provide comprehension assessment opportunities (Figure 2–7).

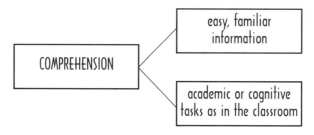

FIGURE 2–7: WAYS OF ASSESSING COMPREHENSION

The GASP Subtest 3

The GASP Subtest 3 (Erber, 1982) is a comprehension screening tool that can serve as an initial assessment instrument. In Figure 2–8, the original items on the GASP Subtest 3 Scoring Form have been augmented with examples to characterize both home and academic settings. Words that appear in brackets could be replaced with words known to the students being assessed.

The procedure for using the GASP Subtest 3 is similar to the identification tasks described in the previous section. That is, the adult first ensures that a student can repeat each sentence correctly

Student: _____ Date: _____

Sentence Comprehension (Questions)	Indicate:				
Practice Items (A-V):	A-V			Number of presentations	√ if correct (auditory alone)
(a) How many [pencils] do you have?	Emphasis (Gesture)				
(b) Where is your [eraser]?					
(c) What color is the [ocean]?					
	Response	Comments			
Test items (auditory alone):					
(1) What's your name?					
(2) What color is [the ocean]?					
(3) How many [students are in the room]?					
(4) Where's your [hearing aid]?					
(5) When is your [P.E. class] ?					
(6) What is your [art teacher's] name?					
(7) What number comes after [seven]?					
(8) How many legs does [an elephant] have?					
(9) Where does [your grandma live]?					
(10) How old is [your sister]?					
			Score		
A-V = auditory + visual [ ] = age-appropriate school/home vocabulary					

FIGURE 2–8: GASP SUBTEST 3 SCORING FORM (SENTENCE COMPREHENSION)

From *Auditory Training* (p. 67), by N. Erber, 1982, Washington, DC: Alexander Graham Bell Association for the Deaf. Copyright 1982 by Alexander Graham Bell Association for the Deaf. Adapted with permission.

when allowed to speechread and understands all vocabulary. The adult presents the sentences in random order and for a sufficient number of trials to ensure that the student understands the task. After training, the adult uses a screen or sits behind the student and randomly asks for a response to each question (audition only). The adult then marks the scoring guide after the student responds.

Objectives

A student who passes an identification task but does not do well at the comprehension level of assessment needs one or more objectives written for the comprehension level of audition work. For example:

Peta will respond correctly each day to ten auditorially presented questions asked with significant context in academic or home routines.

When simpler comprehension questions can be understood, those that require higher-level thinking skills should be asked. These higher-level questions might involve judging, analyzing, synthesizing, comparing and contrasting, and so forth:

Domonicki will respond correctly each day to ten auditorially presented questions asked during social studies or science classes and involving higher-level thinking skills.

Audition Curricula

The following two curricula provide audition assessment as well as facilitation information. Their descriptions are followed by a listing of additional recommended audition curricula.

The *Developmental Approach to Successful Listening–Revised* (DASL) (Stout & Van ert Windle, 1992) is a sequential listening program to help students who are D/HH develop and use their listening ability. The program focuses on the positive aspect of learning by assessing students and then gradually facilitating the acquisition of difficult listening tasks. The DASL program consists of a hierarchy of listening skills designed to be taught in short, individualized auditory training sessions. The curriculum is divided into three sections: Sound Awareness, Phonetic Listening, and Auditory Comprehension. Several listening skills are taught simultaneously from the three sections.

The *Auditory Skills Instructional Planning System* (Thies & Trammel, 1983) is a tool that also incorporates auditory assessment and training ideas. The most well-known section of it is the Test of Auditory Comprehension (TAC), a placement and progress test. Also included is a curriculum (Auditory Skills Curriculum), which consists of a sequence of objectives in four areas (discrimination, memory-sequencing, feedback, and figure-ground). A section of activities completes the kit. Moeller et al. (1987) cautioned that children under four years of age and others with profound losses may fail the lowest subtest of the TAC. Should this occur, adults can return to detection assessment to ensure that the student can reliably indicate the presence or absence of sound. If so, Moeller et al. recommended that the student receive repeated and systematic exposure to speech (not environmental live or recorded sounds). An example might be *"Jump, jump, jump!"* contrasted with *"Pleeeeease wait a minute."*

Audition Curricula

Graham, T. (1992). *Listening is a Way of Loving.* Atlanta: Humanics Publishing Group.

Maxwell, M. (1981). *Listening Games for Elementary Grades.* Washington, DC: Acropolis Books.

Toomey, M. (1991). *Defining and Describing.* Marblehead, MA: Circuit.

Audition Facilitation

> **Study Guide Question**
> *Compare the audition curricula described. Which do you prefer and why?*

When the principles of optimal input (explained by Luetke-Stahlman, 1998) are reviewed with regard to audition, it is obvious that the only meaningful way for audition facilitation to occur is in genuine contexts throughout the day. In addition, these principles promote the use of speechreading cues, fingerspelled cues, tactile cues, kinesthetic cues, print cues, and so on. It might be argued that the use of such audition supports gives more context to how a word sounds (or is articulated) and is more natural than an audition-only context. Some characteristics of audition facilitation are listed below (Luetke-Stahlman & Luckner, 1991; Robbins, 1994a, 1994b, 1995).

Audition Facilitation Characteristics

1. Assessment to establish stimuli that are slightly challenging to the student who is D/HH.

2. The use of spoken stimuli rather than noise or musical instruments if the outcome for the student is to comprehend auditory information. This does not preclude the inclusion of meaningful environmental sounds (the microwave buzzer, the telephone ringing, etc.).

3. Integration of speech, speechreading, and audition employed:
   - to encourage spoken interchanges
   - to verify auditory reception
   - to practice speech production

4. Expectation that speech and audition skills will be integrated daily into academic areas.

5. Use of the adapted Cummins model to set targets and provide systematic facilitation in this communication area (see below).

6. In addition to continued facilitation of speech articulation, possible instruction in musical instruments such as cello or piano for students who are ready for fine discriminations of sound.

Team members can integrate audition with or without additional cues in school subject areas by phrasing IFSP and IEP objectives to include these skills. Some examples from the IEP of a deaf third grader are:

1. Given a graphic organizer, Marcy will answer true/false statements using audition and tactile cues.

2. When speechreading, Marcy will follow two-level commands containing concepts such as *then, sometimes, before, after, while.*

3. Marcy will follow auditory-only directions and spell the target word during weekly spelling lessons.

The difficulty of stimuli presented auditorially may be increased or decreased by doing one of the following:

- increasing or decreasing the number of items in the set
- using familiar (easier) or unfamiliar (more difficult) vocabulary
- increasing or decreasing the rate of presentation
- increasing or decreasing the amount of acoustic highlighting (how much emphasis is placed in the utterance)
- adjusting the figure-ground ratio (the amount of background noise present)
- increasing or decreasing the number of words in the carrier phrase (to decrease difficulty, allow the student to observe the carrier phrase so that auditory comprehension is required for only one item in the phrase, for example, *"Point to the _____"*)
- using an open or closed set of stimuli

Detection Facilitation

When a student is able to detect real-life sounds, such as those in the following examples, he or she will exhibit a natural response. Such a response indicates that the student is able to perceive but cannot necessarily discriminate the sounds heard. Working with real-life sounds at school and at home is recommended for detection facilitation.

Examples of Real-Life Sounds to Detect	
School	**Home**
■ school alarm ringing indicating the beginning or end of school, period changes, etc. ■ announcements over the public address system ■ music	■ doorbell ringing ■ microwave buzzer going off ■ something falling, making a loud noise ■ dog barking ■ hearing aid whistling

Discrimination Facilitation

To encourage the student's auditory discrimination, team members should begin by facilitating listening to stimuli that are highly contrasted. Reference to the Cummins model adapted for audition (see Figure 2–3) could assist with a task analysis and sequencing of the discrimination skills the student should strive to achieve.

The student should listen to specific sounds during meaningful activities. Estabrooks (1994) listed the "Learning to Listen Sounds" and advocated pairing a sound with a particular object in a young child's environment. He recommended consistently using that object/sound pairing when facilitating discrimination between it and another object/sound pair. For example, the consonant-vowel combination /bu/ can be paired with the use of bubbles. Both a bottle of bubbles and a sleeping baby doll (paired with /shhh/) can be set out. When the child hears /bu/, bubbles are blown as reinforcement for discriminating /bu/ from /shhh/. Pictures can be used in place of real objects for older children. Pair suggestions from this "Learning to Listen Sounds" curriculum are listed below. These could be adapted for older students.

Sound Facilitated	Toy/Associated Activity
a, oo, ah, etc.	farm animals
b	any ball
t	clock
shhh	sleeping baby doll
whee	slide

Discrimination includes both *suprasegmental* and *segmental* information. Discriminating suprasegmental information includes the ability to distinguish differences in the number of syllables, pitch, loudness, and/or duration. Discriminating segmental information includes the ability to differentiate vowel and consonant information.

Suprasegmental features are easier for students to recognize and should always be addressed first during facilitation activities.

Practice with auditory discrimination of suprasegmentals can also facilitate the acquisition of these features in the student's speech. Activities such as those exemplified below should be planned for the student who needs practice in discriminating this type of suprasegmental and segmental information.

Examples of Realistic Discrimination Activities

Suprasegmental Activities

School	Home
The student listens to two different songs with different beats and acts out each song, using different props. The target is to discriminate, for example, a fast beat from a slow beat.	The student listens to and must discriminate the number of syllables in each family member's request for drinks such as "chocolate milk," "soda," or "juice."

Segmental Activities

School	Home
The student serves different cookies at a tea party, depending on which cookie other students request. The target here is not to identify words, but to discriminate, for example, the short vowel sound in "big" cookie from the long vowel sound in "spice" cookie.	While folding laundry, the student must pick out the article of clothing requested. The target is not to identify items of clothing, but to discriminate, for example, the number of syllables in "T-shirt" from the number of syllables in "socks."

Identification Facilitation

Real-life activities can quite naturally become ways to facilitate identification of words or phrases. Team members can use any of numerous activities for this purpose.

Examples of Realistic Identification Activities

School
- calling on student at random to line up
- asking student to get something out of the desk
- asking student to find something in a book, on a map, etc.

Home
- asking child to get something in particular in the home
- asking child to get or take off a particular piece of clothing

---

Comprehension Facilitation

Comprehension activities require the student to understand the spoken message and to respond appropriately. The following are some examples of realistic comprehension activities.

Examples of Realistic Comprehension Activities

School
- having the student participate in telephone training*
- asking the student to discuss a topic in a cooperative learning group
- asking the student to get directions from the librarian and follow them

Home
- doing homework together
- reading a story together and predicting outcomes or otherwise discussing the text
- talking in the car when the student is in the back seat
- having the student place an order at a deli or sub shop or other store where choices must be comprehended (*"Do you want that on* white *or on* wheat *bread?"*)

---

*Erber (1982, 1985) developed a comprehensive auditory program for telephone training with students who are D/HH.

Audition Facilitation and the Cummins Model

Study Guide Question

What other examples of comprehension activities would you add to those listed?

The Cummins model as adapted for audition can assist parents and professionals in identifying ways to help students who are having trouble listening (see Figure 2–3). One question that should come to mind when students cannot respond to a message provided auditorially is, *"Can I supply more context without reducing the level of linguistic or cognitive difficulty?"*

Context might be added to listening skills in several ways. Consider the following techniques and adaptations:

- Improve room acoustics.
- Check current and working FM equipment and systems.
- Reduce class size.
- Clarify or emphasize some aspect of articulation.
- Say it again two or three times.
- Move closer and say it again.
- Provide a closed set (*"Is it x, y, or z?"*).
- Add gestures.
- Reduce the complexity of the grammar.
- Say it another way.
- Say it using graphic support (a picture, a drawing, etc.).
- Provide speechreading before trying audition-only.
- Add cues (Cued Speech, Visual Phonics).
- Add tapping or other kinesthetic cues for syllables.
- Provide a word clue (*"It rhymes with ____."*).
- Sign the parts of the message that you think are the most difficult to understand.

Such adaptations should be noted on scoring grids and lesson plans so that a particular student's abilities are not misinterpreted when assessment results are reviewed.

Use of the Cummins model can also remind team members to be aware of cognitive constraints. Some students might need to have elements of cognitive demand reduced, while others may be ready for higher-level thinking skills. Cognitively challenging auditory tasks can also be planned by referring to activities characterized by the demands of Quadrant D behaviors on a Cummins model. Provided no context, the student could be asked to perform a variety of higher-level cognitive or linguistic skills such as those listed by Luetke-Stahlman (1998). For example, like their hearing peers, third graders who are D/HH might be asked to compare two simple questions, describe how a state is different from a country, sequentially order important historical events, and so forth. Students unable to perform audition tasks that are characteristic of Quadrant D will probably need the assistance of an oral or manual interpreter when enrolled in age-appropriate general classroom activities (history, social studies, science, math, and so on).

When Students Are Ready for Cognitive Challenge——

Robbins (1994a, 1994b) described an approach to the facilitation of auditory development that she labeled "**Thinking While Listening.**" The approach is especially appropriate for students who wear cochlear implants but should be attempted with all students who are D/HH for whom improved auditory abilities are a goal. A year after receiving cochlear implants, subjects in the Robbins sample who participated in Thinking While Listening activities evidenced receptive and expressive English language gains that were 8–9 months higher than what would be predicted by maturation alone. Progress in audition and speech abilities was dramatic for some subjects as well. Robbins (1994a) cautioned that it is especially important that students with implants (and those with comprehension difficulties) be expected to

- interpret what is heard
- do more than imitate and repeat models
- demonstrate the generalization of skills capably performed in routinized tasks

Additional ideas that Robbins (1998, in press) is using in conjunction with a series of games are described below.*

*Game ideas and examples from Robbins, 1998, in press. Adapted with the author's permission. Additional works by Robbins for those interested in reading more about her techniques are listed in the references to this chapter.

What Is It Game

Worthley (1978) provided numerous stimuli for the What Is It game, and Robbins added to them. Students who are D/HH were provided several sentence-length clues to determine what is being described.

Adult: What is it? It is soft. (pause) It keeps you warm. (pause) It is made of cotton or wool. (pause)

Anna: (sometimes repeats the clues) Blanket.

Robbins' facilitation of this game included a hierarchy of contextual clues:
- clarification is provided using repetition (auditory-only), acoustic highlighting, slowing of the speech rate, clearer pronunciation, increased intonation contrasts
- rephrasing is presented
- speechreading is added for one word, then a short phrase, then part of the message, then for the entire message
- fingerspelling is used
- signing is added for one word, several words, and finally for the entire phrase

Robbins described Claire, the mother of a third grader, Rici, using the What Is It game to review science and social studies vocabulary with her daughter. Claire would provide clues to identify simple machines, the solar system, characteristics of communities, and the names of states and countries. The two enjoyed studying in this way and Claire simultaneously facilitated development in two areas—audition and academics.

What Is Happening Game

Robbins described a game, similar to the What Is It game, that targets verbs.

Adult: This happens in the morning. (pause) You use an object with a handle. (pause) You stroke the top of your head.

Rici: You brush your hair!

Robbins explained that the game represents an inclusion/exclusion task; with each clue, more possible items are excluded, and clues grow more specific. Understanding inclusion/exclusion is an important cognitive skill. Again, the game can be made cognitive and academic as well.

Adult: You are using a level. (pause) You move the fulcrum towards the load. (pause) Now you push down on one end of the level.

Rici: You are moving an object.

What Number Is Said Twice Game

For the What Number Is Said Twice game, the adult says several digits:

Adult: 4, 7, 2, 3, 4, 8

The student must decide which number was said twice. To do so requires short-term memory, as well as audition ability. However, linguistic skills are avoided, and the difficulty of the game can be altered using longer or shorter sequences of numbers.

Robbins described how Claire adapted this game to practice categories of vocabulary:

Claire: Which words are simple machines? (pause) A level, a pencil sharpener, a screw, a nail.

Change a Sound Game

Robbins explained that the Change a Sound game is a vocabulary and definitions game that requires students who are D/HH to manipulate a speech sound mentally within a word in order to change one word to another:

Study Guide Question
How would you adapt one of the games described to practice adjectives or review a history lesson?

| Adult: | Change the word *pork* to make it mean a play area [*park*]. |

Claire found that this game helped her child, Rici, to pay attention to the pronunciation and letter sequences of her weekly spelling words. The type of substitution skill required in the Change a Sound game is important for reading proficiency.

Robbins commented that this game can be altered to include constant changes, but these can be more difficult for students. Robbins also incorporated material from *Listening Games for Elementary Grades* (Maxwell, 1981) into this game. She noted that if one of the students she works with is unsuccessful, she relies on the hierarchy of contextual clues (see the What Is It game). Sometimes the adult and the student switch roles, and the adult requires the student to bring words from academic classes to the session as well. Then speech articulation is practiced in addition to audition using academic context.

Solve a Problem Game

In the Solve a Problem game, Robbins posed a problem to the student, Anna, that related to current events or activities that had happened at home or school (as described by Anna's parents):

| Ms. Robbins: | A woman in Kansas drove on a country road in a blizzard and is stranded now in a snowdrift. She has a cellular phone but doesn't know where she is. What can she do? |

As with the What Is It game, Robbins again used the hierarchy of contextual clues with this game; she also sometimes added a picture or drawing if necessary. After Robbins described the problem, she and Anna discussed possible outcomes and weighed the merits of different solutions. Robbins and Anna talked about how to prevent or avoid such problems. Their discussion often incorporated complex grammar and infrequently used vocabulary (*country road, blizzard, stranded, cellular,* etc.).

Hit Parade Game

In the Hit Parade game, Robbins and her student, Anna, sang currently popular songs together and discussed the lyrics. Anna recognized these songs because her family members and peers listened to them and she saw them on MTV with captioning, but she had not always understood the vocabulary or the subtle meanings in the lyrics. The lyrics often required making inferences, an important cognitive-linguistic skill. Anna looked forward to these sessions in which she could learn about familiar songs. After the discussion, Robbins and Anna sang the song on tape, and Anna took it home and listened to it several times. Robbins then asked Anna to write a possible new verse. Robbins (1998, in press) commented that "understanding and enjoying music are culturally important experiences for Anna."

Additional Thinking While Listening Activities

Robbins explained several Thinking While Listening activities that give a student who is D/HH two subtle messages:
- *"I want you to do something meaningful with what you hear."*
- *"There is a lot of unpredictability in what you hear."*

The approach begins with making sure the child can select one stimulus out of a field of at least two stimuli: *"Do you hear A or B?"* In fact, the clinician will sabotage the child by presenting A or B or nothing. The absence of sound is *not* identified as one of the choices since this would simply be a three-choice task. Rather, an expectation is set that the child must identify silence, even when she expects to hear A or B. If the child successfully resists sabotage with a field of two items, the set may be systematically expanded.

An example of a listening task of this nature might be as follows:

| Mr. Stewart: | (no sound but voiceless mouthing of a word behind a screen.) Find the word I said. |
| | (pointing to field of four objects) |

> **Study Guide Question**
>
> *Practice with a friend each of the games Robbins described. Which could you best use to practice new vocabulary from reading, social studies, or science? Give reasons for your choice.*

Spike: I didn't hear any sound.

Mr. Stewart: Good job! I tried to
                    trick you! Listen again:
                    baby.

Changing Predictable Routines

As discussed in the Thinking While Listening activities above, the inclusion of times during listening when a student will hear no sound is a technique called "saboteuring" (or "sabotage"). That is, the adult purposely does not voice what the student is expecting. Saboteuring is a technique that can be employed during any level of audition activity (detection, discrimination, identification, comprehension).

Summary

This chapter has focused on the assessment and facilitation of audition. Practical examples to encourage the inclusion of audition objectives across the curriculum were provided. The importance of always practicing listening skills along with speech, language, and appropriately leveled play or academic skills was stressed.

Study Guide Questions

1. What would be an example of saboteuring during an identification level audition activity? Try the technique with a partner.

2. Robbins (1995) provided the following example of saboteuring. What level of audition is this?

Adult asks: "Which number was said twice?"

Trial 1: 5, 4, 2, 3, 1, 3 [3]

Trial 2: 6, 8, 3, 5, 8, 2 [8]

Trial 3: 5, 9, 8, 4, 1, 7 [none]

Activities

1. Use a suggested auditory assessment procedure to evaluate the listening abilities of a student who is D/HH.
Write a professional report describing this experience and include a plan for using the assessment results.

2. Observe a professional facilitating audition across several contexts.

3. Read the IFSPs or IEPs of several students who are D/HH and discuss the audition objectives written for each.

4. Facilitate auditory skills as you teach a student math, social studies, or science content.

Appendix 2-A

Meaningful Auditory Integration Scale (MAIS)
Amy M. Robbins, M.S.*

Level 1 & Level 2

NAME _____   DATE _____

INTERVAL _____

CONDITION (device) _____

EXAMINER _____

INFORMANT _____

1. Score item 1a if the child is younger than age 5 and item 1b if the child is older than age 5.

1a. Does the child wear the device all waking hours WITHOUT resistance?

Ask the parent, "What is your routine for putting on _____'s device each day?" Have the parent explain how long the child wears the device and determine if the child wears it all waking hours WITHOUT resistance or for only restricted periods of time. Ask, "If one day you didn't put the device on ____ would ____ show any indication that she/he missed wearing it (such as pulling or pointing to her/his ear, going over to where the device is kept when not in use, looking upset or quizzical, etc.)." An additional query would be, "Does your child give any nonverbal indication that she/he is upset when the device is removed (such as crying or fussing)?"

_____ 0 = Never: If parent seldom puts the device on the child because the child resists wearing it.

_____ 1 = Rarely: If the child wears the device for only short periods of time but resists wearing it.

_____ 2 = Occasionally: If child wears device for only short periods of time but without resistance.

_____ 3 = Frequently: If the child wears the device all waking hours without resistance.

_____ 4 = Always: If the child wears the device all waking hours and provides some indication if the parent forgets to put it on one day and/or some indication that she/he is upset or misses the device when it is not on.

cont.

*Developed at Indiana University School of Medicine, Indianapolis, IN. Reprinted with permission. (Available from Amy Robbins, 8512 Spring Mill Rd., Indianapolis, IN 46260)

PARENT REPORT:

1b. Does the child ask to have her/his device put on, or put it on WITHOUT being told?

Ask, "What is _____'s routine for putting on his/her device each day?" Have parent explain if it is the parent or the child who takes responsibility for it. Ask, "If one day, you didn't put the device on _____ and didn't mention it, would _____ ask to wear it and be upset by not having it?" An additional query would be, "Does your child basically wear it according to routine (such as all day at school and one hour at night) or does she/he want it on all waking hours?" (For example, she/he puts it on at night even after her/his bath.) The latter would indicate a child who is more bonded and dependent on her/his device than the former.

_____ 0 = Never: If the child resists wearing it.

_____ 1 = Rarely: If the parent says child wears it without resistance, but would never ask for it.

_____ 2 = Occasionally: If child might inquire about it and is content to wear it with a set time routine.

_____ 3 = Frequently: If the child wears the device all waking hours without resistance.

_____ 4 = Always: Only if child wears it all waking hours and it's part of his body (like glasses would be).

PARENT REPORT:

2.   Does the child report and/or appear upset if his/her device is non-functioning for any reason?

Ask parent to give examples of what the child has done (verbally or nonverbally) when the device was not working. Ask also, "Have you ever checked _____'s device and found it was not working (or headpiece had fallen off), but she/he had not noticed or had not told you?" In the case of the younger child, ask, "Have you ever checked _____'s device and found it wasn't working but she/he had not provided any nonverbal indication (such as crying, reaching for the headpiece, etc.) that it was not working?"

cont.

____	0 = Never:	If the child has no awareness of the device working or not.
____	1 = Rarely:	If parent says child might only notice a malfunctioning device (using verbal or nonverbal indication) once in a while.
____	2 = Occasionally:	If parents can give some examples of when the child would recognize a malfunctioning device (or if headpiece has fallen off) more than 50% of the time and may be beginning to distinguish some device problems from others.
____	3 = Frequently:	If parent gives examples and/or child can often distinguish different types of malfunction (bad cord vs. weak batteries).
____	4 = Always:	If child would never go without immediately detecting and reporting a problem with his/her unit and can easily identify what the problem is.

PARENT REPORT:

3. Does the child spontaneously respond to his/her name in quiet when called auditorially only with no visual cues?

Ask, "If you called _____'s name from behind his back in a quiet room <u>with no visual clues</u> what percentage of <u>the first time</u> would he respond the first time you called?"

____	0 = Never:	If the child never does.
____	1 = Rarely:	If he has done it only once or twice or only with multiple repetitions.
____	2 = Occasionally:	If he does it about 50% of the time on the first trial or does it consistently but only when parent repeats his name more than once.
____	3 = Frequently:	If he does it at least 75% of the time on the first try.

cont.

_____ 4 = Always: If he does this reliably and consistently, responding every time just as a hearing child would. Ask for examples.

PARENT REPORT:

4.   Does the child spontaneously respond to his name in the presence of background noise when called auditorially only with no visual cues?

Ask, "If you called _____'s name from behind his back with no visual cues in a noisy room, with people talking and the TV on, what percentage of time would he turn around and respond to you the first time you called?"

_____ 0 = Never: If the child never does.

_____ 1 = Rarely: If the child has done it only once or twice or only with multiple repetitions.

_____ 2 = Occasionally: If he does it about 50% of the time on the first trial or does it consistently but only when the parent repeats his name more than once.

_____ 3 = Frequently: If he does it at least 75% of the time on the first try.

_____ 4 = Always: If he does this reliably and consistently, responding every time just as a normal hearing child would. Ask for samples.

PARENT REPORT:

5.   Does the child spontaneously alert to environmental sounds (door bell, telephone) in the home without being told or prompted to do so?"

Ask, "Tell me about the kinds of environmental sounds _____ responds to at home and give me examples." Question parents to be sure the child is responding auditorially only with no visual cues. Examples could be asking about the telephone, doorbell, dog barking, water running, smoke alarm, toilet flushing, engines revving, horns honking, microwave bell, washer changing cycles, thunder, etc. Examples must be child alerting spontaneously and not prompted by parent.

cont.

____	0 = Never:	If parent can give no examples or if child responds only after a prompt.
____	1 = Rarely:	If parent can give only one or two examples, or give several examples where the child's responses are inconsistent.
____	2 = Occasionally:	If child responds about 50% of the time to more than two environmental sounds.
____	3 = Frequently:	If child consistently responds to many environmental sounds at least 75% of the time.
____	4 = Always:	If child basically responds to environmental sounds the way a hearing child would. If there are a number of sounds which regularly occur to which the child does not alert (even if he consistently responds to two sounds such as the phone and the doorbell) he would score no higher than occasionally.

PARENT REPORT:

6. Does the child alert to auditory signals spontaneously when in new environments?

Ask, "Does your child show curiosity (verbally or nonverbally) about new sounds when in unfamiliar settings, such as in someone else's home or a restaurant by asking, "What was that sound?" or "I hear something!" A younger child may provide nonverbal indications that she has heard a new sound with eye widening, looking quizzical, searching for the source of the new sound, imitation of the new sound (such as when playing with a new toy). Examples parents have reported are children asking about clanging dishes in a restaurant, bells dinging in a department store, PA systems in public buildings, unseen baby crying in another room.

____	0 = Never:	If parents can give no examples.
____	1 = Rarely:	If parents can give only one or two examples.
____	2 = Occasionally:	If child has done this numerous times and parents can give examples.

cont.

____ 3 = Frequently: If parents can give numerous examples and this is a common occurrence.

____ 4 = Always: If very few sounds occur without the child asking about them (or, in the case of the younger child, showing curiosity nonverbally).

PARENT REPORT:

7. Does the child spontaneously RECOGNIZE auditory signals that are part of his/her school or home routine?

Ask, "Does _____ regularly recognize or respond appropriately to auditory signals in his/her classroom (school bell, PA system, fire alarm) or in the home (running to the window to see which family member is home when he/she hears the garage door opening; going to the table when the bell of the microwave goes off, signaling that the food is cooked and it is time to eat) with no visual cues or other prompts?"

____ 0 = Never: If she/he never does it.

____ 1 = Rarely: If there are one or two instances.

____ 2 = Occasionally: If she/he responds to these signals about 50% of the time.

____ 3 = Frequently: If many examples are given and the child does it 75% of the time.

____ 4 = Always: If she/he has clearly mastered this skill and does it all of the time.

PARENT REPORT:

8. Does the child show the ability to discriminate spontaneously between two speakers, using audition alone (such as knowing mother's vs. father's voice, or parents' vs. sibling's voice)

Ask, "Can _____ tell the difference between two voices, like Mom's or Dad's (or Susie's or John's) just by listening to them?"

cont.

_____ 0 = Never: If parent can give no examples of the child discriminating between two speakers.

_____ 1 = Rarely: If one or two examples are given.

_____ 2 = Occasionally: If several examples are given and the child does this at least 50% of the time.

_____ 3 = Frequently: If many examples are given and the child does this 75% of the time.

_____ 4 = Always: If always done and the child shows no errors in doing this.

PARENT REPORT:

9. Does the child spontaneously know the difference between speech and nonspeech stimuli with listening alone?

Ask, "Does _____ recognize speech as a category of sounds that are different from nonspeech sounds? For example, if you were standing behind your child and a noise occurred, would she/he ever say, 'What was that noise?'" In the case of the younger children, ask, "Would _____ ever run into the next room to search for a family member's voice versus looking out the window for a dog or fire truck?"

_____ 0 = Never: If parent can give no examples of the child discriminating speech from nonspeech.

_____ 1 = Rarely: If one or two examples are given.

_____ 2 = Occasionally: If several examples are given and the child does this at least 50% of the time.

_____ 3 = Frequently: If many examples are given and the child does this 75% of the time.

_____ 4 = Always: If always done and the child shows no errors in doing this.

PARENT REPORT:

cont.

10. Does the child spontaneously associate vocal tone (anger, excitement, anxiety) with its meaning based on hearing alone?

Ask, "By listening only, can _____ tell the emotion conveyed in someone's voice such as an angry voice, an excited voice, etc.?" (For example, Father yells at child to "hurry up" through the bathroom door and the child responds, "Why are you mad?" and yells back at him. In the case of the younger child, the child starts to cry because of the angry sound in his voice. Another example is the parent is reading a new book to a young child while she/he is sitting on the parent's lap and cannot see the parent's face: Mom says, "The boy yelled 'Let's go!'" and the child says, "The boy is happy to go to the park").

_____ 0 = Never: If the parent can give no examples or if the child has never had the opportunity to do this.

_____ 1 = Rarely: If the child does it 25% of the time.

_____ 2 = Occasionally: If the child does it about 50% of the time.

_____ 3 = Frequently: If he/she does it 75% of the time.

_____ 4 = Always: If he/she consistently can identify more than one emotion in the listening alone condition.

PARENT REPORT:

Total points correct: _____ /40

References

Beck, A., & Dennis, M. (1997). Speech-language pathologists' and teachers' perceptions of classroom-based interventions. *Language, speech, and hearing services in the schools, 28*(2), 146-152.

Cummins, J. (1984). *Bilingualism and special education: Issues in assessment and pedagogy.* Clevedon, Avon, England: Multilingual Matters.

Erber, N. (1982). *Auditory training.* Washington, DC: Alexander Graham Bell Association for the Deaf.

Estabrooks, W. (1994). *Auditory-verbal therapy for parents and professionals.* Washington, DC: Alexander Graham Bell Association for the Deaf.

Firszt, J., & Reeder, R. (1996). *Classroom goals: Guide for optimizing auditory learning skills.* Washington, DC: Alexander Graham Bell Association for the Deaf.

Haskins, H. (1949). *A phonetically-balanced test of speech discrimination for children.* Unpublished master's thesis, Northwestern University, Evanston, IL.

Jerger, S., Lewis, S., Hawkins, J., & Jerger, J. (1980). Pediatric speech intelligibility test. *International Journal of Pediatric Otorhinolaryngology, 2,* 217-230.

Kirk, K., Pisoni, D., & Osberger, M. (1995). Lexical effects on spoken word recognition by pediatric cochlear implant users. *Ear and Hearing 16,* 470-481.

Ling, D. (1983). *Speech and the hearing-impaired child.* Washington, DC: Alexander Graham Bell Association for the Deaf.

Ling, D., & Ling, A. (1978). *Aural rehabilitation.* Washington, DC: Alexander Graham Bell Association for the Deaf.

Luetke-Stahlman, B. (1998). *Language issues in deaf education.* Hillsboro, OR: Butte Publications.

Luetke-Stahlman, B., & Luckner, J. (1991). *Effectively educating students with hearing impairments.* New York: Longman.

Maxwell, M. (1981). *Listening games for elementary grades.* Washington, DC: Acropolis Books.

Moeller, M., Osberger, M., & Morford, J. (1987). Speech-language assessment and intervention with preschool hearing-impaired children. In J. Alpiner & P. McCarthy (Eds.), *Rehabilitative audiology for children and adults* (pp. 163-187). Baltimore, MD: Williams and Wilkins.

Novelli-Olmstead, T., & Ling, D. (1984). Speech production and speech discrimination by hearing-impaired children. *The Volta Review, 86*(2), 72-80.

Patterson, M. (1992). *Teaching speech to the deaf: More than an articulation problem.* Paper presented at the Alexander Graham Bell Association for the Deaf International Convention, San Diego, CA.

Robbins, A. (1994a). *A critical evaluation of rehabilitation techniques.* Paper presented at the 5th Symposium on Cochlear Implants in Children. New York, NY.

Robbins, A. (1994b). Guidelines for developing oral communication skills in children with cochlear implants. *The Volta Review, 96*(5), 75-82.

Robbins, A. (1995). *Cochlear implants and "new wave" listening in children.* Paper presented at the Minnesota Speech and Hearing Association, Minneapolis, MN.

Robbins, A. (1998, in press). Lesson plan for Lilly. In W. Estabrooks (Ed.), *Cochlear implants for kids.* Washington, DC: Alexander Graham Bell Association for the Deaf.

Robbins, A., & Kirk, K. (1996). Speech perception assessment and performance in pediatric cochlear implant users. *Seminar in Hearing, 17*(4), 353-369.

Robbins, A., Renshaw, J., Miyamoto, R., Osberger, M., & Pope, M. (1988). *Minimal Pairs Test.* Indianapolis: Indiana University School of Medicine.

Robbins, A., Svirsky, M., Osberger, M., & Pisoni, D. (1996). *Beyond the audiogram: The role of functional assessment.* Paper presented at the Fourth International Symposium on Childhood Deafness, Kiawah Island, South Carolina.

Schow, R., & Nerbonne, M. (1989). *Introduction to aural rehabilitation.* Baltimore, MD: University Park Press.

Stout, G., & Van ert Windle, J. (1992). *Developmental approach to successful listening–Revised* (DASL). Englewood, CO: Resource Point.

Thies, T., & Trammel, J. (1983). Development and implementation of the auditory skills instructional planning system. In I. Hochberg (Ed.), *Speech of the hearing impaired—Research, training, and personnel preparation* (pp. 349-367). Baltimore, MD: University Park Press.

Worthley, W. (1978). *Sourcebook of language learning activities.* Boston: Little, Brown.

Chapter 3

Assessing and Facilitating Speechreading and Speech

Speechreading Assessment

Speechreading and the Cummins Model

Speechreading Facilitation

Speech Assessment

Speech Facilitation

Resources

Appendix: Meaningful Use of Speech Scale

Speechreading can be defined as a process of understanding a spoken message by observing all or part of a speaker's face (O'Neil & Oyer, 1981). An older term for speechreading is lipreading. **Speech** is defined as the oral production of language. In this chapter, topics concerning the assessment and the facilitation of speechreading and speech are presented.

     Speechreading = Lipreading

Speechreading Assessment

Contemporary thinking is that students do not just watch for visual information in the area of the cheeks, nose, mouth, and throat in order to speechread but consider all the variables of gestures, facial expressions, and situational cues together as they watch a speaker (Luetke-Stahlman & Luckner, 1991). Usually a formal goal with regard to speechreading is not written until a student is in the early elementary grades. However, team members often raise questions about students' ability to speechread long before this time.

Speechreading assessment should be question-driven. Team members might begin by asking questions such as the following:
- Is speechreading a strategy used by a particular student who is D/HH?
- How can a student's ability to speechread be enhanced?

Moeller (1982) suggested that students who are D/HH would benefit from a speechreading evaluation that assesses abilities in several settings and provides information about strengths and weaknesses. She, as well as Jeffers and Barley (1971), noted that few tests designed for the *formal* assessment of speechreading abilities are commercially available. One helpful evaluation tool and instructional curriculum, however, is the *Speech Perception Instructional Curriculum and Evaluation* (SPICE) (Moog, Davidson, & Biedenstein, 1995). Another is the *Early Speech Perception Test* (Moog & Geers, 1990) which can be used with children as young as three years. A resource list at the end of this chapter provides additional tools and publisher information.

Informal assessment of speechreading requires the consideration and control of many variables. These variables include the student's ability to integrate auditory and visual information, differences among speakers, and the influence of instruction (Montgomery, 1988). As discussed below, the Cummins model (Cummins, 1984) can be used for speechreading assessment. The Erber (1982) matrix (see Chapter 2), which was designed for audition assessment, can also be adapted as a tool to guide speechreading assessment (Montgomery, 1988).

Speechreading and the Cummins Model

The Cummins Model of Language Proficiency (Cummins, 1984) can provide an informal means of considering the variables in speechreading assessment and can supply information for speechreading facilitation. For example, in facilitation with a student who is having difficulty, an adult might add context, simplify the task, or do both (see Figure 3–1).

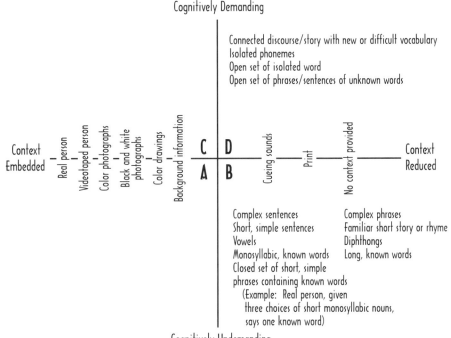

FIGURE 3–1: THE CUMMINS MODEL ADAPTED FOR SPEECHREADING

Cognitive-Linguistic Demand

Study Guide Question
What would you include as an example of a speechreading skill for each of the four quadrants of the Cummins model?

Cognitive-linguistic demand within the Cummins model used for speechreading is defined as the syntactic and semantic difficulty of the stimulus language being speechread. Regarding English, Wozniak and Jackson (1979) found that diphthongs were easier than vowels for adults who were D/HH to identify through speechreading. Erber (1977) reported that students could usually identify longer words and spondees (*baseball*), more easily than shorter, monosyllabic words. The results of studies by Clouser (1976) and Schwartz and Black (1967) suggested that students were able to speechread short, syntactically simple sentences more readily than longer, complex ones. This information has been incorporated into the adapted Cummins model in Figure 3–1. In addition, higher cognitive and linguistic tasks could be used to assess whether students can speechread cognitive academic linguistic information that is representative of Quadrant D behaviors, known as cognitive academic language proficiency (CALP) behaviors (Luetke-Stahlman, 1998).

Research on Speechreading and the Cummins Model*—

The benefit of using an adapted Cummins model in assessing individual speechreading ability in students who are D/HH was tested in a tutorial situation by college students who were studying to become teachers of the deaf (Luetke-Stahlman, 1989). Questions were written to reflect the characteristics of the quadrants as well as the age and interests of each deaf or hard-of-hearing student. Questions included each of the model's combinations of high and low context and high and low cognitive-linguistic demand. Cognitively demanding questions were longer in mean length of utterance than cognitively undemanding questions and involved higher cognitive processing skills (Bloom & Krathwohl, 1977). The questions were presented in individualized tutoring sessions.

---

*From "A Framework for Assessing Speechreading Performance in Hearing-Impaired Children," by B. Luetke-Stahlman, 1989, *The ACEHI Journal*, 15(1), pp. 27-37. Copyright 1989. Adapted with permission of the editor of *The CAEDHH Journal* (previously *The ACEHI Journal*).

Speechreading Questions Based on the Cummins Model

Quadrant A: *Cognitively undemanding, context embedded*
What color is this table?
Who is sitting near you?
Which of these is blue?

Quadrant B: *Cognitively undemanding, context reduced*
Where is your school?
What color is your bedroom?
Who is (teacher's name)?

Quadrant C: *Cognitively demanding, context embedded*
What do you think this textbook is about?
Why are these shoes made of leather?
How does electricity make this light work?

Quadrant D: *Cognitively demanding, context reduced*
How is a state different from a country?
What is similar about Earth and Venus?
Would a suburban area have more residential
land or more farm land?

Each student was asked to speechread the questions, which were presented at random. During the course of three consecutive sessions each question was asked at least three times per session—once without voice in each session. All questions were asked in oral English only (no sign). The results of this assessment were as follows:

- All but one student could speechread and answer all the questions presented without voice that were cognitively undemanding, context embedded (Quadrant A).
- One student could speechread and answer questions that were cognitively undemanding, context reduced (Quadrant B) and that were cognitively demanding, context embedded (Quadrant C).
- One student could speechread and answer questions that were cognitively demanding, context reduced (Quadrant D) (Luetke-Stahlman, 1989).

To summarize the above findings, the following four general types of speechreading abilities using the Cummins model were identified. Facilitation suggestions for each were made (Luetke-Stahlman, 1989).

Study Guide Question

Which of the students described in the speechreading research is (are) most likely not to require the services of an interpreter in at least some general education, public school activities?

1. **Students who cannot speechread even the most familiar expressions:** For these students, team members might pick two typical English expressions to be asked daily, without sign but in context (*"Time for lunch!" "Can I help you?"*).

2. **Students who can speechread Quadrant A material but not phrases or sentences characteristic of Quadrants B and C:** Team members might pick either typical expressions uncued by context (*"Do you have art today?"*) or those that are more difficult and embedded in context (*"Can you compare these two characters?"*).

3. **Students who are ready to speechread material characteristic of Quadrant D:** (*"Please define the word trapezoid"*).

4. **Students who need to have their demonstrated Quadrant D abilities expanded by team members.**

Speechreading Facilitation

Several specific factors that affect the ability and accuracy of speechreading have been identified (Luetke-Stahlman & Luckner, 1991). These factors are essential for team members to consider when a student is learning speechreading (without signs or simultaneous communication):

1. *English language proficiency.* Short phrases known by the student are easier and should be practiced first. Practice individual words later.

2. *Viewing angle of the speaker.* Speechreading at 0 degrees (in front of the student) is easiest and should be practiced first, then 45 degrees, and then 90 degrees (to the student's side).

3. *Visibility of the speaker.* The more visible the upper torso of the speaker, the easier it is to speechread.

4. *Rate of speech.* A slower-than-average rate of speech has been found to be the easiest to speechread. Practice with normal rates of speech should occur later.

5. *Familiarity and age of the speaker.* Knowing the personality of people (relatives and close friends) makes it easier to understand them. Young children with immature language might be more difficult to speechread than those in at least third grade.

6. *Distance from the speaker.* The closer, the better. Training is most meaningful when it is done at distances most representative of typical daily conversational situations (between 4 and 10 feet).

7. *Lighting on the speaker.* Typical classroom lighting is sufficient for optimum speechreading. Bright light, glare, or an overhead projection light behind a speaker can black out or darken his or her face for the student who is D/HH and can make speechreading difficult.

8. *Visual distractions.* Certain characteristics of people or the apparel that they wear can affect speechreading. Adults working with students who are D/HH should not wear dark glasses; have a beard or mustache; wear long, dangling earrings; have long, flowing hair that covers part of the face; move hands or objects in front of the face; or speak with a pencil or other object in the mouth.

Many of the facilitation strategies described in Chapter 1 can be adapted to facilitate speechreading goals and objectives. In fact, it is current practice that the skills of audition, speechreading, and speech articulation are always taught in conjunction with each other.

Ms. Green:	(pointing to a map) What country is this?
Maya:	(having speechread the question) En-an
Ms. Green:	Can you say that again? England.
Maya:	(using speech only) England is that country.
Ms. Green:	You're right. Now, where's France?

The communication games explained by Luetke-Stahlman (1998) can also be adapted for audition, speech, and speechreading.

Speech Assessment

Speech or speech articulation is the oral production of language. "Intelligible speech" is defined here as speech that is understandable. In general, a student who is D/HH and has residual speech or use of an assistive listening device that allows for the hearing of speech across the range of speech sounds will have more intelligible speech than a student who does not have such abilities. Issues concerning speech production by students who are D/HH were reviewed in a special issue of *The Volta Review*, "Speech Production in Hearing Impaired Children and Youth: Theory and Practice" (1992).

A student who is D/HH will be unable to develop intelligible speech or improve speech without systematic and continued assessment. In addition, all team members need to assume responsibility for facilitating needed speech skills across school subjects and activities and within home routines. Teachers and speech-language pathologists agree that the team-teaching of speech articulation is the most appropriate model (Beck & Dennis, 1997). It has the following advantages:

- It increases carryover of skills.
- It keeps students in the most natural environment for service delivery.

■ It provides more appropriate reinforcement of communication behaviors.

Formal Assessment

Formal speech assessment can be accomplished by using Ling's *Phonetic Level Evaluation* and *Phonological Level Evaluation* (Ling, 1976, 1989). Ling's evaluations are examined in the next two sections of this chapter. Some teams also use the tests described below: the *Goldman-Fristoe Test of Articulation* (Goldman & Fristoe, 1986), the *CID Picture Speech Intelligibility Evaluation* (Geers & Moog, 1988), and the *Assessment of Phonological Processes–Revised* (Hodson, 1986). Either the teacher of the deaf or the speech-language pathologist typically administers these instruments. A teacher of the deaf who has a hearing loss might ask the speech-language pathologist to conduct the evaluation and share specific speech targets to be facilitated with the team members. See the resource list at the end of the chapter for addresses of these tests' publishers.

The *Goldman-Fristoe Test of Articulation* (Goldman & Fristoe, 1986) is an articulation test that allows for the sampling of both spontaneous and imitative sound production, including single words and conversational speech. The test is appropriate for ages 2 to 16+ years and has three subtests, each requiring 10–15 minutes for administration. The Sounds in Words subtest uses 35 pictures to elicit articulation of the major speech sounds in initial, medial, and final position. The Sounds in Sentences subtest assesses spontaneous sound production using connected speech. The Stimulability subtest assesses the student's ability to produce a previously misarticulated sound correctly. Scores are given in percentile rankings.

The *CID Picture Speech Intelligibility Evaluation* (SPINE) (Geers & Moog, 1988) uses pictures as stimuli to provide an estimation of the overall speech intelligibility of a student who is D/HH. The evaluation requires 60 minutes for administration. The student says the name of what is pictured on a card, without showing the card to the examiner. Responses are converted to percentages and compared to an interpretive table. The five levels of intelligibility (59% correct and below, 60-69% correct, 70-79% correct, 80-89% correct, 90-100% correct) can be used in the writing of educational objectives.

The Assessment of Phonological Processes–Revised (APP–R) (Hodson, 1986) allows for all speech deviations to be categorized. The manual provides descriptions of more than 30 explicit phonological processes, as well as examples and clear instructions for scoring, a summary form, and two screening forms (Preschool and Multisyllabic). Testing time is 15–20 minutes, and scores are given in percentages for ten basic phonological processes. A computer program for scoring the test is also available and highly recommended.

Phonetic Evaluation

Study Guide Question
Compare the formal speech assessment tools described. Which do you think you would prefer using and why?

Phonetic skills include the control of intensity, duration, and frequency of vocalizations, as well as the ability to produce, repeat, and alternate these features with syllables (Figure 3–2). The purposes of a phonetic level evaluation are

- to determine which motor speech skills the student has mastered or retained
- to specify which phonetic skills should be targeted for development next (Luetke-Stahlman & Luckner, 1991)

In Ling's *Phonetic Level Evaluation* (Ling, 1976), the assessment tasks are sequenced to follow the developmental stages of spoken English acquisition and to represent the abilities needed to produce fluent spoken English (Luetke-Stahlman & Luckner, 1991). As with most formal speech evaluation tools, the adult produces a target sound and asks the student to imitate it. Using Ling's process (1976), students are evaluated for their ability to demonstrate the following sequence of skills:

1. vocalizing on demand
2. making sound patterns loud or soft, long or short, high or low, once or more often
3. producing all diphthongs and vowels with control
5. producing consonants with /u/, /a/, and /i/
6. producing initial and final consonant blends

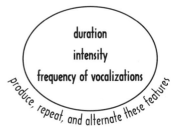

FIGURE 3–2: PHONETIC SKILLS

Team members working with students who are D/HH particularly appreciate the emergent speech skill level tested by this assessment tool, compared to evaluation instruments designed for hearing students.

In Ling's evaluation process, student productions are recorded using a "P" if they are produced consistently, "+" if they are produced inconsistently or "−" if they are not produced at all. As noted in the sequence of skills listed above, students are asked first to vocalize on demand, then to produce some patterns, and then to begin to work on vowel production. After several vowels can be produced, students can begin working on the production of Step 1 consonants as shown in Figure 3–3. At this stage, either the production of /b/ or /p/ is acceptable. Adults continue to administer the phonetic evaluation through the four steps of consonants (see Figure 3–3) in order to determine all the productive phonetic skills in the student's repertoire *or* until five objectives can be written in areas of need.

Figure 3–3 uses several terms which may require explanation. A *fricative* is a manner of articulating a consonant by constricting but not stopping the air flow (examples: *f, s*). An *affricate* is a consonantal sound that starts as a stop but ends as a fricative (example: *ch*). *Liquids* are consonants that are articulated without friction and may be prolonged like a vowel (examples: *l, r*). *Plosives* are sounds made by completely stopping the breath flow and then releasing the air with a relatively strong puff (example: *p, b*).

Sequential Teaching Steps	Plosives	Unreleased Stops	Nasals	Semi-Vowels	Liquids	Fricatives	Affricates
Step 1	[b] or [p]	[b̄] or [p̄]	[m]	[w] or [m]		[h] & [f , θ] or [v ,ʃ]	
Step 2	[d] or [t]	[d̄] or [t̄]	[n]	[i]	[l]	[ʃ , s] or [ʒ , z]	
Step 3	[g] or [k]	[ḡ] or [k̄]	[ŋ]		[r]		[tʃ] or [dz]
Step 4	[b, d, g] versus [p, t, k]	[b̄, d̄, ḡ] versus [p̄, t̄, k̄]	[m]			[f, θ, ʃ, s] versus [v, ʃ,ʒ, z]	[tʃ] versus [dz]

FIGURE 3–3: CONSONANT ASSESSMENT AND FACILITATION

To understand Ling's technique, team members may need to review the International Phonetic Alphabet (IPA) symbols. The IPA symbols representing the 24 consonant phonemes of English are presented in Table 3–1.

Additional information on Ling's *Phonetic Level Evaluation* was presented by Luetke-Stahlman and Luckner (1991). Complete instructions and forms for this technique can be obtained from Alexander Graham Bell Association for the Deaf (see the resource list at the end of this chapter).

TABLE 3–1: IPA SYMBOLS FOR CONSONANT PHONEMES

Phonetic Symbol	Examples	Phonetic Symbol	Examples
/p/	pull	/z/	zip
/b/	bin	/ʃ/	show
/t/	talk	/v/	very
/d/	day	/m/	mine
/k/	kill	/n/	none
/g/	good	/w/	want
/tʃ/	chair	/h/	how
/dʒ/	John	/j/	yet
/f/	fix	/l/	low
/θ/	then	/r/	read
/ʃ/	thin	/ŋ/	thing
/s/	so	/ʒ/	vision

Phonological Evaluation

Phonological skills include the following:

- using vocalizations as communication
- using different voice patterns meaningfully
- using different vowels to approximate real words
- saying some words clearly with appropriate speech quality control
- speaking intelligibly and naturally

Using Ling's *Phonological Level Evaluation* (1976, 1989), five discourse demands are evaluated:

- description
- conversation
- questioning
- explanation
- narration

To administer a phonological level evaluation, all aspects of preparation necessary for collecting *representative samples*—considerations of length, setting, method, and so on— should be included. (See Luetke-Stahlman, 1998, for information on collecting a representative sample.) Long (1986) provided a plan for conducting a phonological assessment (see Luetke-Stahlman & Luckner, 1991). The information gathered using Long's or others' strategies gives team members an idea of what a student's speech is like in running conversation, taking into consideration each of Ling's five areas of discourse demand.

> **Study Guide Question**
> *Invent some data for each of Ling's five areas of phonological evaluation. What would you include in a speech objective for each area?*

Intelligibility Assessment

Speech intelligibility can be defined as how well others can comprehend the speech of a student who is D/HH, regardless of whether they are familiar with the student's speech. When reporting results of intelligibility tasks, however, it is important to note who the listener is and how familiar he or she is with the student who is being assessed. Although formal measures are available, informal measures are also very appropriate to assess this important area.

The following informal methods can be used to assess speech intelligibility:

- Seat one hearing student and one student who is D/HH back to back and ask the student who is D/HH to say single sentences to the hearing student. The hearing student should repeat what is heard while a team member records the results.

- Videotape a representative language sample (see Luetke-Stahlman, 1998) and play only the soundtrack for a panel of listeners. Team members may provide the panel with a randomized list of phrases that are said or simply allow them to write down what they hear.

- Use the *Meaningful Use of Speech Scale* (MUSS) (Robbins & Osberger, 1991). The MUSS is a parent-report and clinician observation tool that assesses three components of speech: volitional control of vocalization, use of speech alone, and ability to modify speech to increase the listener's comprehension. The MUSS appears in Appendix 3–A.

> **Study Guide Question**
> *Administer the MUSS. What would you include in a speech objective for intelligibility based on the results?*

Speech Facilitation

Speech development has been defined as "the acquisition of a variety of skills related to the production and reception of meaningful, spoken language. . . . [including] linguistic competence, auditory comprehension and pragmatics as well as speech production ability" (Nittrouer & Hochberg, 1985, p. 491). Because phonological awareness or understanding the relationship between sounds is necessary for reading, all students who are D/HH deserve the opportunity to receive speech articulation training until they are at least young teenagers.

The following guidelines may be useful to team members as they facilitate speech development:

- Collaboration is paramount in forming questions prior to speech evaluation, choosing appropriate tools, conducting a representative evaluation, scoring and determining priorities, and facilitating skills across environments.
- Phonetic, imitative, and phonological skills should be facilitated simultaneously and should include evaluation by the student as well as the adult.
- Speech evaluation should be conducted twice a year (on students with or without cochlear implants).
- Speech, speechreading, and audition skills should be facilitated simultaneously and should include regular feedback about student performance.
- Speech facilitation should occur throughout the day.
- When five targets can be identified and written as objectives, no further analysis is required until the next team meeting.

An example of a systematic speech facilitation approach, adapted from Ling (1976), is shown in Table 3–2. Using this staged approach, vocalization is facilitated first, followed by the incorporation of voice patterns or suprasegmentals. These stages are discussed on the following page.

Vocalization

When students who are D/HH do not use their voices and it is desired that they do so, they should be encouraged to voice *in abundance!* The desired outcome is a pleasant—not harsh, shrill, or otherwise irritating—voice quality. It will not stop a student from vocalizing if adults request pleasant-sounding productions. Ways to initiate voice include

- tickling the student to evoke laughter
- tickling the student while voicing
- engaging the student in exertion (by pulling, pushing, or lifting a heavy object)
- responding appropriately when the student vocalizes (smiling, patting, giving any verbal response)
- using voice to get others' attention
- expressing emotion

- making comments
- vocalizing in response to a question
- using voice-activated toys

Study Guide Question
Work with a student who does not use voice. Which of the ideas in this section worked best to facilitate vocalization?

Blowing out candles or blowing bubbles should be used prudently as methods to initiate voice. Using these methods can cause the student to associate voicing with overall body tension.

TABLE 3-2: THE LING MODEL OF SPEECH DEVELOPMENT

	Phonetic Level	**Phonological Level**
Stage 1	Vocalizes freely on demand	Uses vocalization as a means of communication
Stage 2	Uses bases of suprasegmentals*	Uses voice patterns meaningfully
Stage 3	Uses all diphthongs/vowels with voice control	Uses different vowels with voice control
Stage 4	Voices consonants* by manner with /a/, /i/, /u/	Says some words clearly and with good voice patterns
Stage 5	Voices consonants by manner and place	Says more words clearly and with good voice patterns
Stage 6	Voices consonants by manner, place, and voicing	Says most words clearly and with good voice patterns
Stage 7	Voices initial and final blends	All speech is intelligible, and voice patterns are natural

*Suprasegmentals and the consonant features of manner, place, and voice are explained later in this chapter.

From *Speech and the Hearing-Impaired Child: Theory and Practices*, by D. Ling, 1976, Washington, DC: Alexander Graham Bell Association for the Deaf. Copyright 1976 by Alexander Graham Bell Association for the Deaf. Adapted with permission.

Suprasegmentals

Suprasegmentals, as discussed in Chapter 2, are physical features of speech such as duration, stress, and pitch. These features are also referred to as "voice patterns." Once voicing is established, team members should discuss realistic ways to incorporate voice patterns (also called "systematic babbling") into the student's communication. Voice patterns may include

- vocalizing for a long or short time
- vocalizing loudly or softly
- vocalizing in a choppy manner rather than a smooth one

Students are often asked to imitate voice patterns such as *lalala* contrasted with *la*, or *LA* (spoken in a loud voice) contrasted with *la* (spoken in a normal or quiet voice), and so on. As soon as a student can produce these vocal gymnastics, known as Ling drills, adults should integrate these sounds into meaningful speech. For example, a student might be encouraged to shout *Mama* to get his or her mother's attention from across the room (Moeller, Osberger, & Morford, 1987).

LING VOICE PATTERN DRILLS IN MEANINGFUL CONTEXTS

"*Boo boo boo,*" says the ghost.
"*Fee fi fo fum,*" says the giant to Jack.
"*Ho ho ho*" says Santa Claus.
"*Waa waa,*" cries the baby.
"*Choo choo,*" goes the train.

Duration is the primary skill being developed; it is unimportant at this point whether the student can imitate specific vowels or phonemes. It is recommended that a student be able to sustain vocalization for a duration of at least three seconds (Luetke-Stahlman and Luckner, 1991). Once that skill has been accomplished, other controls, such as intensity and pitch, can be attempted.

Activities to Develop Precursory Speech Behaviors

Activities that team members might use in working with students who are D/HH to develop precursory speech behaviors include games that involve eye contact and physical availability, activities initiated by the teacher that promote abundant vocalizations, and motor activity imitations (Long, 1986). The form in Figure 3–4 was designed to record data during activities that encourage precursory speech behaviors (Luetke-Stahlman & Luckner, 1991).

	Date of Evaluation	Behavior Emerging	Behavior Consistent

Student Name_____   Your Name _____
Date _____   School _____

Precursory Behaviors for Speech Facilitation

	Date of Evaluation	Behavior Emerging	Behavior Consistent
1. Physical availability			
2. Eye contact			
3. Imitation of motor activities			
4. Abundant vocalizations			
5. Vocal duration			
6. Vocal intensity			
7. Vocal pitch			

List the age-appropriate activities to be used to promote the skills listed above:
1.
2.
3.
4.
5.
6.
7.

FIGURE 3-4: FORM FOR RECORD KEEPING DURING ACTIVITIES THAT ENCOURAGE PRECURSORY SPEECH BEHAVIORS

School situations provide many opportunities during which correct speech production can be generalized. Some activities to facilitate duration, intensity, and pitch are provided by age group in Tables 3–3, 3–4, and 3–5 (Luetke-Stahlman & Luckner, 1991).

"Pitch may be very difficult for profoundly deaf students because it cannot be replicated visibly" (Luetke-Stahlman & Luckner, 1991, p. 191). Without helpful assistive listening equipment, it may be difficult to control pitch. Team members may try the activities in Table 3–5 to facilitate pitch.

Students who are D/HH often confuse pitch with intensity. The adult should stress the difference between these two components during one activity.

TABLE 3–3: DURATION ACTIVITIES

Early Childhood	Elementary Age
■ What does Santa (ghost, etc.) say? *"Brrr, it's cold out!"* ■ Rock a baby doll smoothly; bounce a baby doll. ■ Move a car, truck, animal, and so on, smoothly or roughly across the floor. ■ Play "make me glide/hop/jump" (having the child first move appropriately to your utterances). ■ Pull out a measuring tape in a sustained manner or in jerks. ■ Pull yarn or scarves out of a can that has a hole in the lid. ■ Fingerpaint, color, or manipulate play dough while voicing. ■ Splash water on a doll; drip and pour water into containers. ■ Drop or slide objects through a tube. ■ Turn a faucet on or off; let the water drip. ■ "Paint" with water on a mirror. ■ Walk up the steps of a slide; slide down.	■ Move finger under print in a storybook. ■ Vocalize while someone else counts or while listing chapters in a book or topics for discussion. ■ Imitate the school alarms to signal the beginning/end of the day. ■ Let things drip or stretch during science experiments. ■ Match verbalizations to expressions and colloquialisms to photos or actions: *"You bet!"* *"Give me a break."* (Perusse, Bernstein, & Phillips, 1992).

TABLE 3–4: INTENSITY ACTIVITIES

Early Childhood	Elementary Age
Quiet ■ Sing or talk to a doll. ■ Indicate to the child that you want to be unable to hear his response when you are several feet away.	*Quiet* ■ Politely get a waitress's attention. ■ Talk softly when people in the family are relaxing or are in bed. ■ Calm things down when cooperative learning groups get too noisy. *cont.*

TABLE 3–3, CONT.

Early Childhood	Elementary Age
Loud ■ Throw things far to indicate a loud sound. ■ Pretend to sleep and have the child wake you up with a loud voice, or demonstrate this with a doll. ■ Pop up from behind a barrier on child's production of a loud voice. ■ Use a toy that lights up to sound. ■ Have someone go away from the child and then have the child call that person back. ■ Go outside and call someone from a distance. ■ Get excited about something and shout for joy or in triumph.	*Loud* ■ At recess, yell to a friend. ■ Count sports equipment loudly when outside. ■ In PE, call to a friend to be noticed in a game. ■ Set up an angry situation.
Whisper ■ Put a baby doll to bed. ■ Whisper on a mirror and show the condensation that results. ■ Whisper into tissues or feathers. ■ Play a secretive game or tell a secret.	*Whisper* ■ Give a friend a hint. ■ Tell a friend a secret.
Varied Intensities ■ Tiptoe up to someone talking quietly and then yell, *"Boo!"*	*Varied Intensities* ■ Read *Messy Monsters, Jungle Joggers, and Bubble Bath* (Sobel & Pluznik, 1987) together. ■ Use different loud and soft voices for different story characters.

TABLE 3–5: PITCH ACTIVITIES

Early Childhood	Elementary Age
▪ Make three buildings that vary in height: high, medium, and low. Have Superman fly to the top of and off the buildings. Have the student discriminate or produce an appropriate pitch level to move Superman or while moving him. ▪ Associate the movement of an airplane, bird, car, or roller coaster with pitch by fluctuating your pitch level up and down. ▪ Associate body movement (arms up, lowering of head to chest to force larynx down) with production of lower pitch level. ▪ Incorporate pitch into stories like "The Three Bears," giving Papa Bear a low voice, Baby Bear a high voice, and so on).	▪ Use a blue paper towel roll and a small red tube that fits over the blue roll to represent the larynx. Make associations between your own larynx being up and a high-pitch voice. Move the red tube up and down and have the student produce an associated pitch. ▪ Sing. ▪ Role play characters or read their lines from a book using different voices. ▪ Imitate cartoon characters. ▪ Call a greeting. ▪ Ask a question or tell a joke, changing pitch. ▪ Imitate the calls of animals. ▪ Discuss the pitch changes in Asian languages. ▪ Match a pitch to a gliding movement on a board game or computer (Perusse et al., 1992). ▪ Match pitches to computerized characters on the computer. ▪ Count forward or backward with a rise or lowering in pitch or intensity (Perusse et al., 1992).

Genuine Speech Facilitation

LeBlanc (1997) provided much helpful information about the facilitation of speech when working with students who are D/HH. Her activities have been incorporated into the checklist in Figure 3–5.

___ 1. After Ling's *Phonetic Level Evaluation* has been administered, the target error phonemes are chosen on the basis of the frequency of occurrence and stimulability.

___ 2. Probe to see if the selected targets can be produced in words or phrases at a two-syllable level in the
    ___ initial position of the word
    ___ final position of the word
    ___ medial position of the word: *vocalic releaser* or the target sound (such as /s/) occurring after a vowel (m**y** **s**oup); *abutting releaser* or the target sound occurring after a consonant (ho**t** **s**oup); and *abutting arrester* or target sound occurring in the final position of a word and followed by a consonant in the subsequent word (bu**s** **c**ame)

___ 3. If the probe indicates that the student cannot produce the target phoneme in any of the above positions, then probe for the following nonsense syllables using a variety of vowels. This step determines whether or not there are any vowels that could facilitate correct production of the target phoneme.
    Consonant + Vowel (CV)
    Vowel + Consonant (VC)
    Vowel + Consonant + Vowel (VCV)

___ 4. If the probe in number 3 doesn't provide any nonsense syllables or vowels that facilitate the correct production of the target phoneme, probe the dimensions of the phoneme itself (manner, place, voicing) and determine which feature seems to be most difficult.

___ 5. Teach the student to produce all features of the target phoneme at 90–95% accuracy for three sessions. When this is accomplished, move to single syllables for CV, VC, VCV, and finally to repeated syllables for CV, VC, VCV.

___ 6. Teach words that have the target sound in the initial position and the final position. This will result in a core list of words the student can produce successfully.

cont.

FIGURE 3–5: CHECKLIST FOR FACILITATING SPEECH

FIGURE 3–5, CONT.

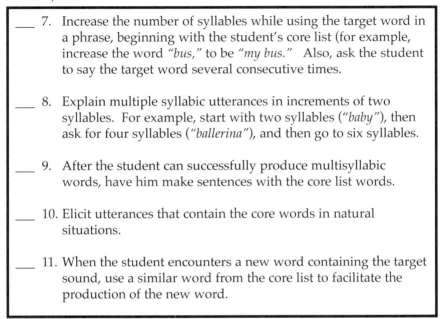

___ 7. Increase the number of syllables while using the target word in a phrase, beginning with the student's core list (for example, increase the word *"bus,"* to be *"my bus."* Also, ask the student to say the target word several consecutive times.

___ 8. Explain multiple syllabic utterances in increments of two syllables. For example, start with two syllables (*"baby"*), then ask for four syllables (*"ballerina"*), and then go to six syllables.

___ 9. After the student can successfully produce multisyllabic words, have him make sentences with the core list words.

___ 10. Elicit utterances that contain the core words in natural situations.

___ 11. When the student encounters a new word containing the target sound, use a similar word from the core list to facilitate the production of the new word.

From *Workshop on the Eclectic Method for Teaching Speech to the Hearing Impaired*, by B. LeBlanc, 1997, a paper presented at the Mississippi Speech-Language-Hearing Association, Biloxi, MS. Adapted with the author's permission.

As team members assess, target, and facilitate the development of speech behaviors, it is important to discuss activities in which these skills have a true purpose. Speech development is most efficiently facilitated when adults

- know that the skill level being targeted is developmentally appropriate
- provide multiple opportunities across settings
- provide pragmatically appropriate feedback (*"I didn't hear that"* rather than *"Can you use your voice?"*)
- keep the affective filter low (do not embarrass the student)
- have a positive attitude about all important features of the process of speech development

Study Guide Question

Using the checklist in Figure 3–5 as a guide, interview a parent or teacher to determine the speech abilities of a student who is D/HH. What objective would you write based on your data?

Several ways to encourage speech development, including genuine requests for repetition or clarification when the speech of a student who is D/HH is not understood, were suggested by Ling (1989):

1. Mending meaning: *"I'm sorry. I didn't get (or understand) that."*
2. Requesting repetition: *"Tell me that again, please."*
3. Specifying difficulty: *"I didn't get what happened to Jim."*
4. Using ellipsis (seeking completion): *"You and Jim went to see . . . ?"*
5. Using open-ended questions (avoiding yes/no questions): *"So then what happened?" "How did Jim like that?" "What do you think Peter will do about that?"*
6. Modeling + imitation: *"Oh! You mean ____. You tell me that.*
7. Modeling + reflection of student's utterance: <u>Student</u>—*"Ppe uh te you hum oh wimme."* <u>Teacher</u>—*"Oh yes, Peter said you come home with me!"*
8. Encouraging continuation: *"Really!" "Uh huh!" "Wow!"*
9. Praising efforts: *"My, you said that well! I understood every word!"*
10. Demanding social elements: *"Tell me what people say when . . . "*
11. Using directions: *"Go to the office and ask Ms. Powers for some more chalk, please. Say: 'Please, Ms. Powers, may I have some more chalk for our class.'"*
12. Using linguistic prompts: *"You should use more breath (talk louder)."*
13. Using nonverbal prompts: holding one's finger in front of one's mouth to prompt the student to increase the breath stream, or pointing to one's chest to indicate that the student should lower voice pitch, and so on

---

From *Foundations of Spoken Language for Hearing-Impaired Children*, by D. Ling, 1989, Washington, DC: Alexander Graham Bell Association for the Deaf. Copyright 1989 by Alexander Graham Bell Association for the Deaf. Adapted with permission.

 Speech development should be facilitated in context.

Study Guide Question
What might you include as additional examples for each of the speech repetition and encouragement suggestions provided by Ling?

Whether in a one-on-one setting or during a small group activity, mediating speech works with other cues. Cues might include speech paired with action:

- kinesthetic
- fingerspelling in syllables near the mouth area
- signing in syllables (for example, AIRPLANE signed three times quickly, as the handshape is moved through the air)

Speech with context should be encouraged until the student is confident in the acquisition of new skills. The mediation material discussed in Chapter 1 can be applied to speech development as well. Task analysis for speech using the Cummins model (adapted from Cummins, 1984) is outlined in Figure 3–6.

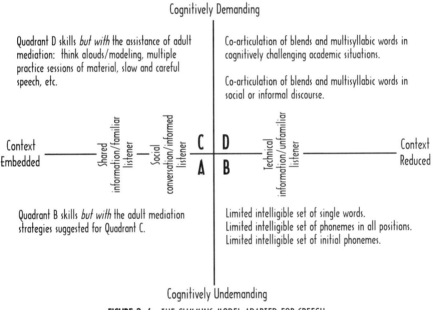

FIGURE 3–6: THE CUMMINS MODEL ADAPTED FOR SPEECH

When Auditory Feedback Does Not Facilitate Speech Development

Team members should use numerous visual and tactile methods to teach sounds if auditory methods have been unsuccessful (Montgomery, 1995). These strategies might include allowing a student to place his or her hand on the throat of an adult to feel the target sound—this strategy emphasizes the presence or absence of voicing.

Additional sounds may also be felt on the face, nose, or throat, so the tactile cue provided should be adjusted accordingly. At times, it may be helpful for team members to place one of the student's hands on the adult's throat and the student's other hand on the adult's mouth. This method supplies information on the manner of placement *and* the voicing concept. Some additional strategies are listed in Table 3–6.

TABLE 3–6: VISUAL AND TACTILE SPEECH STRATEGIES

Sounds Being Learned	Sample Strategies
/k/ and /g/	■ Use a tongue depressor or a candy stick to hold down the front of the tongue. ■ Ask the student to use a finger to hold down the front of the tongue, emphasizing a back placement. ■ Model a wide-mouth production of these sounds to emphasize using the back of the tongue. ■ Try eliciting the /kr/ or /gr/ blends. Since the majority of students produce the /r/ with the back of the tongue, the /r/ may encourage a back production of /k/ or /g/. ■ Try using a lion roar sound leading to a /k/. ■ Place the student's hand on the throat of the team member to emphasize the presence or absence of voicing. This may be referred to as "motor on" versus "motor off," with the student feeling the vibration.
/t/ and /d/	■ Place your finger on the student's upper lip to provide a tactile cue on tongue placement. ■ Place your finger inside the student's mouth right behind the front teeth for a tactile cue. ■ Use peanut butter or honey behind the front teeth for a tactile cue. Instruct the student to get the peanut butter with the tongue. ■ Help the student to feel the slight air release from the /t/ on the back of his or her hand.

cont.

TABLE 3-6, CONT.

	■ Place the student's hand on the throat of the team member to emphasize the presence or absence of voicing. This may be referred to as "motor on" versus "motor off," with the student feeling the vibration.
/f/ and /v/	■ Use a mirror to emphasize the placement of the top teeth on the bottom lip. ■ Place peanut butter or marshmallow cream on the student's bottom lip and instruct him or her to scrape it off with the top teeth. ■ Use the story "Jack and the Beanstalk" for syllable work (*fee, fi, fo, fum*). ■ Place the student's hand on the throat of the team member to emphasize the presence or absence of voicing. This may be referred to as "motor on" versus "motor off," with the student feeling the vibration.
/sh/	■ Visually represent this sound with a long wide line, and contrast it with /ch/ represented by a large dot to illustrate that the /ch/ pops. /sh/ is frequently confused with /ch/. ■ Visually represent the /sh/ by running your whole hand along an imaginary line out in front of your body. Contrast that movement with an explosive gesture that starts with clenched fists and then releases your fingers to illustrate the plosive quality of the /ch/. ■ Use the minimal pair *shoe* versus *chew*. These words are ideal because of the rounded vowel sound.
/s/	■ Visually represent this sound with a skinny line and contrast that with a wide line representing /sh/. This sound is frequently confused with /sh/. ■ Use the key word *see* when eliciting this sound.

Facilitating Vowels*

Students who are D/HH may need help producing all of the vowels and diphthongs of English, producing the vowels in the context of different voice patterns, and producing the vowels in different consonant contexts. These skills were discussed earlier in the Phonetic Evaluation section of this chapter. LeBlanc (1997) noted the following points:

Study Guide Question

Practice providing some of the visual and tactile cues suggested in Table 3–6 while working with a student who is D/HH. Which seem the most helpful?

- Tongue position is an important factor in facilitating vowel production.

- Central vowels should be taught first because they are the easiest to produce and are the most audible.

- Informal strategies for facilitating vowel production can usually be used to assist students to include correct vowel sounds in speech.

- The three most important vowels are *u, a,* and *e* because they serve as reference points for other vowels. In other words, students can learn other vowels by associating the position of the articulators with vowels they can already produce.

- Exaggerated lip movement as a means of facilitating vowel acquisition via speechreading should be avoided. This strategy can promote inappropriate tongue placement.

- If vowels are the target of facilitation, incorrect consonant production should be ignored.

- Diphthongs are adjacent vowels spoken without pausing. To facilitate their acquisition, adults can have students alternate the two vowels involved.

*Text and table on facilitating vowels and consonants from *Workshop on the Eclectic Method for Teaching Speech to the Hearing Impaired*, by B. LeBlanc, 1997, presented to the Mississippi Speech-Language-Hearing Association, Biloxi, MS. Adapted with the author's permission.

Facilitating Consonants

To facilitate the development of consonants, LeBlanc (1997) suggested the following strategies:

- Teach consonants in the order of manner, placement, and then voicing. Manner is the way speech sounds are produced; placement is the location in the oral cavity where the sound is formed; voicing is the presence or absence of vocal fold vibration. Consonant manner and placement information is presented in Table 3–7. In this table, the manner of articulation, similar to the place of articulation, has been treated on a continuum: Stops are closed, continuants are slightly open, and sonorants have greater opening in the oral cavity.

TABLE 3–7: CONSONANT PLACEMENT

Manner	Bilabial	Labiodental	Linguadental	Alveolar	Palatal	Velar	Oral Cavity
Stop	/p, b/			/t, d/	/t, d/	/k, g/	Closed
Continuant		/f, v/	/θ, ʃ/	/s, z/	/ʃ, ʒ/	/h/	Slight Opening
Sonorant	/m, w/			/n, r, l/	/j/	/ŋ/	Greater Opening

- The development of consonants should occur using syllables or short words. However, nasals and fricatives should be taught first in isolation. Teaching new consonants in short segments allows a student who is D/HH to focus on the specific speech feature and helps ensure success.

- Encourage the development or teach unvoiced fricatives (such as /f/) to increase control of the breath stream and timing.

- Teach the following consonants before their voiced or voiceless opposites: voiceless fricatives (such as /f/), voiced plosives (such as /b/), voiceless stops (such as /t/), and voiceless affricates (such as /ch/). Do not teach voiced and voiceless pairs at the same time, but identify and reinforce distinctions when appropriate.

■ Teach manner features for fricatives, nasals, and liquids first in the final position of syllables to avoid intrusive vowels. For example, the words *off*, *on*, and *all* would be good first targets.

■ Avoid attention to the co-articulation of other consonants until the student can produce them in repeated syllables with appropriate duration, voicing, and frequency.

Facilitating Consonant Blends

Co-articulation is a process in which each of the sounds in an utterance is affected by the others with transitions between the sounds smoothed for an overlapping flow of movement (Hudson, 1981). The activities in Table 3–8 might assist team members in facilitating co-articulation of consonants and consonant blends.

TABLE 3-8: ACTIVITIES FOR DEVELOPING USE OF CONSONANTS AND BLENDS

Activity	Example
Phonemes that are common word endings	/s/—possessive, plural, 3rd person singular
Math, counting, and operations— reinforces fricatives and blends	/f/—four, five, fifteen, etc. /s/—six, seven, etc.
Handwriting practice of words that include target sounds— good for developing grapheme/ phoneme association	I *hope* you *had* a *happy holiday.*
Alphabetizing strings of words	School, score, scream, smart, sport, street

cont.

TABLE 3-8, CONT.

Spelling with same initial phoneme; rhyming words	Mouse, mitten, monkey My/by, merry/berry
Reading: pronunciation of words that have silent letters or are exceptions to rules	Debt, foreign
Verbal games	Simon Says I spy with my little eye, something that begins with /ch/. I went on a trip and in my suitcase I packed (all beginning with same sound).
Board games	Any appropriate board game Bingo with sounds on boards and words called out

From "Incorporating Speech Development into an Education Program," by Perusse, Bernstein, and Phillips, 1992, *The Volta Review, 94*(5), p. 89. Copyright 1992 by Alexander Graham Bell Association for the Deaf. Adapted with permission.

Facilitating Generalized Speech Skills

When planning for the facilitation of speech intelligibility, the following list of factors based on the work of Gatty (1992) and Golf (1980) may be helpful to team members:

- Short, intense sessions (e.g., 20 minutes)
- A positive attitude toward oral communication
- Effective and skilled teachers
- Appropriate amplification and maximal development of residual hearing
- A high ratio of known to unknown information
- Development of an effective auditory-kinesthetic feedback system
- Transfer of automatic phonetic skills to the phonological level
- Supportive, informed, and cooperative parents

- An expectation that speech is to be used when communication takes place
- Appropriate modeling of speech for the students
- Goals and objectives based on speech assessment
- Abundant and functional opportunities for using speech
- Encouragement and positive (but realistic) feedback for speech use
- A systematic speech program based on assessment information with continuous attention to the suprasegmental aspects of speech (Luetke-Stahlman & Luckner, 1991).

The activities in Table 3–9 may also assist team members in facilitating generalized speech skills.

TABLE 3–9: ACTIVITIES FOR GENERALIZING SPEECH SKILLS

Target	Activity	Example
Alternations	Tongue twisters: traditional and those written by children	Toy boat, toy boat (5 times) She sells sea shells
	Clapping and skipping songs —also good for rhythm and for releasing tension and acquiring automaticity	Aba daba soda cracker One potato, two potato Miss Mary Mack One little dicky bird Teddy bear, teddy bear
	Words misunderstood in conversation	
Stress and co-articulation in multisyllabic words	New vocabulary in school subjects; names of family members, friends, and teachers	Multiplication, predator / prey
	Literature: words that are less common but are integral to a story or character	*cont.*

TABLE 3–9, CONT.

Target	Activity	Example
Self-monitoring running speech	Show and tell, weekend news: child retells a story he or she has read	On Sunday I walk*ed* with . . . , we play*ed* with . . . , I'*m* go*ing* I liked this story because i*t's* . . . The be*st* part is . . .
	Predictions about an upcoming event	
	Describing science experiments	Student gives hypothesis and steps to proof
	Defining key words and concepts	School subject vocabulary

From "Incorporating Speech Development into an Education Program," by Perusse, Bernstein, and Phillips, 1992, *The Volta Review, 94*(5), p. 90. Copyright 1992 by Alexander Graham Bell Association for the Deaf. Adapted with permission.

As students progress to the pronunciation of single words, it is again appropriate to address relevant applications. The intelligibility of particular names of family members and teachers, kinds of candy bars or breakfast cereals, present/past tense verbs (*said/say, fell/fall*), the names of particular stores or brands of clothing and shoes, food-service words and terms ("*Do you want* white *or* wheat bread"), and other real-life examples can be highly motivating to students who are D/HH.

Many facilitation strategies for language use, meaning, or form (Luetke-Stahlman, 1998) can be adapted for the facilitation of speech. Suggestions presented in Table 3–10, adapted from Calvert and Silverman (1983), can also be helpful.

TABLE 3-10: SPEECH TARGET REMINDERS

Signaling	A signal is invented to remind the student to monitor the speech he or she is capable of producing.
Specifying	Feedback about the correct/incorrect or acceptable/unacceptable pronunciation is provided, using the following techniques: (1) communicate the locus of the deviation (*"I didn't understand the first part of your sentence"*); (2) indicate the type of deviation (*"You left out a sound"*); (3) describe the nature of the error (*"Your voice was too high"*).
Modeling	The speech target to imitate is modeled but not exaggerated. A mirror is often used so the student can see him/herself and the adult model simultaneously.
Demonstration*	Feedback is provided using other sensory modalities in isolation or in combination with the target desired. Luetke-Stahlman & Luckner (1991, p. 197) suggest some specific demonstration techniques.
Manipulation*	The student's articulator is manipulated to provide kinesthetic feedback about what is needed (food, tongue depressor, or feather used to sensitize a student to where in the mouth area to place the tongue, demonstration of rounding the lips, etc.).

*Demonstration and manipulation should be used in private sessions and after other techniques have been tried.

From *Speech and Deafness*, by D. Calvert and S. Silverman, 1983, Washington, DC: Alexander Graham Bell Association for the Deaf. Copyright 1983 by Alexander Graham Bell Association for the Deaf. Adapted with permission.

Keeping Track of Speech Targets

> **Study Guide Question**
> *Facilitate the speech ability of a student who is D/HH using some of the techniques described in Table 3–10. Which seem the most helpful and why?*

Team members might consider writing IFSPs and IEPs to encourage collaboration: Several team members can be made responsible for speech and audition objectives, and objectives can be written to include subject area content.

Some examples from a third grader's IEP include:

- Harold will use phonetic and orthographic word-attack skills during guided and shared reading.
- Harold will pronounce and use ten spelling words correctly in sentences.
- Given a root word, Harold will correctly spell new words by using suffixes, prefixes, and inflection.
- During weekly guided reading, Harold will use appropriate speech.
- During weekly basal reading, Harold will use appropriate speech.

It can be challenging to remember specific speech targets and their incorporation into activities. Creative adults have used the following ideas:

- Write speech targets on a small piece of colorful paper, or make a button for a child to wear (or to attach to the back of a shirt or dress).
- Write speech targets on small pieces of paper that are then stuck on the frames of doors, in planning books, on the covers of textbooks, and so on.
- Write speech targets on bookmarks to be incorporated into a narrative story.

Speech targets are to be practiced briefly (Ah ha! Another activity to do while waiting in line!) or during sessions of no more than ten minutes in length. While one student is speaking, others should be asked to listen (and/or speechread) and imitate what was said. Adults can occasionally sabotage this routine by stating their own opinion of what was said in a slightly incorrect manner and then observing whether students notice or not.

Many teachers of the deaf and speech-language pathologists are familiar with a workbook of task-analyzed phonetic and phonological skills, the *Teacher/Clinician Planbook and Guide to the Development of Speech Skills* (Ling, 1978b). Guidelines in this manual may be helpful in providing a sequence of targets that convert easily into objectives for IFSPs or IEPs.

Summary

Positive change in audition, speechreading, and speech development is most effectively facilitated when a particular student who is D/HH is appropriately assessed, a small set of targets is identified, and facilitation and monitoring are shared among team members, as well as within relevant home and school settings. Students will be motivated to attempt and develop these skills when they receive natural feedback, showing that their efforts produce a response that is meaningful and encouraging to them. Significant adults, peers, and the individual student must *value* audition, speechreading, and speech work. Confidence among team members in contributing to the achievement of desired outcomes in these areas requires collaboration, knowledge, and practice.

Activities

1. Use a suggested speech assessment procedure to evaluate the articulation abilities of a toddler or a student who is D/HH. Write a professional report describing this experience and have a plan for utilizing the assessment results.

2. Observe a teacher of the deaf or a speech-language pathologist teaching speech to a student who is D/HH. Assist with facilitation over several sessions and in several contexts.

3. Choose two phonetic level objectives. Then make a list of phonological-level objectives that you can introduce that will complement the phonetic objectives.

4. Ask a teacher of the deaf or a speech-language pathologist how speech objectives and monitoring requirements are coordinated among school staff and parents.

5. Videotape yourself as you facilitate the speechreading and speech abilities of a student who is D/HH during a school subject area activity. Discuss the session with a peer in terms of how the information provided in this chapter assisted you in planning and facilitating speech.

Activities adapted from *Effectively Educating Students with Hearing Impairments*, by B. Luetke-Stahlman and J. Luckner, 1991, New York: Longman. Copyright 1991 by Longman. Adapted with permission.

Resources for Speech Assessment and Facilitation

Alexander Graham Bell Association for the Deaf
3417 Volta Place, N.W.
Washington, DC 20007
202-337-5220
Ling's Phonetic Level Evaluation
Ling's Phonological Level Evaluation
Teacher/Clinician Planbook and Guide to the Development
  of Speech Skills

Central Institute for the Deaf
818 South Euclid Ave.
St. Louis, MO 63110
314-977-0133
CID *Picture Speech Intelligibility Evaluation* (SPINE)
Speech Perception Instructional Curriculum and Evaluation
  (SPICE)
Early Speech Perception Test

Pro-Ed
8700 Shoal Creek Blvd.
Austin, TX 78757-6897
1-800-897-3202
The Assessment of Phonological Processes–Revised (APP–R)

Slosson Educational Publications, Inc.
P.O. Box 280
East Aurora, NY 14052-0280
1-800-828-4800
Goldman-Fristoe Test of Articulation

Appendix 3-A

Meaningful Use of Speech Scale (MUSS)
Amy M. Robbins, M.S., and Mary Joe Osberger, Ph.D.*

NAME _____   DATE _____

INTERVAL _____

CONDITION (device) _____

EXAMINER _____

INFORMANT _____

1. The child uses vocalizations to attract others' attention. Ask: "Tell me
    about what Johnny does to gain your attention at home. If Johnny wanted
    to get your attention from across the room, what percentage of the time
    would he use:

    a. gestures (stomping, hand waving, etc.)
    b. gestures plus vocalization
    c. vocalization alone

Score question based strictly on percentage of time the child gains attention
using vocalization alone.

_____ 0 = Never: Spontaneously uses voice; uses other means
                            to gain the attention of others.

_____ 1 = Rarely: Vocalizes (less than 50% of the time).

_____ 2 = Occasionally: Uses vocalization alone (at least 50% of the
                            time).

_____ 3 = Frequently: Uses vocalization alone (at least 75% of the
                            time).

_____ 4 = Always: Uses vocalization alone (100%).

COMMENTS:

2. Vocalizes during communicative interactions. Ask: "Tell me about the ways
    Johnny communicates at home. Of the total number of communication
    interactions with Johnny at home, how often would he vocalize during
    them—either using speech plus sign or speech alone (i.e., excluding sign
    alone utterances)"?   *cont.*

*Developed at Indiana University School of Medicine, Indianapolis, IN (1991). Reprinted with
permission. (Available from Amy Robbins, 8512 Spring Mill Rd., Indianapolis, IN 46260)

_____ 0 = Never: Uses voice spontaneously while communicating.

_____ 1 = Rarely: Uses voice spontaneously while communicating (less than half of the time).

_____ 2 = Occasionally: Uses voice while communicating (at least 50% of the time, or uses voice more than 50% of the time but with undifferentiated vocalizations).

_____ 3 = Frequently: Vocalizes (at least 75% of the time) and shows some differentiation of speech sounds and syllable structure.

_____ 4 = Always: Vocalizes with at least approximation of syllable and/or phrase structure of intended message (100%).

COMMENTS:

3. Vocalizations vary with content and message. Ask: "Describe how much control Johnny has in his spontaneous speech over loudness, length of syllables, and the pitch of his voice. If he were relating an event to you (such as retelling a movie plot or story), tell me about the variations in his speech." In the case of the younger child, if he/she were excited about an event, would the pitch of his/her voice reflect that excitement? If he/she were relating an event that happened during the day, would there be variations in the loudness and/or duration of the utterance?

NOTE: Examiner's observations of the child's spontaneous speech are critical here. Appropriate and volitional control of suprasegmentals is the goal of this question, not involuntary changes in pitch, rate, etc.

_____ 0 = Never: All vocalizations are similar re: suprasegmental aspects of speech (i.e., no intentional use).

_____ 1 = Rarely: Child has limited control over volume (loud/soft) and/or duration (long/short) only.

_____ 2 = Occasionally: Child has control over volume and duration at least 50% of the time.

cont.

_____ 3 = Frequently: Child has control of volume and duration of voice at least 75% of the time and may show some variation in pitch.

_____ 4 = Always: Child's spontaneous speech represents appropriate control of loudness, length, and pitch (i.e., speech resembles that of a normal-hearing person).

COMMENTS:

4. Is the child spontaneously willing to use speech only to communicate with parents and/or siblings when the topic of conversation is a known or familiar one? Ask: "If Johnny were talking about a shared event with his family (such as Christmas morning), how much of the time would his communication to his family consist of speech alone?" For the younger child, if he/she were "reading" a favorite book, or reviewing a specific event the family shared that day, how much of the time would he/she use speech alone?

Ask for examples of child's use of gestures, pantomime, drawing, writing. Frequent use of these would suggest a lower score.

_____ 0 = Never: Spontaneously uses speech alone. Only does so with prompting.

_____ 1 = Rarely: Less than half of the time.

_____ 2 = Occasionally: At least 50% of the time.

_____ 3 = Frequently: At least 75% of the time.

_____ 4 = Always: Spontaneously uses speech alone in this situation.

COMMENTS:

5. Is the child willing to use speech only to communicate with parents and/or siblings when the topic of conversation is not a familiar one? Ask:

cont.

"If Johnny were telling his family about an event with which they were unfamiliar (such as something that happened at school that day), how much of the time would his communication consist of speech alone?" Ask about the child's use of gestures, pantomime, writing, and drawing in this situation. Frequent use of these would suggest a lower score.

_____ 0 = Never: Spontaneously uses speech alone.

_____ 1 = Rarely: Less than half of the time.

_____ 2 = Occasionally: At least 50% of the time.

_____ 3 = Frequently: At least 75% of the time.

_____ 4 = Always: Uses speech alone spontaneously.

COMMENTS:

6.   Is the child willing to use speech spontaneously during social exchanges with hearing persons? Ask: "What does Johnny do in social situations when hearing people speak to him?" Would Johnny say "Hello" back to a hearing person who spoke to him, or say "thank you" to a hearing person without being prompted to do so? In the case of the younger child, would she/he say "bye-bye" when waving good-bye without being prompted? Ask about situations where the child is somewhat familiar with the person speaking to her/him, and where her/his parents are present. This avoids evaluating the child's "friendliness with strangers" which is not the goal of this question. Situations to ask about include the child's responses to hearing persons at church, to hearing persons visiting in her/his home, or to speaking with Santa Claus.

_____ 0 = Never: Child never does so, or only with parental prompting.

_____ 1 = Rarely: Less than 50% of the time.

_____ 2 = Occasionally: At least 50% of the time.

_____ 3 = Frequently: At least 75% of the time.

_____ 4 = Always: Uses speech alone spontaneously.

cont.

COMMENTS:

7. Is the child willing to use speech only to communicate with unfamiliar people to get something she/he desires? Ask: "Think about situations outside home and school when Johnny is expected to communicate his needs. How often does Johnny spontaneously use speech alone to order in a restaurant, interact with store clerks, or speak with a cashier (without parent's intervention)?" For the younger child, ask: "Do you see _____ using vocalizations with a new daycare provider when desiring a snack? or when playing on the playground, if she/he wanted another child's ball or toy?" The critical issue here is the child's willingness to do so independently and without prompting.

_____ 0 = Never: Child never does so, or only with parental prompting.

_____ 1 = Rarely: Less than 50% of the time.

_____ 2 = Occasionally: At least 50% of the time

_____ 3 = Frequently: At least 75% of the time.

_____ 4 = Always: Uses speech alone spontaneously.

COMMENTS:

8. Is the child's speech understood by others who are unfamiliar with him/her? Ask: "Suppose Johnny became lost in a store. How well would a security officer or store clerk be able to understand his speech if he tried to explain to them who he was and what he needed?" In the case of the younger child, ask "If _____ were playing on the playground, how well would an unfamiliar person understand one or two word utterances such as "my ball" or "want swing."

_____ 0 = Never: None of the child's speech would be understood.

_____ 1 = Rarely: Adult would understand only single words and gestural or written support would be critical.

cont.

_____ 2 = Occasionally: Adult would understand about half of what
                              the child said. Gestures or writing would aid
                              in the person's comprehension.

_____ 3 = Frequently: Adult would understand most of what the
                              child said, missing only a few details.

_____ 4 = Always: All of the child's speech would be
                              understood with ease by an adult.

COMMENTS:

9.   Child spontaneously uses appropriate oral repair and clarification
     strategies when speech is not understood by people familiar with him/her.
     Ask: "If Johnny is talking to you and you do not understand him, what
     strategies does he use to repair broken lines of communication?" What
     percentage of the time does he use:

                    a. sign or gesture only
                    b. sign/gesture + oral
                    c. oral repair only

Query the parent regarding the various oral strategies the child may have at
his/her disposal. If one is unsuccessful, does he/she try another oral strategy
or immediately resort to a non-oral one? For example, if the child repeats a
word and still is not understood, would he/she pick a synonym, rephrase,
explain the word, spell the word out loud? Evaluate the child's persistence in
using spoken repair strategies.

_____ 0 = Never: Child uses no strategies involving oral
                              communication, or uses them only with
                              prompting.

_____ 1 = Rarely: Less than 50% of the time, child will use an
                              oral strategy such as saying a key word
                              slowly, or emphasizing it in his/her speech.

_____ 2 = Occasionally: Child uses oral strategies at least 50% of the
                              time, and persists when unsuccessful.

_____ 3 = Frequently: Child uses oral strategies at least 75% of the
                              time, and persists when unsuccessful.

_____ 4 = Always: Child uses oral strategies 100% of the time.
cont.

COMMENTS:

10. Child spontaneously uses appropriate oral repair and clarification strategies when speech is not understood by people <u>unfamiliar</u> with him/her. Ask: "If Johnny is talking to someone he does <u>not</u> know and that person does not understand him, what strategies does he use to repair broken lines of communication?" What percentage of the time would he use:

> a. sign or gesture only
> b. sign/gesture + oral
> c. oral repair only

Query the parent regarding the various oral strategies the child may have at her/his disposal. If one is unsuccessful, does she/he try another oral strategy or immediately resort to a non-oral one? For example, if the child repeats a word and still is not understood, would she/he pick a synonym, rephrase, explain the word, spell the word out loud? We're evaluating the child's <u>persistence</u> in spoken repair strategies.

_____	0 = Never:	Child uses no strategies involving oral communication, or uses them only with prompting.
_____	1 = Rarely:	Less than 50% of the time, child will use an oral strategy such as saying a key word slowly, or emphasizing it in her/his speech.
_____	2 = Occasionally:	Child uses oral strategies at least 50% of the time, and persists when unsuccessful.
_____	3 = Frequently:	Child uses oral strategies at least 75% of the time and persists when unsuccessful.
_____	4 = Always:	Child uses oral strategies 100% of the time.

COMMENTS:

Total points correct: _____ /40

References

Beck, A., & Dennis, M. (1997). Speech-language pathologists' and teachers' perceptions of classroom-based interventions. *Language, Speech, and Hearing Services in Schools, 28*, 146-152.

Bloom, L., & Krathwohl, D. (1977). *Taxonomy of educational objectives. Handbook 1: Cognitive domain.* New York: Longman.

Calvert, D., & Silverman, S. (1983). *Speech and deafness.* Washington, DC: Alexander Graham Bell Association for the Deaf.

Clouser, R. (1976). The effect of vowel consonant ratio and sentence length on lipreading ability. *American Annals of the Deaf, 121*, 513-518.

Cummins, J. (1984). *Bilingualism and special education: Issues in assessment and pedagogy.* Clevedon, Avon, England: Multilingual Matters.

Erber, H. (1977). Developing materials for lipreading evaluation and instruction. *The Volta Review, 79*, 35-42.

Erber, N. (1982). *Auditory training.* Washington, DC: Alexander Graham Bell Association for the Deaf.

Gatty, J. (1992). Teaching speech to hearing-impaired children. *The Volta Review, 94*, 49-61.

Geers, A., & Moog, J. (1988). *CID Picture Speech Intelligibility Evaluation* (SPINE). St. Louis, MO: Central Institute for the Deaf.

Goldman, R., & Fristoe M. (1986). *Goldman-Fristoe Test of Articulation* (G-FTA). Circle Pines, MN: American Guidance.

Golf, H. (1980). Principles, objectives, and strategies for speech training. In J. Subtelny (Ed.), *Speech assessment and speech improvement for the hearing impaired* (pp. 143-147). Washington, DC: Alexander Graham Bell Association for the Deaf.

Hodson, B. (1986). *Targeting intelligible speech: A phonological approach to mediation.* Austin, TX: Pro-Ed.

Hudson, A. (1981). *Co-articulation.* Handouts from a workshop, Louisiana State University, Baton Rouge, LA. (Available from B. LeBlanc, 611 N. Burnside, Gonzales, LA 70737)

Jeffers, J., & Barley, M. (1971). *Speechreading.* Springfield, IL: Charles C. Thomas.

LeBlanc, B. (1997, April). *Workshop on the eclectic method for teaching speech to the hearing impaired.* Presented at the Mississippi Speech-Language-Hearing Association, Biloxi, MS.

Ling, D. (1976). *Speech and the hearing-impaired child: Theory and Practices.* Washington, DC: Alexander Graham Bell Association for the Deaf.

Ling, D. (1978a). Speech development in hearing-impaired children. *Journal of Communication Disorders, 11*(2/3), 119-124.

Ling, D. (1978b). *Teacher/clinician planbook and guide to the development of speech skills.* Washington, DC: Alexander Graham Bell Association for the Deaf.

Ling, D. (1989). *Foundations of spoken language for hearing-impaired children.* Washington, DC: Alexander Graham Bell Association for the Deaf.

Long, M. (1986). *Phonologic evaluation.* (Available from Rochester School for the Deaf, 1545 St. Paul St., Rochester, NY 14621)

Luetke-Stahlman, B. (1989). A framework for assessing speechreading performance in hearing-impaired children. *The ACEHI Journal, 15*(1), 27-37.

Luetke-Stahlman, B. (1998). *Language issues in deaf education.* Hillsboro, OR: Butte Publications.

Luetke-Stahlman, B., & Luckner, J. (1991). *Effectively educating students with hearing impairments.* New York: Longman.

Moeller, M. (1982). Hearing and speechreading assessment with the severely hearing-impaired child. In D. Sims, G. Walter, & R. Whitehead (Eds.), *Deafness and communication.* Baltimore, MD: Williams & Wilkins.

Moeller, M., Osberger, M., & Morford, J. (1987). Speech-language assessment and intervention with preschool hearing impaired children. In J. Alpiner & P. McCarthy (Eds.), *Rehabilitative audiology for children and adults* (pp. 162-187). Baltimore, MD: Williams & Wilkins.

Montgomery, A. (1988). Issues and developments in the evaluation of speechreading. *The Volta Review, 90*(5), 193-214.

Montgomery, N. (1995, October). *Strategies for working with students who are deaf/hard of hearing.* Paper presented at the meeting of the Missouri Speech-Language-Hearing Association.

Moog, J., Davidson, L., & Biedenstein, J. (1995). *Speech perception instructional curriculum and evaluation (SPICE).* St. Louis, MO: Central Institute for the Deaf.

Moog, J., & Geers, A. (1990). *Early Speech Perception Test.* St. Louis, MO: Central Institute for the Deaf.

Nittrouer, S., & Hochberg, I. (1985). Speech communication for deaf children: A communication based approach. *American Annals of the Deaf, 130*(6), 491-495.

O'Neil, J., & Oyer, H. (1981). *Visual communication for the hard of hearing: History, research, methods* (2nd ed.). Englewood Cliffs, NJ: Prentice-Hall.

Perusse, M., Bernstein, A. & Phillips, A. (1992). Incorporating speech development into an education program. *The Volta Review, 94*(5), 79-94.

Robbins, A., & Osberger, M. (1991). *Meaningful Use of Speech Scale* (MUSS). (Available from Amy Robbins, 8512 Spring Mill Rd., Indianapolis, IN 46260)

Schwartz, J., & Black, J. (1967). Some effects of sentence structure on speechreading. *Central States Speech Journal, 18,* 86-90.

Sobel, R., & Pluznik, N. (1987). *Messy monsters, jungle joggers, and bubble bath.* Washington, DC: Alexander Graham Bell Association for the Deaf.

The Volta Review (1992). Speech production in hearing impaired children and youth: Theory and practice [Special issue].

Wozniak, V., & Jackson, P. (1979). Visual vowel and diphthong perception from two horizontal viewing angles. *Journal of Speech and Hearing Research, 22*(2), 354-365.

Chapter 4
Social Interaction and Language

The Need for Attention to Social Interaction

Social Interaction Assessment

Available Curricula

Social Integration Facilitation Strategies

The Adult's Role in Students' Social Interactions

Evaluation

Signing in Schools

Resources

Appendix 4–A: Formal Social Assessment Tools

Appendix 4–B: Children's Books about Deafness

Employers indicate that a variety of appropriate social behaviors are necessary in the work world (Chadsey-Rusch, & Heal, 1995). If students who are deaf or hard of hearing are to be appropriately educated and prepared for the workplace, social as well as academic needs must become the responsibility of all team members. It has been reported that "social opportunities exist for [these students] . . . in school programs, but most teachers observed them to be excluded" (Kempton, 1993, p. 64). This is true perhaps in part because "language skills are important in establishing and maintaining successful social relationships" (Fujiki, Brinton, & Todd, 1996).

Adults employed in school settings where students who are D/HH are enrolled can play an important part in facilitating these students' development of mature social interaction—accepting responsibility for actions, having self-awareness, acting with confidence and making decisions, taking initiative, being dependable, adapting behavior, having good interpersonal skills, and so on (White, 1982). Suggestions for social interaction assessment, setting goals and objectives, and social skills curricula are provided in this chapter, as well as suggestions for facilitating social integration, including developing a structured "Circle of Friends," role playing, and direct instruction of social skills. Lastly, a variety of models are described for teaching sign to hearing peers and adults in order to foster improved social integration and communication for everyone.

The Need for Attention to Social Interaction

Peer-related social interaction is the ability of students to select and act on interpersonal skills successfully and appropriately (Guralnick, 1980). The home environments of most students who are D/HH offer a restricted range of interpersonal interactions compared to their hearing peers (Marschark, 1993). Many do not share effective communication with their parents, for instance, and therefore have not been taught how to behave socially.

Because of this inability of parents of many students who are D/HH to explain social skills and manners to their children, adults in school and other social settings can play a vital role in facilitating the acquisition of age-appropriate social skills. In these settings, students engage in peer communication (gossip, self-disclosure, problem solving, self-exploration) "in order to forge an understanding of their own emotions and how these emotions function in relation to other people" (Kluwin & Stinson, 1993, p. 73). Foster (1988) found that the value system of students who are D/HH is identical to that of hearing students: It is important to form friendships, go to parties, share in after-school activities, and so on. However, peer interaction between deaf and hearing students appears to be minimal, and close friendships are not usually established (Farrugia & Austin, 1980; Foster, 1988; Kempton, 1993; Libbey & Pronovost, 1980).

> **Study Guide Question**
> *Ask teachers of students who are D/HH to define social interaction and to rate their students' success in social interactions. How does their students' ability to interact with deaf peers compare with their ability to interact with hearing peers?*

Social Interaction Assessment

To determine whether a goal for increased social interaction should be written into an IFSP or IEP, team members should solicit questions about the student regarding this area of development. Assessment in social interaction should be conducted *before problems arise*. Vernon and Andrews (1990) suggested that an accurate social skills evaluation includes

- a consideration of the student's case history
- the examiner's personal experiences with the student
- student interviews
- observations of social behaviors *by people knowledgeable of deafness*
- formal testing

Formal and Informal Assessment ——————————

Formal social skills assessment instruments allow teachers to identify the extent to which students are deficient in social skills and which hearing and deaf students might need social skills facilitation. The following are examples of formal social assessment tools used with students who are D/HH (Aljundi, 1993; Luetke-Stahlman, 1994; 1995b). The first four are described in Appendix 4–A.

1. *The Battelle Developmental Inventory* (Newborg, Stock, Wnek, Guidibaldo, & Svinicki, 1984)
2. *The Meadow-Kendall Social-Emotional Inventories for Deaf and Hearing Impaired Students* (Meadow, 1983)
3. *Social Skills for Daily Living* (Hazel, Peterson, & Schumaker, 1990)
4. *The Vineland Adaptive Behavior Scale: Classroom Edition* (Harrison, 1985)
5. *Direct Observation of Social Behavior Manual* (Odom, Silver, Sandler, & Strain, 1983)
6. *The Systematic Anecdotal Assessment of Social Interaction* (Odom, Kohler, & Strain, 1987)

Aljundi (1993) surveyed teachers of the deaf in Kansas and found a dismal picture in terms of the measuring of social skills. Many of the instruments used by those responsible for the education of students who are D/HH did not assess social competency to the extent that the term is described in the literature. In addition, seven tools recommended or used by participants did not measure social competency at all—they were self-concept and behavioral tools. Aljundi also compared socialization tools that were used in Kansas to a comprehensive definition of social competence compiled from a thorough review of the literature (see Table 4–1). No single instrument assessed all ten components of social competence, but a combination of two tools did provide a complete battery: *The Battelle Developmental Inventory* (BDI) (Newborg et al., 1984) along with the *Social Skills for Daily Living* (SSDL) (Hazel et al., 1990).

TABLE 4-1: SOCIAL SKILLS ASSESSMENT TOOLS COMPARED TO SOCIAL COMPETENCIES

Social Competence Components										
	Good Communication Skills	Individual Thinking Skills	Self Control & Self Direction	Understands Feelings, Motivations, & Needs of Self & Others	Adapts to the Needs of a Situation	Tolerates Frustration	Tolerates Ambivalence	Relies on and Can Be Relied upon by Others	Understands and Appreciates Culture	Has Skills for Maintaining Relations with Others
BDI	X	X	X	X	X	X		X	X	X
MKSEI-EE	X		X	X						X
MKSEI-PSE	X		X	X						X
SSDL	X	X		X	X		X			X
VABS-CE	X	X	X	X	X			X	X	
VABS-IE	X	X	X	X	X			X	X	X
WPBIC					X					

BDI = *The Battelle Developmental Inventory* (1994)
MKSEI-EE = *The Meadow-Kendall Social-Emotional Inventories–Elementary Edition* (1983)
MKSEI-PSE = *The Meadow-Kendall Social-Emotional Inventories–Preschool Edition* (1983)
SSDL = *Social Skills for Daily Living* (1990)
VABS-CE = *The Vineland Adaptive Behavior Scale: Classroom Edition* (1985)
VABS-IE = *The Vineland Adaptive Behavior Scale: Interview Edition* (1984)
WPBIC = *The Walker Problem Behavior Identification Checklist* (Walker, 1983)

Components of social competence (the column headings on this table) adapted from Greenberg & Kusche, 1993.

Most professionals use informal methods to measure social skills. For example, Torline (1994) surveyed professionals in Kansas who were most responsible for psychosocial assessment and social skills facilitation with students who are D/HH in their school districts. She found the results as bleak as Aljundi's findings about formal assessment. The majority of respondents assessed social behavior through observation even though they were not trained to do so. Other common methods identified as used by professionals were an unspecified interview procedure and school behavior checklists (Torline, 1994).

Study Guide Question
What assessment instruments are team members you know using to identify social interaction skills (not behavioral problems) of students who are D/HH? Ask some team members, and discuss your findings with a peer.

Assessment Checklists and Questionnaires ————

Team members can effectively combine informal and formal measures of social skills assessment. For example, they can use checklists and questionnaires, working from either an existing social skills checklist or devising one of their own. Team members and/or students can also be interviewed.

Masters, Mori, and Mori (1993) suggest that checklists are one of the best ways for adults to gather accurate social skills information. They devised the instrument in Table 4–2, which can be adapted as needed.

TABLE 4–2: SAMPLE TEACHER CHECKLIST FOR SOCIAL SKILLS

	NEVER	SOMETIMES	ALWAYS
PEER INTERACTION			
1. Initiates peer interaction			
2. Interacts positively with peers			
3. Cooperates in group activities			
4. Communicates appropriately with peers			
TEACHER INTERACTION			
5. Seeks attention in an appropriate manner			
6. Reacts appropriately to teacher requests			
7. Interacts positively with teacher			
8. Communicates needs appropriately to teacher			
INTERPERSONAL SKILLS			
9. Views self in positive manner			
10. Understands consequences of behavior			
11. Reacts appropriately to criticism			
12. Reacts appropriately to praise			
13. Has high frustration tolerance			
14. Avoids physical confrontations			
15. Displays appropriate restraint when angry			
16. Requests assistance when necessary			
17. Displays control of emotion			
18. Uses good manners (*thank you, please,* etc.)			

From *Teaching Secondary Students with Mild Learning and Behavior Problems* (p. 280), by L. Masters, B. Mori, and A. Mori, 1993, Austin, TX: Pro-Ed. Copyright 1993 by Pro-Ed. Adapted with permission.

Chadsey-Rusch and Heal (1995) reported on social skills desired of high school students as they made the transition to work environments. Skills highly rated by 228 professionals included the behaviors listed below.* This list could be reformatted for use as a checklist:

- asking for help, offering assistance, providing information, asking questions
- responding to criticism, answering questions
- using appropriate greetings, teasing and joking, social amenities
- initiating, responding to a variety of topics
- advocating for themselves and being persistent problem-solvers
- interpreting and discriminating social situations and cues from others so they know when and with whom to interact in a socially appropriate manner
- having others who like to eat lunch with them or see them after school or work
- having others who consider them to be friends
- having others who like them to attend social events

Fujiki, Brinton, and Todd (1996) developed a set of questions to estimate the number of peer contacts experienced by students with specific language impairments. A sampling of their questions follows; these and other similar questions might be useful to team members working with students who are D/HH.

1. Do you ever play at someone's house? With whom do you play?
2. Do you ever draw or color? With whom do you draw or color?
3. Do you ever play outside at recess? With whom do you play at recess?
4. Do you ever watch TV? With whom do you watch TV?
5. Do you ever play with toys or games? With whom do you play toys or games?
6. Do you ever talk on the phone? Whom do you talk with on the phone?
7. Do you ever eat lunch at school? With whom do you eat lunch?

*List of skills from "Building Consensus from Transition Experts on Social Integration Outcomes and Interventions," by J. Chadsey-Rusch and L. Heal, 1995, *Exceptional Children, 62.* Copyright by the Council for Exceptional Children. Adapted with permission.

• *expectations important!*
• *be realistic*

Goals and Objectives

Social interaction goals and objectives should be included on educational plans if there is evidence of need. For example, objectives for Kent, a three-year-old deaf child, might be written as follows:

1. Kent will work or play with at least one hearing partner for at least five minutes each day.
2. Kent will role play his character (*"I am the bus driver"*) or intended action (*"I'm going downtown"*) to hearing children when encouraged by an adult (using an interpreter, if he chooses).

1. Administer a social skills checklist or questionnaire in a setting involving a student who is D/HH. What are the results?

2. How would you use the Cummins model to design a system for task analyzing a social skill?

Objectives for Eli, a deaf third grader, might include the following:

1. With assistance from an interpreter, Eli will respond to two consecutive requests or comments of a hearing peer during at least one interaction per day.
2. Eli will provide two ideas during a cooperative learning activity with hearing peers.

Available Curricula

Sorensen (1992) emphasized the importance of using social skills curricula within the framework of situations that target friendship, responsibility, and independence. Given the need for social integration curricula, it is unfortunate that materials developed for the general population of students with disabilities have minimized or failed to include strategies that recognize the unique communication differences and needs of students who are D/HH. For example, *The Integrated Preschool Curriculum: Procedures for Socially Integrating Young Handicapped and Normally Developing Children* (Odom et al., 1988) provides many empirically tested social facilitation ideas.

It includes a relevant review of the literature, a rationale for implementing integrative procedures into play contexts, specific goals, an outline of the specific components of the curriculum, and suggested activities to be used in the types of integrated programs mentioned above. Unfortunately, adaptations for students who are D/HH are not included.

The following resources specifically address the needs of students who are D/HH and can be helpful in developing social skills.

- *Providing Alternative Thinking Strategies* (PATHS) by Greenberg and Kusche (1987, 1993) assists students who are D/HH in the acquisition of self-control, emotional awareness, and social problem-solving skills. The results of research conducted by the authors demonstrated that experience in PATHS led to significantly improved social and emotional functioning for both hearing and deaf students. Skills were also shown to transfer to the classroom setting.

- *Access for All: Integrating Deaf, Hard-of-Hearing, and Hearing Preschoolers* by Solit, Taylor, and Bednarczyk (1992) provides relevant information on deafness, a model for interagency collaboration, and strategies for adapting preschool activities to facilitate socialization. However, facilitators in nonmetropolitan areas might have difficulty replicating the approach, which is modeled after a project located at a childcare center on the Gallaudet University campus. The type of program described requires a large number of adult role models who are deaf and a high ratio of staff and children with signing ability.

- *Teaching Social Skills to Hearing-Impaired Students* by Schloss and Smith (1990) provides professionals with a detailed out line of defining, assessing, and facilitating social skills. The social development process, and issues that might impede this process for students who are D/HH, are described, as well as steps for assessing the child's skills, determining objectives, and addressing those objectives through established interventions. Several assessment surveys are provided for children, teachers, and parents.

An additional resource for social skills curricula is Thinking Publications, which publishes *Social Star: General Interaction Skills* (Gajewski, Hirn, & Mayo, 1993), a booklet of lessons that facilitate positive peer interactions. Communication Skill Builders also publishes several curricula to facilitate social skills among students. A booklet entitled *Social Skills Activities for Special Children* (Mannix, 1993) is one example. The Feelings Factory, too, publishes products designed to promote communication and coping skills. The resource list at the end of this chapter provides addresses for these publishers.

It may be that social skills curricula developed for hearing students can be adapted or used as designed with groups of students who are D/HH. Descriptions of some of those that are commercially available were provided by Luetke-Stahlman (1995b).

> ## Study Guide Questions
> 1. *What are some useful additional materials for the facilitation of social competence for a student who is D/HH? Identify and list some materials.*
>
> 2. *Evaluate a student who is D/HH using one of the described materials. Do assessed findings and parent report information match?*

Social Integration Facilitation Strategies

There are a variety of strategies for facilitating social skills. Among them are special early childhood considerations, developing a Circle of Friends, social role playing, and direct social skills instruction.

Early Childhood

Parents of a student who is D/HH who are enrolling their child in a daycare, nursery, after-school care, or similar type of program should visit the program and provide staff with background information such as hearing ability, equipment care, preferred mode of communication, and a copy of educational objectives (Luetke-Stahlman, 1995a). Solit, Taylor, and Bednarczyk (1992) commented that if a child is hard of hearing and using an oral approach, there will probably not be a need to add different personnel to the staff. However, if the family signs in English or uses American Sign Language (ASL), then an English transliterator or an ASL interpreter is a necessity. Engaging teachers, aides, or volunteers who are deaf themselves is recommended, since they can serve as positive role models and provide linguistic access to adult and student exchanges. Solit, Taylor, and Bednarczyk recommended and discussed activities as follows* to facilitate an appreciation for similarities and differences among students.

1. Providing relevant children's books (see Appendix 4–B) and participating in a variety of Deaf Culture activities can reinforce experiences and information directly disseminated in the programs.

2. Teaching basic function signs on a regular basis, using name signs, incorporating signing into routines, and having parts of songs or sections of time where sign only is used, can call attention to manual communications and the acquisition of a simple vocabulary by adults and children.

3. Helping adults become aware of how and under what circumstances they can use their voice to control the class and give information can be explained and monitored. Students who are D/HH may need to be cued to look at speakers or the interpreter. Adults might need to flick the lights in addition to using spoken comments to signal a change in activities. Program participants might need to practice different ways of getting the student's attention.

4. Integrating awareness and respect for Deaf Culture into the program can assist in promoting social awareness and self-esteem. Units such as The Family, How People Are Similar and Different, The Senses, Our Bodies, and so forth, lend themselves naturally to including discussion on deafness, communication, and equipment need. Teachers of older students who are D/HH might include deaf people in units about the Revolutionary War, Civil War, and so on.

---

*From *Access for All: Integrating Deaf, Hard-of-Hearing, and Hearing Preschoolers* (pp. 129-130), by G. Solit, M. Taylor, and A. Bednarczyk, 1992, Washington, DC: Gallaudet University. Copyright 1992. Adapted and reprinted courtesy of Pre-College National Mission Programs, Gallaudet University. Text also incorporates a few suggestions from Masters, Mori, and Mori, 1993.

When parts of the United States and capitals are studied, cities where important events in Deaf History occurred can be discussed. Questions such as the following might bring about interesting discussion of differences between "deaf" and "hearing" homes.

- How many times do you let the telephone ring in your home?
- How do you find out if someone is home when you first walk in?
- Where do your family members sit in a waiting room?
- How are introductions made by your family members?
- What is the job of the passenger when someone in your family is driving?
- How do your family members have a private conversation?

5. During large group activities, students who are D/HH can be helped to feel free to move around to improve their view of information or to move away from noisy distractions. Students who wish to add to a group discussion should raise their hands or in some other way indicate turn-taking so that the student who is D/HH can follow who is contributing. Finally, repetition, rephrasing, and visual support (mime, pictures) may help if a student who is D/HH does not understand a message.

6. Modifying music and movement activities can assist all who wish to participate and enjoy them. How students who are D/HH appreciate and understand music will differ depending on their hearing acuity, interest, and experience. Adults might try increasing the bass on live or recorded music, using review and demonstration before signing and/or acting, making sure the student who is D/HH can see the leader of the activity, and adding signs and visual props to the songs that are taught to everyone. If a student does not wish to be actively involved in musical activities, he or she might assist the leader in some way or be free to choose another activity.

7. Reading stories and discussing them can also facilitate social integration. Team members might choose books about some aspect of social awareness and ask comprehension questions from this perspective. For example:

- How do characters cope with their disappointments and problems?

- How are the characters' problems and needs like yours?
- What are the consequences of the attempted solutions?
- What are some other ways these situations might have worked out?
- What feelings and attitudes are conveyed in this story?

Study Guide Question

Interview deaf adults or teens and share with them the early childhood facilitation ideas. What other strategies can they suggest?

Developing a Circle of Friends

Elementary-age students who are D/HH may lack friends and not be invited to join in weekend sleepovers, parties, shopping trips, and other activities their hearing peers enjoy. School staff working with students who are D/HH of various ages enrolled in public school programs may consider establishing a Circle of Friends (Perske, 1988) if they are concerned about a particular student's opportunities for social interaction. A Circle of Friends meets regularly with the student, parents and family members, peers, and school staff to discuss a social interaction plan. They might brainstorm solutions to situations that present social challenges, such as peers' inability to sign, difficulties in playing board games and signing simultaneously, or frustration at having to repeat comments several times to the students who are D/HH. They might discuss ideas about how to educate schoolmates and parents of hearing peers, make the relay telephone number available to all peers, and so forth, so that opportunities for socialization are increased. Finally, they might plan several fun activities to build the sense of community in the Circle of Friends.

Hearing peers who participate in the Circle of Friends should do so on a voluntary basis and be dependable, caring people, capable of promoting friendship (Perske, 1988). It is also suggested that these peers be able to influence others and be perceived as leaders or independent thinkers. Perske recommended that approximately four or five peers are a sufficient number for weekly meetings at school. Outside Circle meetings, these peers might learn to sign, assist students as needed, and include the students who are D/HH in social activities.

Social Role Playing

Study Guide Question

Discuss the concept of a Circle of Friends with a teacher in a program where students who are D-HH are enrolled. What is his or her opinion of the usefulness of this concept?

Role playing can assist students who are D/HH to gain insight into their social situations. The following role-playing techniques have been adapted from Brammer and Schustrum (1982) by Masters et al. (1993).*

■ In the *role reversal* technique, students assume the roles of significant persons (friend, teacher, parent) in their lives. They then role play a specific situation with emphasis on the perspective of the other person. For instance, the student might role play a friend asking him or her to leave a party because of inappropriate behavior. After the interaction, an adult should specifically ask for clarification of each participant's perceptions and feelings.

■ The *"double" technique* is used to give students insight into personal conflicts. A class member plays the student's "conscience," and a peer verbalizes the problem. The conscience is asked to comment on positive and negative facts, desires, wishes, cautions, and so on.

■ "The *soliloquy* is used to encourage students to reveal their hidden feelings. In this approach, students are permitted to speak their feelings without interruption. Then the teacher asks each student in the group to freeze the action and express how he or she really feels or to discuss what he or she is thinking that was not expressed" (Masters et al., 1993, p. 290). This technique helps students to gain new insights into feelings or to clarify confused thoughts that they might have regarding serious conflicts.

■ "The *mirror technique* is used when the teacher feels that it is a good idea for students to see themselves in action. In this technique, another student in the class sits or stands eye-to-eye with the student and mimics each movement or verbal expression" (Masters et al., 1993, p. 290).

---

*Techniques from *Teaching Secondary Students with Mild Learning and Behavior Problems* (pp. 289-290), by L. Masters, B. Mori, and A. Mori, 1993, Austin, TX: Pro-Ed. Copyright 1993 by Pro-Ed. Adapted with permission.

■ "The *periodic stimuli technique* is used to expose students to a variety of surprise elements that test their adaptive skills. The student is given a particular role to fulfill, for example, a waiter or waitress in a restaurant. At the direction of the teacher, other students are sent in to complain about the service or accuse the 'waiter' of overcharging them on their bill or to provide some other troublesome concerns. The basic situation for the student remains the same, but the problems that are presented change. This is an excellent technique for students with social-affective skill deficits because it forces them to practice adaptive responses to difficult social situations without fear of failure" (Masters et al., 1993, p. 290).

■ For the *hidden theme technique*, the student must interpret the social situation and determine how to relate socially in an appropriate manner to the situation that is being enacted. The student is asked to leave the room or avoid watching while the teacher and the other students set up a social situation, for example, an argument in the cafeteria. When the student returns, he or she must respond socially to the enacted situation.

Students may also learn social skills through roles given them by high status peers or adults. Students who are D/HH can be given status by allowing them to pass out materials, hold needed equipment, lead an activity, or be positioned near the teacher. Adults will need to scrutinize activities to find ways to arrange the environment in order for the student who is D/HH to be given a status role, but without offending hearing students (Brown, Fox, & Brady, 1987).

Direct Instruction of Social Skills

Hops, Walker, and Greenwood (1979) found that students must learn two key social skills:
- Initiating to a peer in a way that is likely to obtain a positive response
- Responding to a peer's initiations in a positive manner in order to continue the interaction or encourage further initiations at a later time

When these two behaviors are evident, social skills instruction has been effective. When they are not, initiating and responding skills can be taught directly to students during individual times. They can be practiced in public school during "Lunch Bunch" activities—while students who are D/HH and hearing students eat lunch with an adult—in cooperative learning groups, and so on. They should be taught throughout the day in a manner that will allow for generalization to other activities.

Antia and Kreimeyer (1992) suggested that adults employ a social skills facilitation package that includes teacher modeling, prompting, phrasing, and reinforcement. Adults and students can be given specific scripts to practice and to role play; the adults gradually retreat, moving from structured practice, to less structured practice, to maintenance practice. Rosenthal-Malek (1997) suggested a social skills facilitation package that includes three strategies in stages:

- Formal self-interrogation training—students are taught to stop and think and ask themselves: *What do I want to do? What will happen if ___? How do I feel? How do my friends feel? What else could I do?*
- Informal strategy training—students practice self-interrogation in a naturalistic session
- Generalization phase—staff members encourage students to use the self-interrogation strategy throughout the day

The Adult's Role in Students' Social Interactions

Initially, an adult will probably be needed to facilitate the development of emerging social interaction behaviors that are desired. This adult might be the general or special education teacher, the teacher of the deaf, an interpreter, or a paraprofessional. Schirmer (1989) found that teacher-structured free play is more beneficial to students who are D/HH than free play in which adults do not participate. Opportunities for such socialization might occur during lunchtime or recess, in the hallways, and during unstructured times in the classroom. Adults should be actively involved during these sessions to

- model appropriate play and use self-talk strategies (Fey, 1986):

"I sure would like to play with someone. I see Lynn over there. Maybe I'll go ask her."

- use comments to direct the student's attention to the appropriate social interactions of others: *"Look over there . . . Lindsey is talking to Amy about lunch."*
- use inform talk (Luetke-Stahlman, 1998): *"Kelly said she liked your illustration and report."*
- interpret and transliterate
- reinforce or encourage the student's social interaction: *"It was nice of you to hand that book to Kerry."*
- present ideas for play, using parallel talk (Fey): *"You are playing with Lynn?"*
- provide question prompts and reverse interpretation or transliteration
- eliminate behaviors that interfere with social interactions, or substitute more acceptable behaviors (Duchan, 1995)
- create environments where nonacceptance is not allowed (Duchan)

> **Study Guide Question**
> *What is the adult's role in facilitating social interaction? Create a web and provide several examples of each role.*

Modeling Appropriate Social Behavior

Gallagher (1988) provided the following guidelines to assist adults in modeling appropriate social behaviors.

Modeling Social Behaviors*

Pretest. Observe the students in a natural environment or in a contrived situation to assess whether they possess the identified social skill.

   a) *Preorganize.* Prior to introducing the lesson, decide who will be the models, have the models practice for the demonstration, and arrange the room.

- Provide a rationale: Students must see how the skill will benefit them.
- Present a modeling situation: Prepare a script that clearly models the desired social skill. It may be necessary to demonstrate it more than once.

- Discuss the modeled skill: Have the students identify the basic components of the skill that was demonstrated. As the students verbalize the responses exhibited by the model, list the responses in the order of their occurrence.
- Make scripts available: Scripts, which contain the skill components, should be distributed to the students. The teacher can also make a chart to post in the room.

b) *Provide behavioral rehearsal time.* Students should be allowed to practice the modeled behavior in order to learn and retain it.

- Provide performance feedback: Feedback, an important part of the training sequence, may include confirmation or disconfirmation of performance, corrective feedback, reteaching, or reinforcement.
- Provide verbal rehearsal time: Students should have the opportunity to practice the role-playing lines verbally. This will eventually lead to skill maintenance.
- Provide reinforcement: It is essential to provide social and group reinforcement at the conclusion of each lesson.

c) *Specify the goal.* Review the criteria that indicate the skill has been mastered.

- Transfer learning: Plan activities that necessitate use of the newly acquired social skill in different settings. This maximizes the chances that the skill will continue to be used when needed.

Facilitating Cooperative Play and Work

As preschool- and elementary-aged students progress in their abilities to play or work cooperatively and interact socially with others, the adult's role becomes one of

- introducing the activity (using more and more of the student's ideas)
- suggesting ideas

- prompting, modeling (via themselves or another student)
- playing or sharing
- interpreting and reverse interpreting
- evaluating progress

Adults should begin cooperative activities by introducing the materials and suggesting themes or uses for them (that is, supplying prompts). Adults could either sign for themselves or use the interpreter. They might assign roles (*"You be the scribe"*) or model a role play using the materials. The adult may need to be encouraging (*"That's a good idea"*) to students who hesitate to interact or communicate. Students may need to be taught that when someone attempts to communicate with them, they should acknowledge them with a smile and appropriate response (Odom et al., 1988). Some students who are D/HH will need other students to tap or wave to them to get their attention before beginning to communicate. Often, turning a student who is D/HH around to face away from other students and asking hearing peers to call his or her name is enough to convince them all that eye contact is paramount to successful linguistic interactions, especially given the noise levels in many learning situations.

As students become more adept in cooperative situations, the adult will need to "fade" his or her role as a social partner but maintain the role of interpreter or reverse interpreter until nonsigning peers have acquired skills in modalities that parallel their spontaneous speech skills. This approach will ensure that students of all ages have *social access* to school activities.

Evaluation

Evaluation data can be used to reconstruct or adapt activities so that the goals and objectives of social integration can be achieved. The evaluation should include a data sheet, systematic observation, written comments, and other helpful information. It should be completed shortly after a play session or a cooperative learning session has ended.

Figure 4–1 illustrates the use of a social integration activity assessment form. In this hypothetical case, five children were involved in an activity (eating and cooking), and an adult observed and took data. Information about the number of times each child played appropriately or inappropriately with peers or materials is coded on the left side, information about whom each child played with is coded on the right.

Activity: Eating and Cooking, Level II

Adult's Name:

Date 3/5 Classroom/Time Integrated/9:45 a.m.

+	−	*	X	N	Children's Names	H	A	B	K	R
5	1	1	0	0	Howard		✓		✓	
3	2	2	0	0	Abby	✓	✓			
0	0	0	2	5	Betsy					
2	1	3	1	0	Kent	✓			✓	
7	0	2	0	0	Rachel	✓	✓	✓	✓	✓

Code:

+ = Plays appropriately with peers: initiates play; shares, trades, interacts verbally or nonverbally; plays cooperatively

− = Plays negatively with peers: takes toys, makes negative statements, threatens nonverbally

* = Plays appropriately with materials by himself or herself

X = Uses materials inappropriately

N = Does not play with materials or with other children

Teacher's Comments:
Betsy doesn't seem to be playing with peers.
Abby and Kent each prefer to play with only one other child.
Few children choose Betsy as a playmate.

FIGURE 4–1: SOCIAL INTEGRATION ACTIVITY ASSESSMENT FORM

Signing in Schools*

As more and more students who are D/HH attend neighborhood schools, a greater number of hearing students and school staff are being exposed to signing. Teaching general education teachers and hearing students to sign deserves serious attention from administrators, especially those whose schools operate on a philosophy of full-inclusion. Some school programs have developed effective approaches to teaching and encouraging the use of sign. The methods, described by Luetke-Stahlman and Beaver (1994), are included here in the hope of building communication among all members of the school community, thereby dramatically increasing the social integration and comfort level of students who are D/HH within public school classrooms.

Recruit Adult Sign Volunteers

In some schools, teachers of the deaf, educational interpreters, parent volunteers, and college students teach sign for 10 to 15 minutes of each school day. Volunteers fan out and visit every classroom, giving the entire student body and staff access to sign instruction. Although few published curricula are available, a good way to teach basic, functional vocabulary is simply by asking the hearing children what they would like to be able to communicate to their deaf peers. A sign curriculum for hearing peers, *Signing with Kids*, has been developed by Diane Schmidt (1997), the mother of a deaf child (see the resource list at the end of this chapter for more information).

It is essential for everyone in school to use the same mode of signing and the same sign dictionary. Sign lessons should occur on a regular and frequent basis. If the adults teach after school, a local agency or community group may be willing to help cover some of the cost.

Have Students Teach Students

When not enough adult sign volunteers are available, another strategy is to select a few students from each classroom to receive

*From "Signing in Schools: It's Elementary," by B. Luetke-Stahlman and D. Beaver, 1994, *Perspectives in Education and Deafness, 12(4)*. Adapted and reprinted courtesy of *Perspectives in Education and Deafness*, Pre-College National Mission Programs, Gallaudet University.

weekly professional sign instruction and then to be responsible for teaching their peers. One teacher can be assigned to monitor the project.

In a pilot program in Illinois, called "A Sign and a Pledge," the selected students taught their classes three signs each morning right after the Pledge of Allegiance. They chose the signs to teach from a worksheet of fifteen signs prepared each week by the professional sign teacher. This worksheet was filed in a booklet in all classrooms for reference. The pilot worked well: The project monitor teacher received college credit for independent study for her monitoring role, and parents of the three deaf students in the school were particularly pleased to see hearing peers converse in sign with their children outside school.

Offer Family Sign Classes

Schools where students who are D/HH are enrolled should offer family sign classes that are supported by the public school administration and teachers of the deaf. Someone who works for the school program should be hired to teach the classes, using the same sign system or language that is used by the school program. Interested hearing students and their parents, as well as neighbors and relatives of the students who are D/HH, can be instructed either by age or skill level. A ten-week course taught twice a year should be sufficient, given the demands on today's families. One family sign class organized a no-host dinner at a local restaurant each week before sign classes so that class members could socialize, practice, and really converse in sign with friends, both hearing and deaf.

Incorporate Sign into the Daily Routine

It takes a conscientious teacher to incorporate the signing of functional words or phrases throughout the school day. However, some teachers stop to do just that, or to review key words and phrases in conjunction with routine activities. They sign the days of the week during the opening activities when the date is discussed; use the signs during "show and tell" for cartoon characters, favorite foods, and popular activities; teach the signs for school supplies as they wait for students to get their pencils out for a lesson; and so forth. One educational interpreter in Kansas schools teaches a sign a day that corresponds to the first letter of the month. In November, for example, students learn about twenty words beginning with the letter N (*noun, necklace, now, night*, and so on).

It is helpful to teach signs for introductory phrases such as *"Do you have some," "I want,"* or *"I need."* Then students can try incorporating the word of the day into sentences and have the other children try to interpret them. Thus being able to put signs for new vocabulary into immediate use and to sign practical sentences makes it possible for all children, deaf and hearing, to be included in informal classroom chatter.

Give Hearing Students Name Signs

All students attending schools with students who are D/HH should have name signs. Boys' names are sometimes initialized on the forehead (at the place where the sign for *boy* is made) and, similarly, girls' names near the cheek. If two boys have the same first initial, then one could be made on the forehead and the other on the heart, the middle of the chest, down the arm, from heart to opposite waist location, or some other typical name sign location.

Deaf adults at one public school give all first grade teachers name signs on the chin, all second grade teachers name signs on the heart, and so forth. They sign the librarian's name in the space where *library* is signed, the counselor's name in the *counselor* space, and so on. These clues help all students to remember not only names but functions of school staff members. Deaf adults or students who are D/HH can assist in giving name signs.

Label the School with Sign Print and Words

One way for students to learn vocabulary and help increase reading skills is to label all common objects at the school with sign print. At Scarborough School in Olathe, Kansas, items such as fire extinguishers, trash cans, door knobs, windows, and tables are labeled with the printed word and a drawing of how to make that object's sign.

Sign/Print sentence strips, such as those that appear in *The Signed English Schoolbook* from Gallaudet University Press, can also be posted in appropriate areas of the classroom. For example, the phrase "WASH YOUR HANDS" can be taped near the sink; "LINE UP" can be taped to the outside door.

Signed Story Time

There are many excellent story/sign books now available that have been written especially for young children. They can be read during shared reading time and then left for students to enjoy during silent reading periods. These books can be purchased for individual classrooms as well as the school library. Some signed and captioned videotapes of children's stories are also now available. Again, a parents' organization or a local community group might help cover the cost of these support materials.

Organize Schoolwide Activities

Remember the old-fashioned spelling bee? A signing bee can be organized in a similar manner. Students in each class sign words from a list developed by a teacher or interpreter who selects words from the sign dictionary used in the school. Those who win classroom signing bees proceed on to schoolwide competition. Two levels of competition may be appropriate, one for kindergarten to third grade and one for third to sixth grade. The school's parent group or local businesses can be asked to donate prizes.

Caldwell School in Wichita, Kansas, has declared a "Silent Lunch" Day each week. On this day, students are encouraged to use sign during lunchtime conversations such as "who is having what for lunch," "who wants to trade food items," and so on. This school also has an active Singing Hands Choir. Twice a week, students who are D/HH meet with the music teacher to practice singing and signing songs, which they then perform at school and in the community.

Encourage Positive Teacher Attitudes

As any parent of an elementary-age student can tell you, students respect and emulate the attitude of their teachers. If teachers are positive about learning to sign, model their own attempts to learn, use what they know without embarrassment about mistakes, show excitement for the learning process, and reinforce any appropriate attempts to sign by the students, they will create a healthy learning environment in which many hearing children will truly want to— and will—learn to sign. While it can be frustrating for general education teachers to see that some hearing students would prefer to watch the educational interpreter, the positive and respectful attitude of the hearing teacher is a key to transforming that frustration into rapid learning.

Summary

All students should have friends at school and feel safe and comfortable in the academic environment. Ideas presented in this chapter can make the tasks of team members easier when it comes to improving socialization and facilitating interaction in a variety of social settings. The challenge of creating a community of learners who are hearing, deaf, and hard of hearing requires thoughtful assessment, goal setting, facilitation, evaluation, and re-evaluation by significant adults.

Activities

1. Work with a school team to identify the social interaction needs of one or more students who are D/HH.

2. Review commercial social skills assessment or facilitation materials and share your findings with a peer.

3. Read and discuss a story for the purpose of facilitating social interactions.

4. Conduct an activity that focuses on Deaf Culture or similarities and differences. Share your perceptions of the outcome with a peer.

5. Videotape yourself explaining and monitoring a cooperative learning group designed to encourage social interaction.

Resources for Facilitating Social Skills

Communication Skill Builders
3830 E. Bellevue
P.O. Box 42050-C54
Tucson, AZ 85733
602-323-7500
- *Social Skills Activities for Special Children* (Mannix, 1993)

Feelings Factory
508 St. Mary's Street
Raleigh, NC 27605
- materials to promote communication and coping skills

Thinking Publications
P.O. Box 163
Eau Claire, WI 54702
1-800-225-4769
- *Social Star: General Interaction Skills* (Gajewski, Hirn, & Mayo, 1993)

Modern Signs Press
P.O. Box 1181
Los Alamitos, CA 90720
1-800-572-7332
- *Sign with Kids* (Schmidt, 1997)

Appendix 4-A

Formal Social Assessment Tools:
Descriptions of Tools Most Frequently Used*

The Battelle Developmental Inventory

The Battelle Developmental Inventory (BDI) is a standardized, individually administered assessment battery of developmental skills for children from birth to eight years of age, and was developed for the purpose of early childhood screening and diagnosis. It is designed mainly for use by special educators and teachers working with preschool and primary-aged students who are D/HH. Student development is characterized by attainment of critical skills or behaviors in a hierarchical sequence. Use of the tool can assist in writing short and long-term goals and objectives.

The BDI assessment instrument consists of 341 items grouped into five domains. The domains are further divided by subdomains. The domains and their respective subdomains are as follows: Personal-Social Domain—adult interaction, expression of feelings, self-concept, peer interaction, coping, and appropriate and varying social roles; Adaptive Domain—attention, eating, dressing, personal responsibility, and toileting; Motor Domain—muscle control, body coordination, locomotion, fine muscle and perceptual motor; Communication Domain—receptive and expressive; Cognitive Domain—perceptual discrimination, memory, reasoning and academic skills, and conceptual development (administered in 60 minutes). Domains dealing specifically with social competency skills and communication include the Personal-Social Domain, the Adaptive Domain, and the Communication Domain. The Personal-Social Domain consists of 85 items and measures abilities and characteristics that allow the child to engage in meaningful social interactions. The Adaptive Domain consists of 59 items and measures self-help skills and task-related skills. The Communication Domain consists of 59 items and measures verbal and nonverbal reception and expression of information, thoughts, and ideas. The BDI also includes a screening test consisting of 96 of the 341 test items (administered in 10 to 30 minutes).

cont.

*From *Assessing the Social Skills of Children Who Are D/HH in the State of Kansas* (pp. 96-108), by J. Aljundi, 1993, Unpublished Master's Thesis, Kansas City: University of Kansas Medical Center. Adapted with permission.

The BDI has procedures designed to collect data through presentation of a structured test format; interviews with parents, caregivers, or teachers; and observations of the child in natural settings. Items can be administered to children having various handicapping conditions by using modifications that are provided for this purpose. Scores are available for subdomains as well as total domain scores. Scores obtained are standard scores, percentile ranks, and age equivalents.

The Meadow-Kendall Social-Emotional Inventory: Preschool and Elementary Editions

The Meadow-Kendall Social-Emotional Inventory (MKSEI) is a rating scale that provides information in three categories: (a) sociable, communicative behaviors, (b) impulsive, dominating behaviors, and (c) special items related to deafness. This tool may assist professionals and parents in determining behaviors considered typical for students who are D/HH at specific chronological periods. It is the only social-emotional assessment tool designed specifically for children who are D/HH. Some of the areas covered in the preschool edition (PSE) include sociable, communicative behaviors; impulsive, dominating behaviors; developmental lags; anxious, compulsive behaviors; and special items related to deafness. The elementary edition (EE) covers the areas of social adjustment, self-adjustment, and emotional adjustment. Some items included on the MKSEI-EE and the MKSEI-PSE tests relate to the assessment of social competence. These items appear mainly in the sections on sociable-communicative behaviors, emotional adjustment, social adjustment, and self-image. Less than half of the items on these two tests are directly related to the assessment of social competence.

Social Skills for Daily Living

The *Social Skills for Daily Living* (SSDL) is intended for three groups of students 12 to 21 years of age: those with mild learning disabilities, mild mental retardation, and mild emotional disturbance. The tool is used to help adolescents and young adults with mild disabilities to build confidence and independence with social skills. A variety of instructional formats to stimulate acquisition and application of targeted social skills are used (Baechle, 1991).

The tool consists of a unique series of comic book adventures. Depending on students' needs, professionals may choose from specific

cont.

social skill modules: conversation and friendship skills, skills for getting along with others, and problem-solving skills. The comprehensive tool includes 30 different social skills that are identified most often by special educators as common problem areas for students with mild disabilities. Formats that aid in the transfer of social skills include comic books, skill books, workbooks, quizzes, and role-play practice.

The Vineland Adaptive Behavior Scale–Interview Edition

The Vineland Adaptive Behavior Scale–Interview Edition provides general assessment information dealing with adaptive behavior (adapting to various situations; controlling one's feelings, emotions and needs; building coping skills; and so on). The tool may be useful in determining strengths and weaknesses in the areas of communication, socialization, motor skills, and daily social living skills. The tool covers a wide range of adaptive behaviors and domains, followed by their respective subdomains: Communication—receptive, expressive, written; Daily Living Skills—personal, domestic, community; Socialization Skills—interpersonal relationships, play and leisure time, coping skills; Motor Skills—gross and fine.

There are three editions of this scale: the Expanded Form, the Survey Forms/Interviews, and the Classroom Edition. All three editions assess communication, daily living skills, socialization, and motor domains. The two interview editions also assess maladaptive behavior. The Adaptive Behavior Component summarizes performance in all four domains. Social and behavioral maturity is measured by the examiner's evaluation of responses to 117 items in six major areas: self-help, locomotion, communication, self-direction, occupation, and socialization. Scores are expressed as social-age values, and the age scores are converted to ratios to produce a social quotient.

Appendix 4-B

Children's Books About Deafness

Arthur, Catherine (1979). *My Sister's Silent World*, Children's Press.

Cocoran, Barbara (1974). *A Dance to Still Music*, Atheneum.

Costello, Mary Rose (1970). *My Friend's Big Talk and Little Talk*, Phillips Co.

Curtis, Patricia (1981). *Cindy, A Hearing Ear Dog*, Dutton.

DeGering, Etta (1964). *Thomas Hopkins Gallaudet*, McKay.

Felfand, Ravina & Letha Paterson (1962). *They Wouldn't Quit*, Lerner.

Greene, Laura & Eva Dicker (1988). *Discovering Sign Language*, Kendall Green.

Henry, Marguerite (1948). *King of the Wind*, Rand.

Luetke-Stahlman, B. (1996). *Hannie*, Butte Publications.

Luetke-Stahlman, B. (1998). *Martha's Vineyard*, Butte Publications.

Starowitz, Annie M. (1988). *The Day We Met Cindy*, Kendall Green.

These books and catalogs of additional books, videos, and software are available from:

Butte Publications
P.O. 1328
Hillsboro, OR 97123-1328
1-800-330-9791

Gallaudet University Bookstore
800 Florida Avenue, NE
Washington, DC 20002-3695
202-651-5450

References

Aljundi, J. (1993). *Assessing the social skills of children who are D/HH in the state of Kansas.* Unpublished master's thesis, University of Kansas Medical Center, Kansas City.

Antia, S., & Kreimeyer, K. (1992). *Project interact: Final report.* Washington, DC: U.S. Department of Education.

Baechle, C. (1991). *Learning disabilities and social skills deficits.* Paper presented at Pensacola Junior College, Pensacola, FL.

Brammer, L., & Shustrum, E. (1982). *An introduction to special education* (2nd ed.). Boston: Little, Brown.

Brown, W., Fox, J., & Brady, M. (1987). Effects of spatial density on 3- and 4- year-old children's socially directed behavior during play: An investigation of a setting factor. *Education and Treatment of Children, 10,* 247-258.

Chadsey-Rusch, J., & Heal, L. (1995). Building consensus from transition experts on social integration outcomes and interventions. *Exceptional Children, 62*(2), 165-187.

Duchan, J. (1995). *Supporting language learning in everyday life.* San Diego, CA: Singular.

Farrugia, D., & Austin, G. (1980). A study of social-emotional adjustment patterns of H.I. students in different educational settings. *American Annals of the Deaf, 12*(6), 535-541.

Fey, M. (1986). *Language intervention with young children.* San Diego, CA: College-Hill Press.

Foster, S. (1988). Life in the mainstream: Reflections of deaf college freshmen on their experiences in the mainstreamed high school. *Journal of Rehabilitation of the Deaf, 22,* 37-56.

Fujiki, M., Brinton B., & Todd, C. (1996). Social skills of children with specific language impairments. *Speech, Language, Hearing Services in the Schools, 27,* 195-202.

Gajewski, N., Hirn, P., & Mayo, P. (1993). *Social star: General interaction skills* (Book 1). Eau Claire, WI: Thinking Publications.

Gallagher, P. (1988). *Teaching students with behavior disorders: Techniques and activities for classroom instruction* (2nd ed.). Denver, CO: Love Publishing.

Greenberg, M., & Kusche, C. (1987). Cognitive, personal, and social development of deaf children and adolescents. In M. Wang, M. Reynolds, & H. Walberg (Eds.), *Handbook of special education; Research and practice: Vol. 3* (pp. 95-129). New York: Pergamon.

Greenberg, M., & Kusche, C. (1993). *Promoting social and emotional development in deaf children: The PATHS project.* Seattle, WA: University of Washington.

Guralnick, M. (1980). Social interaction among preschool handicapped children. *Exceptional Children, 46,* 248-253.

Harrison, J. (1985). *The Vineland Adaptive Behavior Scale: Classroom Edition.* Circle Pines, MN: American Guidance Service.

Hazel, J., Peterson, J., & Schumaker, J. (1990). *Social skills for daily living.* Circle Pines, MN: American Guidance Service.

Hops, H., Walker, H., & Greenwood, C. (1979). PEERS: A program for remediating social withdrawal in school. In L. Hamelynck (Ed.), *Behavioral systems for the developmentally disabled: School family environments* (pp. 48-86). New York: Bruner/Mazel.

Kempton, V. (1993). *General education teachers' perceptions of the signing abilities of hearing children.* Unpublished master's thesis, University of Kansas Medical Center, Kansas City.

Kluwin, T., & Stinson, M. (1993). *Deaf students in local public high schools. Springfield, IL: Charles C. Thomas.*

Libbey, S., & Pronovost, W. (1980). Communication practices of mainstreamed H.I. adolescents. *The Volta Review, 82*(4), 197-220.

Luetke-Stahlman, B. (1994). Facilitating social integration of preschoolers who are hearing, deaf, and hard-of-hearing. *Topics in Early Childhood Special Education, 14*(4), 472-487.

Luetke-Stahlman, B. (1995a). Classrooms, communication, and social competence. *Perspectives in Education and Deafness, 13*(4), 12-16.

Luetke-Stahlman, B. (1995b). Social interaction: Assessment and intervention with regard to students who are deaf. *American Annals of the Deaf, 140*(3), 295-300.

Luetke-Stahlman, B. (1998). *Language Issues in Deaf Education.* Hillsboro, OR: Butte Publications.

Luetke-Stahlman, B., & Beaver, D. (1994). Signing in schools: It's elementary. *Perspectives in Education and Deafness, 12*(4), 15-19.

Mannix, D. (1993). *Social skills activities for special children*. West Nyack, NY: The Center for Applied Research in Education.

Marschark, M. (1993). *Psychological development of deaf children*. New York: Oxford University Press.

Masters, L., Mori, B., & Mori, A. (1993). *Teaching secondary students with mild learning and behavior problems*. Austin, TX: Pro-Ed.

Meadow, K. (1983). *The Meadow-Kendall social-emotional assessment inventories for deaf and hearing impaired students: Manual*. Washington, DC: Gallaudet University.

Newborg, J., Stock, J., Wnek, F., Guidibaldo, J., & Svinicki, A. (1984). *The Battelle Developmental Inventory*. Dallas, TX: DLM Teaching Resources.

Odom, S., Bender, M., Stein, M., Doran, L., Houden, P., McInnes, M., Gilbert, M., Deklyen, M., Speltz, M., & Jenkins, J. (1988). *The integrated preschool curriculum, procedures for socially integrating young handicapped and normally developing children*. Seattle, WA: University of Washington Press.

Odom, S., Kohler, F., & Strain, P. (1987). *Social interaction skill curriculum*. Unpublished manuscript, University of Pittsburgh.

Odom, S., Silver, F., Sandler, S., & Strain, P. (1983). *Direct observation of social behavior manual*. Pittsburgh, PA: Early Childhood Research Institute, University of Pittsburgh.

Perske, R. (1988). *Circle of friends*. Nashville, TN: Abingdon.

Rosenthal-Malek, A. (January/February 1997). Stop and think: Using metacognitive strategies to teach students social skills. *Teaching Exceptional Children 29*(3), 29-31.

Schirmer, B. (1989). Relationship between imaginative play and language development in hearing-impaired children. *American Annals of the Deaf, 124*(3), 219-222.

Schloss, P., & Smith, M. (1990). *Teaching social skills to hearing-impaired students*. Washington, DC: Alexander Graham Bell Association for the Deaf.

Schmidt, D. (1997). *Signing with kids*. Los Alamitos, CA: Modern Signs Press.

Solit, G., Taylor, M., & Bednarczyk, A. (1992). *Access for all: Integrating deaf, hard-of-hearing, and hearing preschoolers*. Washington, DC: Gallaudet University Press.

Sorensen, D. (1992). Facilitating responsible behavior in deaf children. *Journal of the American Deafness and Rehabilitation Association, 25*(3), 1-7.

Torline, J. (1994). *Availability of psychosocial services for students who are deaf/hard-of-hearing in the State of Kansas.* Unpublished master's thesis, University of Kansas Medical Center, Kansas City.

Vernon, M., & Andrews, J. (1990). *The psychology of deafness: Understanding deaf and hard of hearing people.* New York: Longman.

Walker, J. (1983). *The Walker Problem Behavior Identification Checklist.* Los Angeles: Western Psychological Services.

White, K. (1982). Defining and prioritizing the personal and social competencies needed by hearing impaired students. *The Volta Review, 84*(6), 266-274.

Chapter 5

Reading to Students

Language and Reading

Reading Assessment

Facilitation of Text Reading and Comprehension

Adults Get Ready to Read

The Essential Practices

Examples of the Adult Reading Practices

Appendix 5–A: Making the Most of an
    Adult-Read Session

Appendix 5–B: Examples of Text Structure
    Graphic Organizers

"Reading is the intellectual and emotional perception of a printed message" in which

- *intellectual* is defined as "cognitive, rational, and meaning-driven"
- *emotional* is defined as recognizing that "feelings and connotations prompted by the topic . . . color the reader's perception"
- *perception* is defined as a "personal construction of the message," a construction that differs among readers
- *message* is defined as "communication, intentionality, and organization" (Harris & Smith, 1986, p. 5)

A good reading program for *all* students (see Figure 5–1) should involve three components: adults reading to students, students reading to adults, and students reading independently (Harris & Smith, 1986).

The adults involved in reading with students who are D/HH might be general or special education teachers, teachers of the deaf, speech-language pathologists, paraprofessionals, parents, or relatives. The students involved might be emergent, beginning, or on-grade-level readers. Students who do

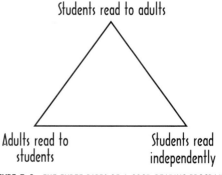

Students read to adults

Adults read to students

Students read independently

FIGURE 5–1: THE THREE PARTS OF A GOOD READING PROGRAM

not understand or express language or read as well as their same-age peers should be read to frequently by adults (Adams, 1995; Hoggan & Strong, 1994).

In the last several years, deaf educators have stressed the importance of adult "read alouds" (Andrews & Mason, 1991; Luetke-Stahlman & Luckner, 1991; Schleper, 1995a). Parents and school staff can make a significant difference in the language and literacy abilities of students who are D/HH *of all ages* if they will read *narrative stories and expository texts* (school subject texts) to them regularly (Luetke-Stahlman, Hayes, & Nielsen, 1996; Marschark,

1993; Webster, 1986; Williams, 1994). This chapter provides guidelines and practices to achieve these aims.

Language and Reading

The language difficulties and differences of students who are D/HH can have consequences for their language and reading development. Some young students who are D/HH might have "extensive knowledge of written language despite severe language delay" (Williams, 1994, p. 150), but most do not. (Refer to Brasel & Quigley, 1975; Paul & Jackson, 1993; Paul & Quigley, 1990; Kampfe & Turecheck, 1987; and Lane & Grosjean, 1980 for information on the language/reading difficulties of students who are D/HH). Figure 5–2 illustrates the effect of language difficulties and differences on development.

In addition, reading activities become complicated when adults cannot communicate in the dominant language or system used by the student. Cummins (1989) suggested that parents and teachers be encouraged to use the student's dominant language when reading. Important English

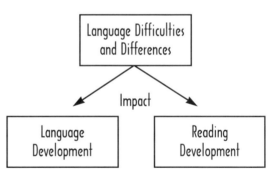

FIGURE 5–2: THE IMPACT OF LANGUAGE DIFFICULTIES AND DIFFERENCES ON DEVELOPMENT

vocabulary and figurative expressions should be incorporated when the student is retelling text. The challenge, at the very least, is to provide students who are D/HH of all ages with *accessible* language while facilitating the development of cognitive academic skills.

 Students with immature language development typically do not read and write proficiently.

Researchers have explored both student and adult variables in cognitive/language development and facilitation that contribute to problems in literacy development. *Student variables* include

- difficulty in processing English syntax (Geers & Moog, 1989; Hanson, 1991; Kelly, 1996; Luetke-Stahlman, 1988; Quigley & Power, 1972)
- difficulty in accessing phonological processing (Hanson, 1991; Leybaert, 1993)
- difficulty in using short-term memory efficiently (Bellugi, Klima, & Siple, 1975; Kelly, 1995)
- difficulty in understanding and expressing comprehension of the text by applying higher-level thinking skills (deBot, 1996)

Adult variables focus in part on instructional practices—for example, when attention is paid to students' weaknesses in the areas of phonology and syntax rather than on their strengths in the area of semantics (Ewoldt, 1981, 1985; Gormley & McGill-Franzen, 1978; Rodda, Cummings, & Fewer, 1993; Williams, 1994; Yurkowski & Ewoldt, 1986). Yet, when adults are aware of and implement the changes they need to make to mediate reading activities effectively, they can contribute significantly in assisting students to become proficient readers (Luetke-Stahlman, Griffiths, & Montgomery, 1998a, 1998b). Activities to mediate reading are described in this chapter.

> **Study Guide Question**
> *Review the language needs of a particular student who is D/HH on the IFSP or IEP. How do the linguistic needs of this student compare to the student variables described?*

Although persuasive text and other genres of writing may be studied, narrative stories and expository texts are particularly emphasized in education. Howard (1991) has argued that narrative story development, in fact, is the foundation of human thinking. Importantly for students who are D/HH, Dickinson and Snow (1987), Lindfors (1987), and McCabe and Rollins (1994) noted that analytical conversational ability can provide a critical bridge to both narrative and expository print literacy, while weak conversational skills about challenging topics and concepts adversely affect students' print literacy and, hence, academic success.

☛ **Weak analytical conversational skills = Poor academics**

Inability to comprehend the expository text structure of content (subject area) logically affects academic success as well. Unfortunately, expository text is especially difficult for students who are D/HH because they often lack background knowledge about topics (deVilliers, 1995). To "lack background knowledge" does not usually mean that a student who is D/HH has not been exposed to a particular action, object, or process; it means that no one has described it, discussed its critical elements, and explained or referred to it linguistically in subsequent conversations with the student. It is a lack of access to language that deprives students of background knowledge. Text structures of expository text are usually new to these students, and grammatical forms complex (deVilliers, 1995). Many students come to school lacking both narrative and expository text experiences (Ewoldt, 1986; Feitelson & Goldstein, 1986; Heath, 1982; Williams, 1994).

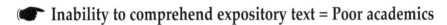 **Inability to comprehend expository text = Poor academics**

Reading Assessment

Most team members are aware that students who are D/HH do not in general read proficiently (Karchmer, Milone, & Wolk, 1979; Allen, 1986), yet standardized (formal) as well as informal or process evaluation of reading is necessary for the same reasons assessment is needed for other abilities (to compare students who are D/HH to hearing peers, to document annual progress, to identify strategies to be used, and so on).

Formal Assessment

Formal tools typically used to assess the reading abilities of students who are D/HH are provided below, approximately ordered by student age.

The Test of Early Reading Ability–Deaf or Hard of Hearing (TERA–D/HH) (Reid, Hresko, Hammill, & Wiltshire, 1991) is administered individually to students who are D/HH between the ages of 3 and 14. It was normed on deaf and hard-of-hearing students from 20 different states, with hearing losses ranging from 41 dB to 91 dB+. It has two equivalent forms that are useful for pre-and post-testing.

Woodcock-Johnson Psycho-Educational Battery–Revised (Woodcock & Johnson, 1989) is a norm-referenced measure that is individually administered. The reading subtests include Letter-Word Identification, Passage Comprehension, and Reading Vocabulary. Both grade equivalent and percentile scores are given. This battery was normed with hearing individuals from 3 to 80 years of age in both urban and rural communities.

Peabody Individual Achievement Test–Revised (PIAT–R) (Dunn & Markwardt, 1988) was normed with a balanced representation of gender, racial, and SES backgrounds of hearing students in kindergarten through twelfth grade. It has two subtests for reading: Reading Recognition and Reading Comprehension. It is individually administered.

The Test of Reading Comprehension–3 (TORC–3) (Brown, Hammill, & Wiederholt, 1995) is a norm-referenced test that is individually administered. It is appropriate for students from ages 7 to 18. It was normed on hearing children. The TORC–3 has eight subtests including Vocabulary, Science Vocabulary, and Reading Directions.

Stanford Achievement Test for Hearing Impaired Students (SAT–HI) (Gallaudet University, 1983) was normed specifically for students who are D/HH. The test allows for comparison of students who are D/HH with other students who are D/HH and with hearing students across the United States. The test itself is the same one given to hearing students, but the screening, administration procedures, scoring, and norms are based on the needs of students who are D/HH. The reading subtests include Word Reading/Reading Vocabulary and Sentence Reading/Reading Comprehension.

The Gates-MacGinitie Reading Test (MacGinitie & MacGinitie, 1989) is an easy-to-administer test consisting of two parts: Vocabulary and Comprehension. The Vocabulary portion asks students to choose a synonym for target words. The Comprehension portion requires students to read from a wide range of unfamiliar test genres and answer questions that require analyzing and interpreting meaning. The Gates-MacGinitie can be given to students in kindergarten through 12th grade. It requires about 30 minutes to administer. Percentile rank, grade equivalent, and extended scale scores are obtained.

Curriculum-based assessment (CBA) is especially useful if a basal series is being used. CBA and criterion-referenced assessment allow for a determination of whether a student who is D/HH is learning the assumed skills from the current reading program. Running records are useful in determining whether students are able to decode a percentage of words in material being used.

Visual Needs Assessment

Harris and Smith (1986) cautioned that visual assessment is critical to the reading facilitation process. Young students especially are often farsighted. Because they see well at a distance, they are usually able to pass school vision checks such as the Snellen Chart. They may have difficulty, however, seeing close up. Signs of visual problems (Harris & Smith) include

- complaints of headaches or blurry vision
- squinting
- holding books too close or too far away
- closing one eye in order to read
- tilting the head
- red or watery eyes

> **Study Guide Question**
>
> *Before continuing, take the quiz in Appendix 5–A. How do you rate when it comes to including these practices? As you read this chapter, try to pay closer attention to the discussion of practices that you do not currently include in your read-aloud sessions with students who are D/HH.*

Facilitation of Text Reading and Comprehension

The practice of adults' reading to students of all ages has been highly acclaimed by educators and researchers alike (Adams, 1995; Hoggan

& Strong, 1994). Research has documented that such mediated experiences

- aid semantic and syntactic language development (Chomsky, 1972; Elley, 1989; Holdaway, 1979; Irwin, 1960; Karweit, 1989; Ninio, 1980; Peterman, 1988)
- enhance the understanding of text structure and the forms, functions, and conventions of print (Applebee, 1978; Cochran-Smith, 1984; Dickinson & Snow, 1987; Stein & Glenn, 1979; Teale, 1984)
- have a positive effect on comprehension (Green & Harker, 1982; Morrow, 1986)

Figure 5–3 graphically represents these benefits.

Observations of deaf parents (Schleper, 1995a) and of parents who are hard of hearing (Andrews & Taylor, 1987) showed that these adults provided positive, interactive environments while reading to their children.

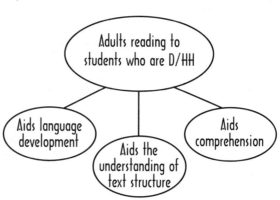

FIGURE 5–3: POSITIVE EFFECTS OF READING TO STUDENTS

Sometimes they engaged in activities such as clarifying specific vocabulary and expanding concepts. Other times they provided a mutually rewarding atmosphere that encouraged creative interpretation of the text. Accounts of parents using some kind of English-based signing have demonstrated that hearing parents of children who are D/HH can create positive reading sessions as well, sessions similar to those experienced by hearing children (Lartz & Lestina, 1993; Maxwell, 1984; Schlesinger & Meadow, 1972). Figure 5–4 shows how all parents can help to facilitate reading.

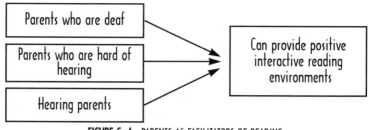

FIGURE 5–4: PARENTS AS FACILITATORS OF READING

Gelzer (1988) found that when students who are D/HH are read to by adults, they can experience the joy of playing with new vocabulary, detecting rhythmical language patterns, and encountering new ideas that stimulate and reinforce their imagination and curiosity. *Yet many adults do not know **how** to mediate reading effectively to make it an enjoyable experience.* Hearing abilities differ among students who are D/HH, but most cannot access discussion about stories and text solely through listening and speech. Instead, they need cues or signs (alone or in conjunction with what is being said) to make conversation about text understandable and to discuss what they have read in a critical manner (making judgments and analyses). Without such cues, students may not find reading enjoyable.

> It is not surprising that when elementary- and middle-school-aged deaf and hard-of-hearing students were interviewed by Ewoldt (1986), only 20% reported ever having read with their parents. Schleper (1995b) found that undergraduates interviewed at Gallaudet University did not enjoy having stories read to them as youngsters and remembered reading as an unpleasant experience.

Adults should read to students often and in a systematic manner. Unlike proficient readers who typically interact pleasurably as they share text frequently with their parents (Adams, 1995; Clark, 1976; Durkin, 1966), students who are D/HH often are not read to and, therefore, miss out on this interaction. Students who are D/HH also often lack the social opportunities hearing students have for obtaining important literacy experiences (Marschark, 1993; Webster, 1986). Their reading is often limited to reading groups at school, where they might *only observe the reading of other poor readers* if adults do not read to them. Yet adults can facilitate the reading and comprehension of both narrative and expository text when read alouds or guided reading occur daily and in a systematic manner.

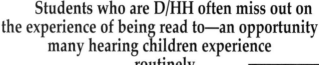

Students who are D/HH often miss out on the experience of being read to—an opportunity many hearing children experience routinely.

Daily and systematic guided reading or read alouds must include the elements of both *access* and *mediation* (Adams, 1995). The term "access" addresses the quantitative: who is being read to, how often, and whether the language or mode used is understood. The term "mediation" addresses the qualitative: who is involved in the process and what they are communicating to each other (Luetke-Stahlman, Hayes, & Nielsen, 1996). A high degree of access to and mediation of higher-level thinking skills using the language of the text is of paramount importance to students who are D/HH. Providing these elements involves negotiating the meaning of the text together by encouraging students to discuss text structure, the meaning of words and phrases, the grammar used to explain and summarize, and concepts of print. Through this process, students are helped to paraphrase, question, predict, and clarify material. The method of reciprocal teaching can also be employed so that students begin to take responsibility for comprehension (Andrews & Mason, 1986; Palincsar & Brown, 1986). Using this method, language and reading are facilitated through a conversational approach which encourages students to become gradually responsible for their own learning.

> **Study Guide Question**
> *Survey the parents or caretakers of the students who are D/HH with whom you work. How often do they read to their children? Would they like help in finding ways to read with their children more often and in learning how to make reading an enjoyable experience? Ask the adults who work with a student who is D/HH at school how often they read with the student. Compare your findings to your personal memories of access to text as a child.*

> **Study Guide Question**
> *How would you define the elements of access and mediation? Share your descriptions with a peer.*

Adults Get Ready to Read

Adults need to plan their reading sessions with students who are D/HH carefully. They should have a particular goal in mind (attention to schema, a unit theme, a specific vocabulary word or phrase, ease in signing, phonemic awareness, student's interest, and so on). Before reading to students, adults should review the material several times and think about it on a variety of levels (Barrentine, 1996). They should identify

- the time allotted for the read aloud or guided reading and how to structure the reading activity to minimize time constraints
- the text structure, including any component themes
- the main characters' point of view
- the purpose of illustrations and parts of text (clarifying concept development, creating text structure components, and so forth)
- how questions could be asked about the material (analytical rather than literal conversation)
- how students might respond and how to handle excessive student contributions
- what extension activities would be appropriate

Choosing an Appropriate Narrative or Expository Text. Books written at the students' independent or recreational level or books written at a language level that is frustrating to students may not sustain their attention. "High-interest books with rich language, absorbing plots, lively characters, and multiple layers of meaning will simultaneously promote pleasure and opportunity for learning" (Barrentine, 1996, p. 36).

 Adults should read texts that are of high interest to students or that focus on their experiences.

Level + 1 Reading. Carlsen (1985), Luetke-Stahlman and Luckner (1991), and Stewart and Cegelka (1995) noted that for the greatest gains in obtaining literacy, material should be meaningful, connected text that is *slightly above the vocabulary and syntactic maturity*

of the students (this is known as "**level + 1**" or "**input + 1**"). That is, adults should choose text to read that is challenging but within the student's zone of proximal development (Vygotsky, 1978; also see Luetke-Stahlman, 1998).

Signability. Stewart, Bennett, and Bonkowski (1992) developed a "signability" index for children's books. They provide criteria and a list of recommended books for students who are D/HH from preschool through second grade. They considered variables such as reading rate, sentence length, quantity of text used to express thoughts, word imagery, and ease of translation. Deaf storyreaders at the Kansas School for the Deaf (KSD) reviewed over 250 storybooks. Based on their comments, Hayes and Shaw (1993) developed guidelines for selecting read-aloud books for students who are D/HH from preschool through eighth grade. Books were evaluated on the basis of five main categories: illustrations, plot, characters, setting, and English language and vocabulary. Those books determined to be appropriate were videotaped, the tapes were placed in the KSD library with a copy of the book, and the packages were made available for sale.

Holding a Book While Signing or Cueing. Sometimes it is challenging to sign or cue a book and simultaneously hold it so that illustrations, graphics, or the print itself can be seen. Adults have found some creative ways to hold the book:
- use a plastic recipe holder
- use a string around the neck with alligator clips attached at each end
- use a music stand and clips
- use a plastic or wooden book holder
- have a hearing student hold the book

Additional Tips. Webster (1986) suggested that reading sessions be short, that adults be focused, that praise and encouragement be given in a quiet, relaxed situation, and that enjoyment be emphasized. Gelzer (1988) provided parents with basic tips for developing reading appreciation in students who are D/HH, including signing considerations, English language considerations, using expression, establishing rapport, asking questions, and engaging in follow-up activities. Hafer, Richmond-Hearty, and Swann (1991) wrote a similar article for teachers.

The Essential Practices*

Study Guide Question

Before parents or school staff begin to read to students, what three or four points should they consider? How could you help a parent get ready to read?

Winzer (1985) found little consensus about the best way to teach students who are D/HH to read. Thus, to assist school personnel and parents in reading to students efficiently, Luetke-Stahlman, Hayes, and Nielsen (1996) conducted a broad review of the literature in related fields. From their findings they developed a rationale and description of ten practices that were empirically documented as being essential to include when reading to students if those students are to become proficient readers themselves.

These essential practices do not support either a phonics or a whole language approach. They are research-based practices that have been found to develop proficient readers. Using them, team members may be able to facilitate positive change in the reading skills of the students in their care. Descriptions and examples of the essential practices follow.

 It is not special materials that are required, but materials used in special ways (adapted from McCoy, 1995).

1. Focus on Purpose and Enjoyment

Adults should focus on the purpose and enjoyment of reading.

Purpose. Research evidence (Beauchamp, 1925; Shores, 1960; Harris & Smith, 1986) has supported stating the purpose for reading overtly and has documented that this affects comprehension and retention positively. However, some researchers (Wiesendunger & Wollenberg, 1978) have cautioned that stating the purpose or mutually agreeing on the purpose may help some students but be inappropriate for others, especially if students lack the experience or perception to

*Essential Practices section from "Essential Practices as Adults Read to Meet the Needs of Deaf or Hard of Hearing Students," by B. Luetke-Stahlman, P. Hayes, and D. Nielsen, 1996, *American Annals of the Deaf, 141* (4), pp. 309-320. Copyright 1996 by *American Annals of the Deaf*. Adapted with permission.

relate to purposes stated by others (Harris & Smith). In another study, the researcher found that teachers used "not even one minute" to develop a purpose for reading (Durkin, 1984).

Enjoyment. Adults should read text that stimulates students' internal responses—their interests, motivations, attitudes, beliefs, and feelings (Harris & Smith, 1986). "It is not just reading to children that makes the difference, it is enjoying the books with them and reflecting on their form and content . . . developing and supporting curiosity . . . encouraging the students to examine the print . . . and showing them that we value and enjoy reading and that we hope they will, too" (Wigfield & Asher, 1984; quoted by Adams, 1995, p. 87).

Practice #1

Practice Defined	Adult Actions
Adults focus on the purpose of reading. They might overtly state this purpose (enjoyment, unit theme, and so on) or ask students to deduce it.	Adults should read enthusiastically and demonstrate that reading is enjoyed and valued.

Multimedia Books. Well-designed electronic books are enjoyable and highly motivating for some students who are D/HH. Electronic books are available from numerous publishers including Broderbund, Scholastic, Simon and Schuster, and Voyager. Most companies will allow the return of material after a 30-day trial period.

2. Engage in Interactive Dialogue

Adults should use the student's dominant language in an interactive dialogue aimed at increasing understanding. Adults should ask open-ended questions, allowing for prediction and encouraging risk-taking such that students move out of their present comfort zone and acquire new insights. Adults should work to create an environment in which each student can make "cognitive leaps" (Hayden, 1987), connecting what is already understood about life-to-text and text-to-life constructions with what they can understand of the components of the text structure given adult support.

"Adult-child proximation" is a form of interactive dialogue. It is a term coined by Webster (1986) to refer to those times when adults help students construct accounts of events in terms they understand. Adults guide students, eventually leading them to formulate their accounts without guidance. Interactive dialogues, such as these, are a key element in the text reading experience (Adams, 1995). They have been recommended for use with students who are D/HH by Andrews (1984) and Andrews and Mason (1986).

☞ *Dialogue* among participants is as important as the *information* provided by the text in terms of what is remembered by the student.

Vygotsky (1978) noted that reading to students is an example of a social event that is essential for intellectual development. Adult behaviors of supporting, modeling, and scaffolding responses and questions build a bridge between what a student knows and what a student is coming to know in his or her dominant language, as well as between that language and English. Mediated, interactive dialogue moves the student from dependence to independence. Thus, from a Vygotskian perspective, the adult is the mediator between the familiar, contextualized (spoken, spoken and signed, or signed) language and the decontextualized English language of texts and instructional conversations.

Team members may find the Directed Reading–Thinking Activity (DRTA) useful in stimulating interactive dialogue with students who are D/HH (Stauffer, 1980). With this program, students are encouraged to engage in honest discussion, critical thinking, concept formation, and to use a basic problem-solving strategy: formulate a problem statement, collect data, accept or reject the hypothesis, and revise the original statement. Although an adult leads the students through this process, the students are encouraged to take responsibility for discussions.

Study Guide Question
Which parts of the essential practices would work especially well with students with whom you work? Flag or list these as you study the descriptions and examples in this section.

Practice #2

Practice Defined	Adult Actions
Adults use the student's dominant language in an interactive dialogue and create an environment in which each student can make cognitive leaps, bridging what is already known and what can be understood with adult support.	Adults can match the language or system that is used as they read with the student's dominant language. They can use scaffolding strategies to provide mediated dialogue and make reading both a social event and a meaning-making process. Adults should take appropriate breaks before, during, and after the reading of the text to engage students in discussion.

3. Introduce the Text

Adults should provide a "preparatory set" or text introduction (Hoggan & Strong, 1994; Clay, 1985). Adults begin by showing the material to be read to the students and assessing what is known and unknown about it. DeFord, Lyons, and Pinnell (1991) recommended that adults discuss the text, using the specific vocabulary and figurative expressions that appear in the work, while encouraging students to use background knowledge and make predictions.

Gelzer (1988) delineated three steps to introduce a story to a student who is D/HH:
- look at the cover and title and make predictions
- discuss the topic and characters, relating them to past experiences
- decide how the book will be held

Satchwell (1993) defined the strategy of making predictions as one in which students who are D/HH quickly preview material to be read and state what they already know or might guess about the text: "This is considered to be very important as it helps give a mindset to what will be read" (p. 40). Providing such a preparatory set was one of the strategies found by Satchwell (1993) to have the most positive effect on reading ability. Similarly, Andrews, Winograd, and DeVille (1996) found that when seven eleven- and twelve-year-old students who are D/HH were provided signed summaries of stories prior to reading them, their retell of the stories improved.

Practice #3

Practice Defined	Adult Actions
Adults create a preparatory set or text introduction. During these activities, adults deduce what is known and unknown as they discuss the story line or main theme with students. They review the material to be read, using specific vocabulary and figurative expressions that appear in the work.	Adults can summarize stories prior to reading them or page through the material and discuss vocabulary, pictures or graphs, and various text structure components.

4. Relate Text to Life

Adults should relate the student's life to the text, the text to the student's life, and the text to the world beyond the book through interactive dialogue (Cochran-Smith, 1984; Heath, 1983). Students will attend better when the topic is one to which they have a personal association, and they in turn will then comprehend the text better. Students may be able to read every word on a page, but if access to the words and concepts has not been provided, or if personal experiences with the thoughts, motivations, perceptions, and problems of the characters have not been discussed, students generally cannot bring the appropriate understanding to the text.

> An early-childhood teacher told of a little girl, Sky, who was hard of hearing and enrolled in the general education kindergarten: *"Oh, boy . . . oh, boy,"* Sky *yelled at Mary, "the teacher said we are going to the circus. . . . What's a circus, Ms. Bilson?"*

Cochran-Smith (1984) coined the terms "life-to-text" and "text-to-life" in reference to adult mediation behaviors during reading that relate the text and the students' personal experiences. She found that during these interactions, adults taught the students how to make sense of text by bringing to life related extra-textual information. This was done by calling up broad sources of prior knowledge (lexical labels, narrative structure, literacy and cultural heritage, and conventions) needed in order to make inner-textual sense. She also witnessed text-to-life interactions where text was connected with students' lives.

Research shows that many teachers do make life-to-text and text-to-life connections, and that doing so aids the development of reading ability. Williams (1994) found in an ethnographic study of the literacy development of three young (three- and five-year-old) students who are D/HH that teachers routinely made life-to-text, text-to-life, and life-to-(previously read) text connections. Bilson (1995) surveyed residential school (preschool to fourth grade) teachers of the deaf and found that 72% included life-to-text and text-to-life discussions during read-aloud sessions. Satchwell (1993) found that the reading abilities of five elementary-aged deaf students improved when they were helped to use the strategies of associating and inferring. Kelly (1995) found that older, proficient and average deaf readers used their world knowledge to comprehend texts.

Many students lack text-to-life experiences with narrative and expository text when they come to school (Ewoldt, 1986; Feitelson & Goldstein, 1986; Heath, 1982; Williams, 1994). Ninio and Bruner (1978) and Heath found that some students who were read to at home focused on text structure and meaning, behaviors that facilitated success in school literacy experiences; other students, however, focused on discrete pieces of information—separate letters of the alphabet, and random shapes, colors, and labels—behaviors that were at odds with the demands at school. Heath found students in this latter group were not asked to make connections between text and real-world experiences and thus could not decontextualize (shift into other experiences) their knowledge of events. The students experienced difficulty in discussing and comprehending text. They evidenced progressive difficulty in tackling literacy tasks, which was particularly noticeable around fourth grade. Students who are

D/HH have also been found to experience difficulties with reading at about this age (research reviewed by King & Quigley, 1985).

Paul and Jackson (1993) cautioned that text-to-life and life-to-text experience be discussed in *both* ASL and English when students who are D/HH are ASL-dominant language users: "Without a command of the English language, ASL students, like other poor readers, will rely heavily on prior knowledge and not what they are presently reading" (p. 138). This may result in a misinterpretation of the text, which is written in English.

Traditionally, teachers of the deaf have used notebooks that are sent home and back to school again to share passages about events that can be linked to life. Copies of books used at school have also traveled back and forth between families and teachers so that text-to-life connections can be enhanced. Students also benefit when connections are made across school subject texts and discussions by a consistent educator throughout the school day.

> **Study Guide Question**
> *What other activities can you suggest to encourage text-to-life and life-to-text connections?*

Practice #4

Practice Defined	Adult Actions
Adults relate the student's life to the text, the text to the student's life, and the text to the world beyond the print through interactive dialogue. Adults should view misconceptions or gaps about knowledge as opportunities for learning and should build on what a student already knows, no matter how insufficient.	Adults can help students to link knowledge, narrative structure, cultural heritage, and conventions to the text. Each of these areas should be considered. Adults can help students to shift their knowledge of fictionalized events to their own lives or to situations in the real lives or writings of others. They can discuss the history of the period in which the story occurs and note whether the work is fact or fiction. Finally, they can tie together experiences throughout the school day so that information is linked in a meaningful way.

5. Model Concepts of Print

Adults should model concepts of print using authentic materials. Concepts of print are those basic understandings about how English print works (left-to-right, return sweep, stop at a period, and so on). These concepts include how sentences are written; the language used in talking about print; punctuation; structure; the concept of letter versus that of word; and book parts such as the table of contents and glossary. A checklist of concepts of print for primary-aged children is provided in Chapter 6.

Andrews and Akamatsu (1993) stated that it is critical that adults use correct signs for concepts of print. Obviously, students who rely on sign still need labels for terms such as exclamation point, silent *e*, and so forth, as well as for any technical vocabulary used. Cues or fingerspelling might also be used for these purposes. Luetke-Stahlman, Griffiths, and Montgomery (1998b) found that one deaf student, studied intensively as she developed early reading skills, was able to learn the basic concepts of print when they were paired with specific signs. As a second grader, the child was learning the difference between a paragraph and a chapter (highly similar signs in the manual code she was using), identifying a sentence as compared to a paragraph, and using the table of contents and glossary. Kretschmer (1989) has called for direct instruction of "typography cues" such as headings and subheadings with students who are D/HH (p. 213).

> **Study Guide Question**
> *Look at the concepts of print checklist in Chapter 6. What would you add to it?*

Practice #5

Practice Defined	Adult Actions
Adults model concepts of print.	Adults can use specific signs, fingerspelling, or cueing to label concepts of print so that students have access to exact terms.

6. Discuss Text Structure

Adults should discuss the text structure or schema of a story (characters, setting, problems or goals, conclusion or resolution) **or an expository text** (compare and contrast, cause and effect). Adults should plan writing activities that allow for the development of each student's inner appreciation and comprehension of text structure (McAnnally, Rose, & Quigley, 1994).   Adults can model "think alouds," talking through how the reader deciphers information about text structure, recognizes words, decodes content, and so on.

Marshall (1983) suggested that questions be asked to link comprehension to text structure. For example, questions could be asked about story text structure as illustrated in Figure 5–5.

Text Structure	Comprehension Questions
Stories have a theme.	What do you think the theme of this story might be?
Stories have a plot.	Can you describe the plot of this story in about three sentences?
A complete episode contains a setting and a series of events.	What is an example of an episode from this story?
The setting includes the time and place.	What is the setting of this story? What information in the text tells you about the setting?
The series of events includes (a) an initial event that sets a goal or problem; (b) attempts at resolution; (c) attainment of goal or resolution of problem; (d) reactions of the characters.	Describe the events in the story. What was the problem? How did the character attempt to solve it? How did characters react when the problem was solved?

FIGURE 5–5: TEXT STRUCTURE AND COMPREHENSION QUESTIONS

Text structure is a mental framework that guides understanding and helps students comprehend material. Comprehension of text structure develops over time when opportunities for repeated experiences with narrative or expository text occur. Students' experiences with plots and themes will help them to anticipate events and characters' actions in more complicated stories and to understand the grammar used to convey the information.

Students' comprehension of text structure is generally tapped by having them retell or rewrite a piece. For example, Yoshinaga, Itano, and Snyder (1984) used a model of story development to analyze written language samples from students who are D/HH; they found that 50% of the subjects did not retell the basic story components accurately (compared with 7% of the normal-hearing participants). Kluwin and Papalia (1989) found that the ability of younger students to answer comprehension questions and make predictions about a text was related to their ability to retrieve the salient elements of the text's structure.

Graphic organizers (word webs, charts, Venn diagrams, and so forth) can assist students in retelling story elements by organizing information from the text visually (Luetke-Stahlman & Luckner, 1991). Examples of graphic organizers that might be helpful appear in Appendix 5–B. Specific reading activities to enhance enjoyment, understanding of text structure, and comprehension of English use and form have been explained by Maxwell (1986), who advised that "if ASL is one of the languages used, the signed words will not match the print, but the episodic (event) units will" (p. 16).

Practice #6

Practice Defined	Adult Actions
Adults discuss text structure and expository elements. Writing activities that allow students to respond to text can assess comprehension of structure so that facilitation can be planned if needed.	Adults can facilitate an appreciation of story schema by labeling and discussing text structure elements or by using a story map to highlight them. Likewise, they can coach students to use graphic organizers to delineate text structure components. Adults can retell the story or reread the expository piece several times to heighten students' awareness of and appreciation for the structure of the material.

7. Model Word Recognition or Decoding Skills ————

Adults should facilitate word recognition or decoding skills by modeling the use of phonic, visual, meaning, and/or structural cues. These skills require phonological aware-ness, or the ability to think about features of words. Phonological awareness can be facilitated through phonics, structural awareness, or a combination of these strategies. Numerous studies have documented a positive correlation between phonological awareness and reading proficiency (Adams, 1995; Ball & Blachman, 1991; Bradley & Bryant 1983; Hanson & Fowler, 1987; Liberman, Shankweiler, & Liberman, 1989; Torgesen, 1994; Torgesen, Morgan, & Davis, 1992).

> **Study Guide Question**
>
> *Compare and contrast the materials and methods that can be used to clarify text structure and to assess comprehension. What other materials and methods can you add?*

Phonemic Cues (Sound-System Cues)

While some profoundly deaf students will not be able to use auditory and speech training to decode words, many will (Dodd, 1987; Hanson, 1991). Hanson (1989) clarified that phonological lin-guistic units "are not sounds, but rather a set of meaningless primitives out of which meaning units are formed" (p.73). One interpretation of this perspective then is that phonological awareness can be accessed auditorially, visually, or by using a combination of both senses.

Given individual differences, adults should model a variety of word recognition strategies when they read to students. Stanovich (1994), for instance, promoted explicit instructions rather than self-discovery as a more effective way for poor readers to learn word recognition skills. Adults should accept the possibility that students who are D/HH might use an auditory approach, a visual approach, or a combination of the two (labeled as learning styles 1, 2, and 3 in Figure 5–6).

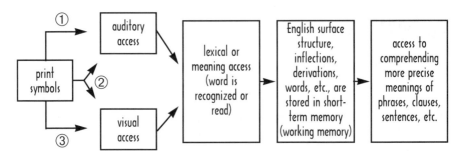

FIGURE 5–6: APPROACHES TO PHONOLOGICAL AWARENESS

Students who are D/HH may be able to develop an awareness of English phonology (phonological awareness) through speech articulation, production movements (subvocalization), and speechreading. Some studies, however, have illustrated that phonological awareness (speech recoding, phonological recoding, phonemic recoding) is *not* dependent on speechreading or speech articulation abilities (Conrad, 1979; Hanson, 1982; Kelly, 1995; Lichenstein, 1983, 1985; Marschark, 1993; Reynolds, 1986). The important point is that regardless of whether a student uses an auditory style, a visual style, or a combination of the two, he or she should be assisted in developing subvocalization and phonological coding (the mental representation of how words are formed), with the goal of achieving phonological awareness (see Figure 5–7).

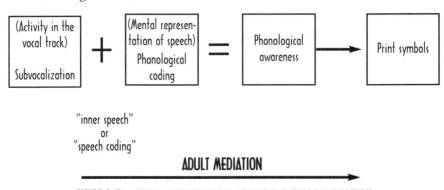

FIGURE 5–7: ASSISTING DEVELOPMENT TO ACHIEVE PHONOLOGICAL AWARENESS

Given training, some students with hearing loss will be able to master phonological awareness skills, which will support their word recognition efforts as readers (see, for example, Dodd, 1987; Hanson, 1989; Hanson & Fowler, 1987). This mastery is especially possible for the large number of students who are hard of hearing (Schein &

Delk, 1974; Schildroth, 1996). It is even more possible when hearing aids, cochlear implant equipment, and FM systems are used and when learning occurs in quiet environments.

Schaper and Reitsma (1993) studied 73 orally educated students, 6 to 13 years of age, and found that older students tended to differentiate and prefer either a speech-based or a visual strategy when reading and recalling written words. "The [speech-based strategy] was found to be associated with better performance in reading tasks" (p. 46). High school and college-aged deaf readers with good skills were found to use auditorily accessed phonological coding, compared to deaf readers with poor skills, who did not (Conrad, 1979; Hanson, Goodell, & Perfetti, 1991; Kelly, 1995; Schaper & Reitsma). (For further review of this topic, see Wandel, 1989). For these reasons, it is recommended that facilitation of sound-letter(s) training, and not just visual training, be included when it is determined that a student who is D/HH is capable of benefiting from it (Luetke-Stahlman & Luckner, 1991).

Structural or Orthographic Cues

Structural analysis or orthographic awareness can be especially helpful to profoundly deaf students as they learn the predictable sequences of letters that form word parts and wholes (*unused, unbutton, undone*). Cunningham and Stanovich (1990, 1993) found that hearing third and fourth graders demonstrated orthographic processing ability, which contributed in part to their success with word recognition. Students who are D/HH might also logically benefit from having adults model structural analysis or orthographic awareness as they read to them.

Word Work. Adams (1995) and Hanson, Liberman, and Shankweiler (1984) advocated that "word work" be modeled by adults as they read to students and be based on recently read text or portions of a text. Word work activities include all or some of the following types of activities:
- playing "Odd One Out"—several words with similar properties are presented, and students are asked to explain how the words are similar and dissimilar (e.g., *beat, boat, meat*)

- comparing the sounds in words with how the words are spelled (*fork, phone, laugh*).
- segmenting (breaking a word from the text into its component sounds)
- blending (combining isolated sounds to make a word from the text)
- discussing accent
- discussing rhyme
- detecting—students are asked what sound is heard when a word is pronounced by an adult
- identifying alliteration—students are asked to find a word that begins or ends with a specific sound
- identifying word families or pattern words (*fat, hat, mat, rat*) that visually rhyme—this might also provide clues to the meaning of unknown words, especially if the student has some hearing ability
- performing syllabication (orally, via fingerspelling, or with cues)
- discussing the meaning of root words
- discussing the meaning of prefixes and suffixes
- discussing the meaning of the parts of compound words
- identifying word derivations (*happy, happiness, happily*) and inflections (*come, coming, came*)
- sentence diagramming (in context)

PHONEME = a single speech sound; the smallest unit that can be distinguished from one word to another. The critical sound elements that distinguish the word *bat* from the word *cat* are the phonemes /b/ and /k/. Phonemes are enclosed by slashed lines; see *grapheme* below.

GRAPHEME = a printed symbol that represents a phoneme. For example, the sound /k/ is often represented by the letter *c*. A single grapheme may be italicized.

The ability to segment and blend sounds appears to enable initial reading, whereas reading itself appears to help develop the skill of deletion (*skill* minus the /sk/ sound is *ill*). *The ability to segment is considered to be the best predictor of reading success* (see, for example, Perfetti, Beck, Bell, & Hughes, 1987). Luetke-Stahlman, Griffiths, and Montgomery (1998a, 1998b) studied word work with a deaf child as she progressed from first to second grade and found that her progress was slow but steady. Despite a four-year English language delay, the girl read on grade level. In 5th grade, she evidenced a two-year English delay and read a year below grade level.

Practice #7

Practice Defined	Adult Actions
Adults facilitate word recognition by assessing each student's ability to apply phonological or orthographic knowledge to decode words that are difficult to read. Word recognition skills include the development of strategies so that an adult does not simply inform the student when a word cannot be read.	Adults can model the application and reinforcement of word recognition skills while reading. They can do this by stopping at difficult words and studying them collaboratively, looking carefully at the sound and structural patterns involved.

8. Discuss Word and Text Meaning

Adults should discuss several levels of text meaning. They should discuss the meaning of specific words and phrases by calling attention to picture cues; explaining, defining, paraphrasing; and providing synonyms and antonyms. The meaning of paragraphs can be discussed with students after whole chunks of text have been read. Adults should model repeated readings of difficult words, sentences, paragraphs, or pages (Adams, 1995; Engen, 1995; Snow, 1993; Topol, 1995) to aid text comprehension. Reference skills can also be facilitated within the genuine context of discussing an unknown or partially understood semantic feature and using glossaries or dictionaries as meaning is discussed.

Discussion of word and text meanings should be held in

English as well as in ASL when students who are D/HH are ASL-dominant language users. This is because "there is *no* evidence that first and second language learners can achieve high levels of literacy through exposure to the written form only of the language (i.e., English). . . . " (Paul & Jackson, 1993, p. 138). Thus, it is important for ASL-dominant students to achieve high levels of competency in cognitively challenging academic English so that they can access print. Figure 5–8 illustrates how to maximize English acquisition with ASL-dominant language users.

With regard to accessing print, the whole language movement has been misapplied in the field of deaf education. Proponents of this approach to reading "assume readers have intuitive knowledge of sound-letter correspondence and other bottom-up skills because of their command of conversational language (now used in print form) prior to learning to read" (Paul & Jackson, 1993, p. 139).

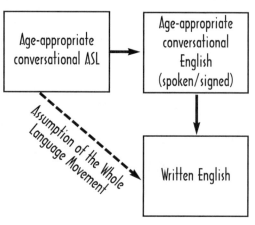

FIGURE 5–8: READING ENGLISH AS A SECOND LANGUAGE

Adapted from Paul & Jackson

Marschark (1993) clarified that "at its most essential level, competent reading requires recognition of the words on a printed page" (p. 208). Gartner, Trehub, and Mackay-Soroka (1993) studied 104 students from 4 to 14 years old who were both hearing and D/HH. They found that the students who are D/HH had considerably more difficulty distinguishing between words and their referents than did their hearing peers; they also had greater difficulty defining words (see also reviews in Paul & Jackson, 1993; Paul & Quigley, 1990). Moores (1967) and Paul and Quigley confirmed that the largest reading-related deficits of students who are D/HH were in the area of vocabulary knowledge. These were in sign, oral, and written productions (Everhart & Marschark, 1988; Griswold & Cummings, 1974; King & Quigley, 1985). Other areas of meaning found to be impaired in samples of students who are D/HH include anaphoric relationships within conjoined sentences (Wilbur & Goodhart, 1985), figurative English (Giorcelli, 1982; Paul, 1984; Payne, 1982; Payne & Quigley, 1987), inferences (Wilson, 1979), and multiple meanings (Blackwell, Engen, Fischgrund, & Zarcadoolas, 1978).

The semantic needs of students who are D/HH can have an effect on how adults read to them. As adults change their reading styles according to suggestions in this chapter, they may find that they become less controlling, less dominant with the dialogue, and better able to facilitate discussion; students, in turn, will show an increased willingness to take turns and share opinions, and will be less frustrated as more of the text is truly comprehended.

To assist in facilitating the development of meaning, adults need to engage students who are D/HH in dialogue and discuss concepts as they read to them, just as they do with hearing students. Use of the dictionary and encyclopedia may be appropriate at such junctures. At an early age, students can learn the function of these tools and how to use them.

> **Preteaching of difficult vocabulary should be replaced by discussion of specific vocabulary and figurative phrases, using strategy talk and instructional mediation either during the discussion of text or after it has been read.**

Dickinson and Smith (1994) suggested that the type of mediation used by adults to facilitate comprehension of text as they read to students is as important as the cognitive concepts presented. For example, Hoggan and Strong (1994) found that extensions were recommended by many researchers "to clarify meanings, guide students in more abstract interpretations of particular words, and invite the student to add comments and examples" (p. 80). "Analytical talk," in which adults ask students to think beyond the information provided, has been found to be critical to academic success (Cummins, 1989; Dickinson & Smith). Along these same lines, Hoggan and Strong recommended that adults question students as they read to them "whenever opportunities arise for making predictions, drawing inferences, classifying information, justifying actions, or assuming the role (perspective) of the characters" (p. 81). Adults might also model rereading as a strategy to aid comprehension (Andrews & Mason, 1991), a practice that has been found to affect the depth of student response (Hickman, 1981) and literacy achievement (Cochran-Smith, 1984; Flood, 1977; Morrow, O'Connor, & Smith, 1990; Nielsen, 1993).

Hoggan and Strong (1994) recommended that story mapping be modeled by adults as they read, an idea supported by a number of other researchers (see Hoggan & Strong for a review). They clarified that both episode mapping (focusing on individual aspects) and text mapping (focusing on the piece as a whole) are beneficial and can be used interchangeably. Luckner and Humphries (1992) and Luetke-Stahlman and Luckner (1991) recommended that pictures and word webs, flow charts, and graphic organizers be used to aid comprehension.

Practice #8

Practice Defined	Adult Actions
Adults discuss the *meaning* of specific words and phrases and model how to infer meaning. They encourage repeated readings of difficult words, sentences, paragraphs, and text.	Adults can provide vocabulary instruction to increase a student's word knowledge and reading comprehension. Methods in which students are given *word definitions* and *examples of word usage* in context result in the largest English language gains. Adults can model how to define words to include categorical information and distinguishing details, as well as how to supply synonyms and antonyms. Adults should use specific signs or finger-spelling, cueing, or writing for technical vocabulary and figurative English.

9. Model and Discuss Syntactic Structures

Adults should model and discuss the grammar (form, syntax) of the story and the structural rules as needed for comprehension. Adults also should encourage repeated readings of difficult words, sentences, passages, or whole texts (Adams, 1995; Andrews & Mason, 1991; Engen, 1995; Topol, 1995).

Study Guide Question

What would you include in a web showing all the ways adults might facilitate the meaning of text?

Paul and Jackson (1993) lamented that "most [students who are] D/HH do not learn English at a highly competent level, which results in inadequate English form, which contributes to poorly developed literacy skills" (p. 127). Kelly (1996) noted that the direct influence of lack of syntactic competence on the low reading comprehension of many deaf readers has been substantiated by the research of, for example, Berent (1988), Geers and Moog (1989), Isrealite (1981), Kelly, and Robbins and Hatcher (1981). Syntactic English competence as a component of reading proficiently may be far more important than is generally recognized.

As noted by Harris and Smith (1986), English syntactic structures include
- word order
- form or arrangement of sentences
- surface compared to deep structure (*"He drew a brown bear"* compared to *"He drew a bear that was brown."*)
- sentence combining (*"It was black. It was a bear"* to *"It was a black bear."*)
- relational phrases: subject-predicate, coordinate, complement, and modifiers

Many students who are D/HH, when reading or writing, do not comprehend or use syntactic properties such as affixes, function words, morphology, subordinate structures, verb inflections, pronouns, and question formations (see Paul & Quigley, 1994, for details). When adults are cognizant of specific student syntactic needs, they can choose reading materials for sharing that are both of interest to students and that include specific linguistic structures.

The adults can use those materials to reinforce structures emerging in the student's English language ability (Weintraub, 1984).

Andrews and Akamatsu (1993) stated that it is important for adults to make sign-to-print relationships explicit when they read to students. They found that students who are D/HH, and for whom such relationships were made explicit, acquired significantly greater letter-, word-, and story-reading abilities than did students for whom these associations were not made. Luetke-Stahlman (1990) found that the more closely the speech, sign, and written morpheme match, the better students read as a group; in her study, elementary-aged students with severe and profound hearing losses who were exposed to grammatically complete and literally communicated modes of communication (oral English, Seeing Essential English, Signing Exact English) scored higher on English vocabulary, grammar, and reading tests than did students exposed to manual forms of English that do not encode the grammar of the language.

Engen (1995) recommended that the direct instruction of the fragile properties of English grammar (those that are difficult or unacquired by the student) should occur in meaningful context with explicit attention to the literate use of these properties. For example, an adult might explain the use of the past perfect tense (*has had*) to indicate a flashback. Once the content of the text is understood by the student, the adult should focus on form, allowing imitation of linguistic models (Huang & Hatch, 1978), grammatically expanding the student's utterances, and using syntax that is only slightly more developmentally complex than what the student is using to discuss the text (Luetke-Stahlman, 1993, 1998).

Rogers (1989) reported that students who are D/HH at a residential school demonstrated improvement in English language ability when adults systematically read to them. She reported that ten students showed receptive gains in English, as well as gains in expressive skills for prompted and imitated production. These students scored higher on assessment tests than did the deaf norming population, although lower than the norms for hearing

Study Guide Question

Review a text to identify inverted or complex sentences. How might you use the text to explain these grammatical structures?

peers. In addition, Rogers confirmed that the students particularly enjoyed having text reread.

Practice #9

Practice Defined	Adult Actions
Adults discuss the English grammar within the text and its structural rules as needed in order to understand the text (for example, the use of the past perfect tense to indicate a flashback). They encourage repeated readings of difficult word combinations, sentences, passages, or whole texts to assist student comprehension.	Adults can call attention to grammar within the reading context. They can model the reading of particular structures, and they might ponder aloud about how English structure compares with that of American Sign Language.

10. Use a Variety of Response Modes

Adults should employ a variety of modes of responding to text both to deepen students' comprehension and to facilitate their English cognitive academic language skills (Gelzer, 1988; Hickman, 1981; Weintraub, 1984). Interaction and co-construction of ideas during response activities are as important as all the mediation activities that have been mentioned up to this point. If a team's goal is to facilitate reading development, the use of output, or language to communicate responses to the text, can be particularly effective (Swain, 1985).

deBot (1996) explained the importance of allowing students the opportunity to struggle consciously to make expressive decisions by manipulating shades of meaning between words. Harris and Smith (1986) supported encouraging students to manipulate degrees of meaning: "A competent reader can distinguish between the dictionary definition of a word or phrase (i.e., denotation) and the images and implications suggested by the word (i.e., connotation)" (p. 309). The ability to access different forms of words (such as derivations, verb tenses, singular or plural) is dependent on frequency of use in the text as well as frequency of use by the student (deBot).

To produce a thought as a hearing student would, a student who is D/HH requires opportunities to respond to text and to

- conceptualize the meaning of a message
- match thought to language in general
- activate grammatical procedures
- activate word forms and grammatical structures
- plan articulation of the sentence in speech and sign
- execute the plan to express the response to text in English (deBot, 1996)

Noticing matches and mismatches between production and an "internal norm" causes the student to acquire aspects of language that can be used initially only in specific linguistic contexts. Through frequent use, these facts and rules get formalized and become procedures. When the student can "proceduralize," constantly tuning and restructuring, he or she can automatically process increasingly larger units of information (deBot). Response activities can allow students who are D/HH opportunities to acquire the English needed to comprehend and express those larger units required for academics.

There are many strategies for practicing language skills while discussing reading material. Students who are D/HH can be asked to reread sections of a text and locate words with similar meanings (for example, a story set in a meadow for which the descriptive words *green, fern, lime,* and *forest* are used). Older students can read advertisements and find words that appeal to the senses (Harris & Smith, 1986). Students can be encouraged to create a speech for a particular character or dramatize a larger section of the story to practice using grammar.

Verbal activities completed after an adult has finished reading a story or text are the best methods for facilitating student's achievement of some literacy-related objectives. Such activities include using the cloze procedure, asking cognitively-demanding academic questions, oral (sign and/or speech) retelling, and so forth (Harris & Smith, 1986). For example, given stories with repetitive and rhyming words that provide a structure for creating new versions, adults might encourage students to substitute sounds and letters from the original. Using the book *Down By the Bay* by Raffi (1987), for instance, students can be guided in creating their own nonsense rhymes, such as "Did you ever see a dog riding a hog?" Likewise, students can be asked to retell a story, changing several details to stump the audience.

Students can be asked to invent new endings for stories or discuss what would happen if a situation were changed. For example, in a science experiment, what would happen if a different ingredient were added? Students can also write parallel stories—stories that grow from the original plot but may follow a minor character into full development or expand on an event only briefly mentioned—to assist English language development (Harris & Smith). Students can be encouraged to reread text independently or with a peer during free time. They can also be asked to orally (sign or speech) retell or write about a story or text, using a graphic organizer as an aid.

Hoggan and Strong (1994) recommended that students be taught four types of questions that can be asked at the end of reading: "right here," "think and search," "author and you," and "on my own." Developing potential test questions and discussing other possible outcomes are also beneficial activities. Older students might employ the SQ3R approach explained further in Chapter 10: survey the text, ask questions, read, respond to questions, and review the material. Miller and Rosenthal (1995) found that summarizing text particularly assisted ASL users.

Smaller copies of shortened versions of stories or a second set of school subject books can be taken home for additional experience with familiar text. Videotaped signed versions can be sent home to assist parents in rereads. Parents can be encouraged to watch story videotapes with their child and to read or look at pictures of the same story in a storybook.

Practice #10

Practice Defined	Adult Actions
Adults employ a variety of response modes to reading text.	Adults can encourage qualitative shifts in students' responses by providing a variety of verbal (sign/speech) activities.

Examples of the Adult Reading Practices

Study Guide Question
Which response activities would be most helpful to a student who is D/HH with whom you work?

Examples of the ten essential practices for adults to model when reading to students who are D/HH are presented in Figure 5–9. Two narrative stories (labeled Story 1 and Story 2) and one expository text have been used as models.

Narrative Story	Expository Text
1. Purpose/Enjoyment *Story 1.* How many of you enjoyed the other Arthur stories we've read? Today we are going to read about a problem Arthur had and then talk about how he solved it. I hope we'll also have time to talk about how *we* solve problems today. *Story 2.* Historical events are easier to understand if we read about people who lived during those times. This story will help us understand the Southerners' perspective during the Civil War.	This chapter is about alligators. We are reading it because we'll be going to the zoo on Thursday. One of the caretakers there is going to meet our group and help us to compare alligators and crocodiles. There are some charts in the story that will help us discuss what is similar and dis-similar about these two reptiles.
2. Text-to-Life, Life-to-Text, Text-to-World, Text-to-School Day *Story 1.* This fiction book is entitled *Arthur's Eyes.* We have read other books about him, right? In this one, Arthur gets glasses. How many of you wear glasses? Why do you wear them?	This is a nonfiction story. Does that mean the information is true and real, or pretend? (Students respond.) Yes, and so some of what we read about in this story, we might expect to see at the zoo. *cont.*

FIGURE 5–9: EXAMPLES OF THE ADULT READING PRACTICES

FIGURE 5-9, CONT.

Narrative Story	Expository Text
Story 2. Mr. Rex and you have been talking about the Civil War during history class. Today we are going to begin reading *Gone with the Wind*. It's a fictional story about the Civil War period. Most of the main characters live on plantations. Has anyone here ever visited a Southern plantation?	
### 3. Preparatory Set Let's look through this Arthur book before we read it. I'll cover up the words, and let's just look at the pictures. Let's guess or predict what we think the story will be about, OK? (Students review the illustrations, and the adult uses some of the essential vocabulary that is challenging.)	Let's look at some of the charts and pictures in this chapter before we read more of it. Just ignore the words for now. Look on pages 24–25. David, which of those pages has a chart on it? (He responds.) Good. Judy, how are alligators and crocodiles compared on that chart? (She responds.) Good. Who can tell me one detail you expect the text to mention about how these two reptiles are similar? As we turn the pages of the chapter, let's make a list of what you all know about alligators, OK?
### 4. Interactive Dialogue Let's list the things that happened *before* Arthur got his new glasses. (The adult involves the children, who offer ideas based on the story. After each idea, the adult reads the part from the book that confirms that idea.) Yes, Janie, Arthur got headaches. On the first page it says "Sometimes he got headaches." (After the possibilities are listed and confirmed by consulting the text, the adult asks what Arthur did next. His visit to the optometrist might be discussed in terms of other occupations that end with *-ist* and what the optometrist and other workers, such as dentists, orthodontists, and so on, do.)	

cont.

FIGURE 5–9, CONT.

Narrative Story	Expository Text
5. Concepts of Print (The adult begins to read, modeling in speech, cues, and/or signs, moving his or her eyes from left to right and describing his or her thoughts. Big books might be used so that students can see clearly as concepts of print are referenced. Referencing can occur by pointing and moving a finger under a word, phrase, or punctuation mark, and by asking rhetorical questions.) Do you think this bold print means to shout or whisper? Let's look at the first sentence in this Arthur book. This is a *period*. It tells us we are at the end of the sentence. Sometimes we pause at a period and take a breath of air.	Let's look back at the table of contents for our science book. Lindsey, what page is that on? (She identifies.) Good, now let's find the chapter that we are reading today. (A student finds it.) Good. Now, here is a heading in the middle of the page. It tells me that a new topic is going to be discussed here when we have finished this section about reptiles. (Adult reads heading.) Look at *My Big Backyard*, our science magazine, and find a heading or a subheading. (They do.) Great, now you can guess what I want to see when you write your science report. A subheading! Right!
6. Text Structure Can you tell me who the main characters in this story are? (They do.) Let's point to the *names of the main characters* together. Good, and where does the story happen? (No response.) Does the story take place in a zoo, a forest, or a city? (Children guess correctly.) Good, yes, a city. OK, and what is Arthur's problem? Let's use your worksheet now.	We're going to divide into three groups now and do three different things. Group 1, you're going to make a word web about alligators, OK? Group 2, you are going to make a chart for us that tells how alligators and crocodiles differ. Group 3, I want you to use this visual picture to describe what happens when people tease alligators.

cont.

FIGURE 5–9, CONT.

Narrative Story	Expository Text

<u>A Story Frame</u>
The problem was _____
_____.

It began when_____
_____.

After that_____
_____.

The problem was solved when
_____.

The story ends when _____
_____.

A different title might be _____
_____.

When people tease alligators →
[Couldn't see math problems]
[Arthur hid his glasses.] →
  → [Couldn't see math problems]
  → [Went into the Girl's Bathroom]
  → [ ]

When Arthur *hid* his glasses, what happened?

7. Word Recognition Skills

Now that we've read this, let's go back and look at this one sentence on page 6. It says, "No one wanted to play with Arthur." Can you tell me another word on the page that starts like *wanted*?

Let's look at this sentence on page 11. It says, "Everything looks clearer through this lens." If I wasn't sure how to say that first word, what could I do? (Students suggest strategies: *cont.*)

FIGURE 5-9, CONT.

Narrative Story	Expository Text
(Students list words. They can supply words by using either phonic awareness and thinking of the /w/ sound or by using orthographic awareness and thinking of words that start with the letter *w*.) Let's divide the word *wanted* into syllables. You write *wanted* on your paper and decide how many syllables there are, OK? How many other words can you think of that have the word *want* in them? (Students list *wants, unwanted,* etc.) Correct! Good job. What are some words that are in the word family that *play* is in? If you need help, look on our word wall.	sounding it out, dividing it into syllables, etc.) What two words can you find in the word *every-thing*? (Students tell.) Good. Let's look at the word *look*. What words with the same root do you know? (Students suggest *looked, looking.*) Wow, great. Turn to a partner and talk about the words you know that look a lot like *clearer*. Write them down for me. (Students write.) But you know what happened to me as I read the word *looks*? I almost said *books* instead. Would that be right? (Students respond.) What are some other words in that family? Let's all reread this sentence together. (Students read.) I want to ask one more question about a word on page 1 of this science book. Let me read you this sentence. (Adult reads it.) How would you sign the word *couldn't* ? (Both ASL and SEE-II versions are offered.) Yes, good. Where else did you see that word? (Students respond.) Yes, so let's all picture it in our minds and then fingerspell the word *couldn't*.
8. Meaning It says here that Arthur had to consider how his glasses helped him. At first I wasn't sure if that word was *concern* or *consider*. If it said "Arthur had to concern how his glasses helped," would that make sense? What do you	What is similar and dissimilar about the alligator and the croco-dile? Let's make a diagram and write in things where they belong.

cont.

FIGURE 5–9, CONT.

Narrative Story	Expository Text
think *consider* means? Let's write down your ideas. 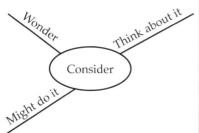 Yes, the word *consider* means to think about something. What is Arthur considering in this story? Lynn, come and point to the word *consider* for us. (She does.) Diane, can you define *consider* for us? (She does.) If you didn't take the time to consider something, you might make a quick decision and regret it later, right? Can everyone copy the word *consider*? You trace each letter as I say it. (They do.) I'm going to add *consider* to our spelling list and ask you to spell it again for the spelling test. OK, let's look on this page. What is Arthur doing in this picture? (Students respond.) Yes, good, and see, it says here . . . (reads a sentence). Let's all read this sentence again. (Choral reading) Wow, that was much smoother that time! You really sound like readers. Let's talk again about what this paragraph means. What is Arthur considering?	Alligators: Broad noses, Lower teeth don't show Crocodiles: Narrow noses, Teeth show, Fiercer Similar Reptiles Live in swamps Ancient ancestry Now that we have finished reading this chapter, let's go back and look on the third page. The author has said that alligators are "fascinating." What fascinating characteristics do alligators have? (Students read parts from text that describe fascinating characteristics.) *cont.*

FIGURE 5–9, CONT.

Narrative Story	Expository Text
9. Grammar Tell me if this sentence is in the right order. (Reads a sentence from the text.) What does the word *he* stand for in this sentence? Who is the author talking about? Here the author writes "he had problems" as Arthur is telling about his problems. Let's figure out why. Here's a long sentence (complex, multiclausal sentence). Let's break it down into smaller sentences or phrases and decide what they mean.	Let's reread this sentence on the bottom of page 15. It says, "Alligators aren't crocodiles, and crocodiles aren't alligators, although they belong to the same family." Hannah, look at the diagram we drew above. Can you explain this sentence to me? (No response) What does the author mean by saying that alligators are reptiles? (Hannah answers.) Good, and what does she mean when she writes that crocodiles are in the same family, Lynn? (Lynn responds.) Good. What about the phrase "although they belong to the same family"? What's another word you could use for the word *although* in that sentence?
10. Variety of Response Modes Let's divide into several cooperative learning groups and retell this story. This group will write a book report; this group will design a skit to retell the story; this group will videotape themselves retelling the story; and this group will use puppets to act out the story. I've listed the words here I want each group to use in the retelling. Every student is to contribute and help make decisions. Tomorrow you'll get a chance to rotate.	We are going to share what we have learned about alligators in some new ways. Here are some choices. Some students can draw pictures of alligators and their habitat. Others can go to the library and choose some books for us to look at tomorrow that have some good descriptions of reptiles. Still others can use our computers to word process a two- or three-page report about reptiles.

Summary

An impressive amount of quality research has substantiated how beneficial it is to students when parents read to them at home. When parents do not read, read infrequently, or read in a manner that is not comprehensible to a student, adults at school can intervene and provide frequent and systematic reading activities. Adult reading in the manner described in this chapter should include both access to information and mediated dialogue and should use a variety of texts. The examples and survey in Appendix 5–A can help to identify inservice needs in this important school subject area.

Activities

1. Design a lesson plan that would be useful to adults who wish to include the ten essential practices for reading with a student who is D/HH.

2. Videotape yourself reading to a student who is D/HH and include the ten essential practices. Label each practice on the videotape so that a viewer can identify your work.

3. Provide an inservice to an adult or group using the information provided in this chapter.

4. Consult a professional journal, such as *The Reading Teacher*, *Journal of Reading Research*, or the *Journal of Reading Behavior* and review a research article on reading that is relevant to your interests.

Appendix 5-A

Making the Most of an Adult-Read Session: How Do You Rate?

Reading to students is an activity during which an adult such as a teacher, parent, or librarian reads the contents of a chosen book or story to a student or group of students by speaking, cueing, and/or signing the printed text. The reader can serve as a role model in demonstrating important aspects of the reading process to the audience. Yet, recent research has demonstrated that while many teachers of the deaf are providing read-alouds for their students, they are not always including important components of the process (Bilson, 1995). To see if you are including the essential practices when you read an expository or narrative selection, take the quiz that follows. Your task is to respond to each question and check your response against the information provided at the end of the quiz. Give yourself one point for each correct answer. Good luck!

1. When choosing an appropriate book or story, I might make my selection because the content (a) uses a particular story structure; (b) calls attention to a unit theme; (c) includes a specific vocabulary word or phrase that was experienced in another story; (d) is easy to sign; (e) has systematically introduced phonemic content; (f) is of interest to the student; (g) all except (e); (h) all of the above.

2. When I read, I model that I enjoy reading and value the experience (a) with each story that I read; (b) some of the time; (c) only on rare occasions.

3. I relate the student's life to the text, the text to the student's life, or the text to the world beyond the story (a) often; (b) sometimes; (c) only on rare occasions.

4. When choosing a story for an individual, I try to ensure that the syntax (form) and semantics (meaning) are (a) at his or her linguistic maturity; (b) slightly above his or her linguistic maturity; (c) slightly below his or her linguistic maturity; (d) I do not assess the student's comprehension of the syntax and semantics of English, so I do not pick stories based on this information.

cont.

5. When I read aloud, I (a) don't stop to talk much for fear of losing the story line; (b) engage the students before, during, and after in an interactive dialogue about the story; (c) discuss the story with the students at the end of the reading.

6. As I read, I call attention to (a) the title of the story only; (b) sentences that are statements and those that are questions; (c) a systematic list of "concepts of print."

7. I usually discuss (a) the main characters; (b) the main characters, setting, and conclusion of the story; (c) all the story structure elements (characters, setting, problem or goal, conclusion or resolution, and so forth).

8. When I come to a somewhat difficult word that is important to the story line, I (a) skip the word; (b) sign, fingerspell, or cue the word; or (c) replace the word with an easier word.

9. I (a) often; (b) sometimes; or (c) rarely read the same story twice.

10. I (a) often; (b) sometimes; or (c) rarely plan a response activity (role play, written response, etc.) to a story I have read.

Answers (Give yourself one point for each correct response.)

1. (h) "All of the above" is the correct answer unless *every* student in your audience has absolutely no ability to hear speech (then "g" would be the correct answer). Stories should be selected based on a particular literacy goal. If students have some hearing ability, adults might call attention to some initial and final sounds, rhyming patterns, the blending of sounds to form words, and the names of sounds compared to the names of letters. They might facilitate the student's knowledge of words that cannot be sounded out easily (such as the word *night*) and to the similarity of spelling of words (*back* as compared to *black*).

2. (a) Books and stories that adults particularly enjoy are the same materials that students want to read and discuss. Teachers and parents can increase the enjoyment of read-alouds by using a language or system that is easily understood by the student and by choosing stories for which the student has the required background knowledge or interest.

cont.

3. (a) Adults should always take the time to introduce the story and link it to the student's life, helping students to make these connections by activating thought about the title of the story, explaining the historical period in which the story occurs, or discussing the book as fact or fiction. Adults often need to help students shift from events in the story to those in their own lives or the real lives of others (*"Have you ever felt embarrassed, as Denise did in this story?"*)

4. (b) Stories should be chosen that are within the student's "zone of proximal development" (Vygotsky, 1978)—challenging but not frustrating to comprehend—and in accordance with the goals of the adult (story structure, unit theme, ease of signing, etc.). Reading assessments can be conducted so that the student's level of English comprehension is known. Based on this information, a story should be chosen that is written at a slightly more difficult grammatical and semantic level than is understood by the student.

5. (b) Adults need to mediate the story, making it a meaning-making experience. Conversation in the student's first language should occur through an interactive dialogue, using questions, strategy talk (*"I knew that word was* necktie *because I looked at the picture"*), and predictions. As the story unfolds, relevant ideas should be emphasized and irrelevant predictions discarded. Plenty of open-ended questions should be asked so that the student is not attending to relatively unimportant details of the story. The atmosphere should be one that encourages risk-taking on the student's part to use English structures, to discuss the text with regard to his or her own life, and to respond cognitively (summarize, provide a new title, and so forth).

6. (c) Adults should use fingerspelling or signs to label the "concept of print" used in a story (Clay, 1985). These might include basic concepts such as the direction of the print, or what an exclamation point is, as well as understanding more sophisticated terms such as *chapter* and *subheading*. See Andrew and Akamatsu (1993).

7. (c) Adults should model an appreciation of the complete schema for the story. Adults might label and discuss each of the elements (character, setting, problem, solution in narrative; cause or effect in expository, and so on). They can have the student retell the story using puppets, role play, or use graphic organizers such as story maps, networking, and word webs. The goals are for the story elements to be clarified and for students to realize that these elements are an important part of every story. *cont.*

8. (b) Novel or challenging vocabulary should be signed, cued, or fingerspelled and should not avoided. Instead of preteaching vocabulary that is important to the story line, adults can discuss it in context when they introduce the story, again during the reading of the story, and once again after the story has been read. If the students understand English signing, then signs and markers can be used to further discuss the form and meaning of the word or phrase (for example, *unworkable*). If the students use ASL, then the adult can facilitate discussion that compares and contrasts the meaning of the English word(s) and the ASL equivalent(s). Paul and Quigley (1994) suggested that special attention should be given to text that includes pronouns (including *this* and *that*, and making sure that students can identify their antecedents), variations of verbs (*break, breaking, broke, broken*), the meaning of clauses, the shades of meaning that modals represent *(can, could, might,* and so on), and inferences.

9. (a) When teachers repeat read alouds, students are the beneficiaries of multiple exposures to story structure and specific grammar and vocabulary. Hickman (1981) noted that repeated readings affect the depth of student responses, their ability to make more complicated predictions, and their literacy achievement. Teachers are encouraged to reread the same stories, and parents may find it a relief to know that it is beneficial to recue or sign a story that they have read several times before.

10. (a) Adults should provide a variety of verbal (retell or paraphrase) and nonverbal (art, mime) responses to read alouds. Such activities can deepen the students' comprehension of the story and their ability to discuss the form and meaning of the text. Students might be asked to decide on a new title, develop test questions, or invent a new ending.

Tallying Your Score

Count up your points. How did you do?

9–10 Points
Congratulations! You are effectively reading aloud to students and should continue to include the components discussed above in your read alouds. You might assist other adults, using this tool to conduct inservices.

cont.

> **6–8 Points**
> You've made a good start, but there is room for improvement! You are including many of the essential components when you read aloud, but your skills need polishing. Students could benefit a great deal more from your read-aloud efforts.
>
> **1–5 Points**
> Perhaps the information provided in this chapter will give you specific ideas for ways to improve your read alouds.

Appendix 5-B

Examples of Text Structure Graphic Organizers*

*Graphic organizers from "Using Graphic Organizers to Develop Critical Thinking," by J. Cassidy, 1989, *Gifted Child Today*, 12(6), pp. 34-36. Copyright 1989 by Prufrock Press. Reprinted with permission.

STORY MAP

Title: _____

Setting: ┌───┐
         │   │
         └───┘

Problem: ┌───┐
         │   │
         └───┘

Event 1 _____

Event 2 _____

Event 3 _____

Event 4 _____

Event 5 _____

Solution: ┌──┐
          │   │
          └──┘

Characters:

_____   _____

cont.

STORY MAP

Title:_____

Setting:

Problem:

Difficulty #1 _____

Difficulty #2 _____

Difficulty #3 _____

Difficulty #4 _____

Difficulty #5 _____

Climax (Difficulty) _____

Resolution:

Protaganist: _____

Antagonist: _____

X = Difficulty or Obstacle

Protagonist

Conflict

Climax

Resolution *cont.*

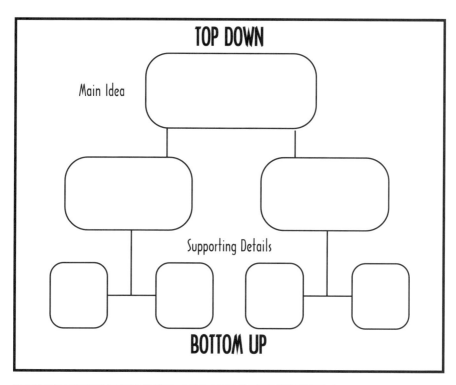

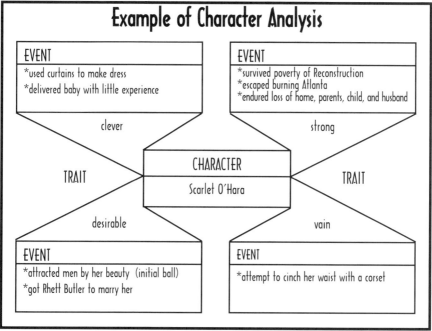

238

References

Adams, M. (1995). *Beginning to read: Thinking and learning about print.* Cambridge, MA: MIT Press.

Allen, T. (1986). Patterns of academic achievement among hearing impaired students: 1974 and 1983. In A. Schildroth & M. Karchmer (Eds.), *Deaf children in America* (pp. 161-206). San Diego, CA: Little, Brown.

Andrews, J. (1984). *How do young deaf children learn to read? A proposed model of deaf children's emergent reading behaviors.* (Technical Report #329. ED 250 674)

Andrews, J., & Akamatsu, T. (1993). Building blocks for literacy: Getting the signs right. *Perspectives in Education and Deafness, 11*(3), 5-9.

Andrews, J., & Mason, J. (1986). Childhood deafness and the acquisition of print concepts. In D. Yaden & S. Templeton (Eds.), *Metalinguistic awareness and beginning literacy: Conceptualizing what it means to read and write* (pp. 277-290). Portsmouth, NH: Heinemann.

Andrews, J., & Mason, J. (1991). Strategy usage among deaf and hearing readers. *Exceptional Children, 57,* 536-545.

Andrews, J., & Taylor, N. (1987). From sign to print: A case study of picture book "reading" between mother and child. *Sign Language Studies, 56,* 261-274.

Andrews, J., Winograd, P., & DeVille, G. (1996). Using sign language summaries during prereading lessons. *Teaching Exceptional Children, 28*(3), 30-34.

Applebee, A. (1978). *The child's concept of story.* Chicago: University of Chicago Press.

Ball, E., & Blachman, B. (1991). Does phoneme awareness training in kindergarten make a difference in early word recognition and developmental spelling? *Reading Research Quarterly, 26,* 49-66.

Barrentine, S. (1996). Engaging with reading through interactive read-alouds. *The Reading Teacher, 50*(1), 36-43.

Beauchamp, W. (1925). A preliminary experimental study of techniques in mastery of subject matter in elementary physical science. *Supplemental Elementary Monograph.* No. 24 (pp. 47-87). Chicago: University of Chicago Press.

Bellugi, U., Klima, E., & Siple, P. (1975). Remembering in signs. *Cognition, 3*, 93-125.

Berent, G. (1988). An assessment of syntactic capabilities. In M. Strong (Ed.), *Language, learning and deafness* (pp. 133-161). New York: Cambridge University Press.

Bilson, M. (1995). *Reading aloud with children who are deaf and hard of hearing: A survey of teachers working in state schools for the deaf.* Unpublished master's thesis, University of Kansas Medical Center, Kansas City.

Blackwell, P., Engen, E., Fischgrund, J., & Zarcadoolas, C. (1978). *Sentences and other systems.* Washington, DC: Alexander Graham Bell Association for the Deaf.

Bradley, L., & Bryant, P. (1983). Categorizing sounds and learning to read—A causal connection. *Nature, 301*, 419-421.

Brasel, K., & Quigley, S. (1975). *The influence of early language and communication environments on the development of language in deaf children.* Urbana-Champaign: University of Illinois, Institute for Research on Exceptional Children.

Brown, V., Hammill, D., & Wiederholt, J. (1995). *Test of Reading Comprehension–3* (TORC–3). Austin, TX: Pro-Ed.

Carlsen, J. (1985). Between the deaf child and reading: The language connection. *The Reading Teacher, 38*(4), 424-426.

Cassidy, J. (1989). Using graphic organizers to develop critical thinking. *Gifted Child Today, 12*(6), 34-36.

Chomsky, C. (1972). Stages in language development and reading exposure. *Harvard Educational Review, 42*, 1-33.

Clark, M. (1976). *Young fluent readers.* London: Heinemann Educational Books.

Clay, M. (1985). *The early detection of reading difficulties* (3rd ed.). Portsmouth, NH: Heinemann.

Cochran-Smith, M. (1984). *The making of a reader.* Norwood, NJ: Ablex.

Conrad, R. (1979). *The deaf schoolchild: Language and cognitive function.* London: Harper & Row.

Cummins, J. (1989). A theoretical framework for bilingual special education. *Exceptional Children, 56*(2), 111-119.

Cunningham, A., & Stanovich, K. (1990). Assessing print exposure and orthographic processing skill in children: A quick measure of reading experience. *Journal of Educational Psychology, 84*(2), 733-740.

Cunningham, A., & Stanovich, K. (1993). Children's environments and early work recognition subskills. *Reading and Writing: An Interdisciplinary Journal, 5*(2), 193-204.

deBot, K. (1996). The pycholinguistics of the output hypotheses. *Language Learning: A Journal of Research in Language Studies, 46*(3), 529-555.

DeFord, D., Lyons, C., & Pinnell, G. (1991). *Bridges to literacy: Learning from reading recovery.* Portsmouth, NH: Heinemann.

deVilliers, P. (1995). *Expository writing, extended discourse and science: Towards an integrated curriculum for deaf students.* Paper presented at the 10th Annual Issues in Language and Deafness Conference, Nebraska City, NE.

Dickinson, D., & Smith, M. (1994). Long-term effects of preschool teachers' book readings on low-income children's vocabulary and story comprehension. *Reading Research Quarterly, 29*(2), 104-122.

Dickinson, D., & Snow, C. (1987). Interrelationships among pre reading and oral language skills in kindergartners from two social classes. *Early Childhood Research Quarterly, 2,* 1-25.

Dodd, B. (1987). Lip-reading, phonological coding and deafness. In D. Dodd & R. Campbell (Eds.), *Hearing by eye: The psychology of lipreading* (pp. 177-189). Hillsdale, NJ: Erlbaum.

Dunn, L., & Markwardt, F. (1988). *Peabody Individual Achievement Test–Revised* (PIAT–R). Circle Pines, MN: American Guidance Service.

Durkin, D. (1966). *Children who read early.* New York: Teachers College.

Durkin, D. (1984). Is there a match between what elementary teachers do and what basal reader manuals recommend? *The Reading Teacher, 37*(8), 734-744.

Elley, W. (1989). Vocabulary acquisition from listening to stories. *Reading Research Quarterly, 24*(2), 174-187.

Engen, E. (1995). *English language acquisition in deaf children.* Final report to the National Institute on Disability and Rehabilitation Research (Grant No. HI33A80070). Providence, RI: Rhode Island School for the Deaf.

Everhart, V., & Marschark, M. (1988). Linguistic flexibility in the written and signed/oral language productions of deaf and hearing children. *Journal of Experimental Child Psychology, 46,* 174-193.

Ewoldt, C. (1981). A psycholinguistic description of selected deaf children reading in sign language. *Reading Research Quarterly, 17*(1), 58-89.

Ewoldt, C. (1985). A descriptive study of the developing literacy of young hearing-impaired children. *The Volta Review, 87*(5), 109-126.

Ewoldt, C. (1986). What does "reading" mean? *Perspectives for Teachers of the Hearing Impaired, 4*(3), 10-13.

Feitelson, D., & Goldstein, Z. (1986). Patterns of book ownership and reading to young children in Israeli school-oriented and non-school oriented families. *The Reading Teacher, 39,* 924-930.

Flood, J. (1977). Parental styles in reading episodes with young children. *The Reading Teacher, 30,* 864-867.

Gallaudet University. (1983). *Stanford Achievement Test for Hearing Impaired Students.* Washington, DC: Gallaudet University. (Available from the Center for Assessment and Demographic Studies, Gallaudet University; 800 Florida Avenue, NE; Washington, DC 20002-3695)

Gartner, G., Trehub, S., & Mackay-Soroka, S. (1993). Word awareness in hearing impaired children. *Applied Psycholinguistics, 14,* 61-73.

Geers, A., & Moog, J. (1989). Factors predictive of the development of literacy in profoundly hearing-impaired adolescents. *The Volta Review, 91*(2), 69-86.

Gelzer, L. (1988). Developing reading appreciation in young children. *Perspectives for Teachers of the Hearing Impaired, 6*(2), 13-16.

Giorcelli, L. (1982). *The comprehension of some aspects of figurative language by deaf and hearing subjects.* Unpublished doctoral dissertation, University of Illinois, Urbana-Champaign.

Gormley, K., & McGill-Franzen, A. (1978). Why can't the deaf read? Comments on asking the wrong question. *American Annals of the Deaf, 123*(5), 542-547.

Green, J., & Harker, J. (1982). Reading to children: A communication process. In J. Langer & M. Smith-Burke (Eds.), *Reader meets author/bridging the gap: A psycholinguistic and sociolinguistic perspective* (pp. 196-221). Newark, DE: International Reading Association.

Griswold, E., & Cummings, J. (1974). The expressive vocabulary of preschool deaf children. *American Annals of the Deaf, 119*(1), 16-28.

Hafer, J., Richmond-Hearty, E., & Swann, M. (1991). Sowing the seeds of literacy. *Perspectives in Education and Deafness, 10*(1), 7-10.

Hanson, V. (1982). Short-term recall by deaf signers of ASL: Implications for order recall. *Journal of Experimental Psychology: Learning, Memory, & Cognition, 8*, 572-583.

Hanson, V. (1989). Phonology and reading: Evidence from profoundly deaf readers. In D. Shankweiler & I. Liberman (Eds.), *Phonology and reading disability: Solving the reading puzzle* (pp. 69-89). Ann Arbor, MI: University of Michigan Press.

Hanson, V. (1991). Phonological processing without sound. In S. Brady & D. Shankweiler (Eds.), *Phonological processes in literacy: A tribute to Isabelle Y. Liberman* (pp. 153-161). Hillsdale, NJ: Erlbaum.

Hanson, V., & Fowler, C. (1987). Phonological coding in word reading: Evidence from hearing and deaf readers. *Memory and Cognition, 15*,199-207.

Hanson, V., Goodell, E., & Perfetti, C. (1991). Tongue-twister effects in the silent reading of deaf college students. *Journal of Memory & Language, 30*, 319-330.

Hanson, V., Liberman, I., & Shankweiler, D. (1984). Linguistic coding by deaf children in relation to beginning reading success. *Journal of Experimental Child Psychology, 37*, 378-393.

Harris, L. (1996). Grab a good e-book. *Electronic Learning.* New York: Scholastic.

Harris, L., & Smith, C. (1986). *Reading instruction: Diagnostic teaching in the classroom.* New York: Macmillan.

Hayden, R. (1987). *Mediating storybook experience.* Paper presented at the annual meeting of the International Reading Association. (ERIC Document Reproduction Service No. ED 283 138)

Hayes, L., & Shaw, P. (1993). Guidelines for selecting read-aloud books for deaf children. In B. Snider (Ed.), *Post Milan ASL and English literacy: Issues, trends, and research* (pp. 105-116). Washington, DC: Gallaudet University Press.

Heath, D. (1982). What no bedtime story means: Narrative skills at home and school. *Language in Society, 11*, 49-76.

Heath, S. (1983). *Ways with words: Language, life, and work in communities and classrooms.* New York: Cambridge University Press.

Hickman, J. (1981). A new perspective on response to literature: Research in an elementary school setting. *Research in the Teaching of English, 15*, 343-354.

Hoggan, K., & Strong, C. (1994). The magic of "once upon a time": Narrative teaching strategies. *Language, Speech, and Hearing Services in Schools, 25*, (pp. 76-89).

Holdaway, D. (1979). *The foundations of literacy.* Portsmouth, NH: Heinemann.

Howard, G. (1991). Culture tales: A narrative approach to therapy in cross-cultural psychology and psychotherapy. *American Psychologist, 40*, 187-197.

Huang, J., & Hatch, E. (1978). A Chinese child's acquisition of English. Reprinted in D. Durkin (Ed.), *Language issues: Readings for teachers* (pp. 117-129). New York: Longman.

Irwin, O. (1960). Infant speech: Effect of systematic reading of stories. *Journal of Speech and Hearing Research, 3*, 187-190.

Isrealite, N. (1981). *Direct antecedent context and comprehension of reversible passive voice sentences.* Unpublished doctoral dissertation, University of Pittsburgh, PA.

Kampfe, C., & Turecheck, A. (1987). Reading achievement of prelingually deaf students and its relationship to parental method of communication: A review of the literature. *American Annals of the Deaf, 132*(1), 11-15.

Karchmer, M., Milone, M., & Wolk, S. (1979). Educational significance of hearing loss at three levels of severity. *American Annals of the Deaf, 124*, 97-109.

Karweit, N. (1989). *The effects of a story reading program on the vocabulary and story comprehension of disadvantaged prekindergarten and kindergarten students.* Baltimore, MD: Center for Research on Elementary and Middle Schools. (ERIC Document Reproduction Service No. ED 313 655)

Kelly, L. (1995). Processing of bottom-up and top-down information by skilled and average deaf readers and implications for whole language instruction. *Exceptional Children, 61*(4), 318-334.

Kelly, L. (1996). The interaction of syntactic competence and vocabulary during reading by deaf students. *Journal of Deaf Studies and Deaf Education, 1*(1), 75-90.

King, C., & Quigley, S. (1985). *Reading and deafness.* San Diego, CA: College-Hill Press.

Kluwin, T., & Papalia, J. (1989, March). *The relationship between knowledge of story structure and question comprehension in young, hearing impaired children.* Paper presented at the Annual Meeting of the American Educational Research Association, San Francisco, CA. (ERIC Document Reproduction Service No. ED 328 048)

Kretschmer, R. (1989). Pragmatics, reading, and writing: Implications for hearing impaired individuals. *Topics in Language Disorders, 9*(4), 17-32.

Lane, H., & Grosjean, F. (1980). *Recent perspectives on American Sign Language.* Hillsdale, NJ: Erlbaum.

Lartz, M., & Lestina, L. (1993). *Introducing deaf children to literacy: What deaf mothers can teach us.* Paper present at the 56th Biennial Meeting of Council of American Instructors of the Deaf, Baltimore, MD.

Leybaert, J. (1993). Reading in the deaf: The roles of phonological codes. In M. Marschark & M. Clark (Eds.), *Psychological perspectives on deafness* (pp. 269-309). Hillsdale, NJ: Erlbaum.

Liberman, I., Shankweiler, D., & Liberman, A. (1989). The alphabetic principle and learning to read. In D. Shankweiler & I. Liberman, (Eds.), *Phonology and reading disability: Solving the reading puzzle* (pp. 1-33). Ann Arbor, MI: University of Michigan Press.

Lichenstein, E. (1983). *The relationships between reading processes and English skills of deaf students.* Unpublished manuscript, National Technical Institute for the Deaf, Rochester, NY.

Lichenstein, E. (1985). Deaf working memory processes and English language skill. In D. Martin, (Ed.), *Cognition, education & deafness: Directions for research and instruction* (pp. 111-114). Washington, DC: Gallaudet University Press.

Lindfors, J. (1987). *Children's language and learning.* Englewood Cliffs, NJ: Prentice-Hall.

Luckner, J., & Humphries, S. (1992). Picturing ideas through graphic organizers. *Perspectives in Education and Deafness, 11*(2), 8-9.

Luetke-Stahlman, B. (1988). The benefit of oral English-only as compared with signed input to hearing-impaired students. *The Volta Review, 90*(7), 349-361.

Luetke-Stahlman, B. (1990). Types of instructional input as predictors of reading achievement for hearing-impaired students. In C. Lucas, (Ed.), *Sign language research: Theoretical issues,* (pp. 325-336). Washington, DC: Gallaudet University Press.

Luetke-Stahlman, B. (1993). Research-based language intervention strategies adapted for D/HH children. *American Annals of the Deaf, 138*(5), 404-410.

Luetke-Stahlman, B. (1998). *Language issues in deaf education.* Hillsboro, OR: Butte Publications.

Luetke-Stahlman, B., Griffiths, C., & Montgomery, N. (1998a). *Text structure development in the oral (signed and spoken) retells of text by a deaf student.* Unpublished manuscript, University of Kansas Medical Center, Kansas City.

Luetke-Stahlman, B., Griffiths, C., & Montgomery, N. (1998b). *A deaf child's language acquisition verified through text retelling.* Unpublished manuscript, University of Kansas Medical Center, Kansas City.

Luetke-Stahlman, B., Hayes, P., & Nielsen, D. (1996). Essential practices as adults read to meet the needs of students who are deaf or hard of hearing. *American Annals of the Deaf, 141*(4), 309-320.

Luetke-Stahlman, B., & Luckner, J. (1991). *Effectively educating students with hearing impairments.* New York: Longman.

MacGinitie, W., & MacGinitie, R. (1989). *Gates-MacGinitie Reading Tests* (3rd ed.). Chicago, IL: Riverside.

Marschark, M. (1993). *Psychological development of deaf children.* New York: Oxford University Press.

Marshall, N. (1983). Using story grammar to assess reading comprehension. *The Reading Teacher, 36*(7), 616-620.

Maxwell, M. (1984). A deaf child's natural development of literacy. *Sign Language Studies, 44,* 191-224.

Maxwell, M. (1986). Beginning reading and deaf children. *American Annals of the Deaf, 131*(1), 14-20.

McAnnally, P., Rose, S., & Quigley, S. (1994). *Language learning practices with deaf children.* Austin, TX: Pro-Ed.

McCabe, A., & Rollins, P. (1994). Assessment of preschool narrative skills. *American Journal of Speech-Language Pathology: A Journal of Clinical Practice, 3*, 45-56.

McCoy, K. (1995). *Teaching special learners in the general education classroom.* Denver: Love.

Miller, K., & Rosenthal, L. (1995). Seeing the big picture: Deaf adults' development of summarization through book discussions in ASL. *Journal of Adolescent & Adult Literacy, 39*(3), 200-206.

Moog, J., & Geers, A. (1985). *Grammatical analysis of elicited language.* St. Louis, MO: Central Institute for the Deaf.

Moores, D. (1967). *Educating the deaf: Psychology, principles, and practice.* Boston: Houghton Mifflin.

Morrow, L. (1986). Effects of structural guidance in story retelling on children's dictation of original stories. *Journal of Reading Behavior, 18*, 135-152.

Morrow, L., O'Connor, E., & Smith, J. (1990). Effects of a story reading program on the literacy development of at-risk kindergarten children. *Journal of Reading Behavior, 22*, 255-275.

Nielsen, D. (1993). The effects of four models of group interaction with storybooks on the literacy growth of low-achieving kindergarten children. In C. Kinzer and D. Leu (Eds.), *Examining central issues in literacy research, theory, practice* (pp. 279-287). Chicago: National Reading Conference.

Ninio, A. (1980). Picture-book reading in mother-infant dyads belonging to two subgroups in Israel. *Child Development, 51*, 587-590.

Ninio, A., & Bruner, J. (1978). The achievement and antecedents of labeling. *Journal of Child Language, 5*, 1-15.

Palincsar, A., & Brown, A. (1986). Interactive teaching to promote independent learning from text. *The Reading Teacher, 39*(8), 771-777.

Paul, P. (1984). *The comprehension of multimeaning words from selected frequency levels by deaf and hearing subjects.* Unpublished doctoral dissertation, University of Illinois, Urbana-Champaign.

Paul, P., & Jackson, D. (1993). *Toward a psychology of deafness: Theoretical and empirical perspectives.* Boston: Allyn & Bacon.

Paul, P., & Quigley, S. (1990). *Education and deafness.* New York: Longman.

Paul, P., & Quigley, S. (1994). *Language and deafness* (2nd ed.). San Diego, CA: Singular.

Payne, J. (1982). *A study of the comprehension of verb-particle combinations among deaf and hearing subjects.* Unpublished doctoral dissertation, University of Illinois, Urbana-Champaign.

Payne, J., & Quigley, S. (1987). Hearing-impaired children's comprehension of verb-particle combinations. *The Volta Review, 89*(3), 133-143.

Perfetti, C., Beck, I., Bell, L., & Hughes, C. (1987). Phonemic knowledge and learning to read are reciprocal: A longitudinal study of first grade children. *Merrill-Palmer Quarterly, 33,* 283-319.

Peterman, C. (1988). *Successful storyreading procedures: Working with kindergarten teachers to improve children's story understanding.* Tucson, AZ: Paper presented at the annual National Reading Conference. (ERIC Document Reproduction Service No. ED 314 739)

Quigley, S., & Power, D. (1972). *The development of syntactic structures in the language of deaf children.* Urbana-Champaign: University of Illinois, Institute for Research on Exceptional Children.

Raffi. (1987). *Down by the bay.* New York, NY: Crown Publishers.

Reid, D., Hresko, W., Hammill, B., & Wiltshire S. (1991). *Test of Early Reading Ability–Deaf or Hard of Hearing* (TERA–D/HH). Austin, TX: Pro-Ed.

Reynolds, R. (1986). Performance of deaf college students on a criterion-referenced modified cloze test of reading comprehension. *American Annals of the Deaf, 131*(5), 361-364.

Robbins, H. & Hatcher, L. (1981). The effects of syntax on the reading of hearing impaired children. *The Volta Review, 3,* 165-115.

Rodda, M., Cummings, C., & Fewer, D. (1993). Memory, learning, and language: Implications for deaf education. In M. Marschark & M. Clark (Eds.), *Psychological perspectives on deafness* (pp. 339-352). Hillsdale, NJ: Erlbaum.

Satchwell, S. (1993). Does teaching reading strategies to deaf children help increase their reading levels? *Association of Canadian Educators of the Hearing Impaired (ACEHI), 19,* 38-48.

Schaper, M., & Reitsma, P. (1993). The use of speech-based recoding in reading by prelingually deaf children. *American Annals of the Deaf, 138*(1), 46-54.

Schein, J., & Delk, M., Jr. (1974). The deaf population. Silver Springs, MD: *National Association of the Deaf.*

Schleper, D. (1995a). Read it again and again . . . and again. *Perspectives in Education and Deafness, 14*(2), 16-19.

Schleper, D. (1995b). Reading to deaf children: Learning from deaf adults. *Perspectives in Education and Deafness, 13*(4), 4-8.

Schlesinger, H., & Meadow, K (1972). *Sound and sign: Childhood deafness and mental health.* Berkeley: University of California Press.

Shores, H. (1960). Reading of science for two separate purposes as perceived by sixth grade students and able adult readers. *Elementary English, 37*(7), 461-468.

Snow, C. (1993). Families as social contexts for literacy development. *New Directions for Child Development, 61*, 11-24.

Stanovich, K. (1994). Constructivism in reading. *Journal of Special Education, 28*(3), 259-274.

Stauffer, R. (1980). *The Language-Experience Approach to the Teaching of Reading.* New York: Harper & Row.

Stein, N., & Glenn, C. (1979). An analysis of story comprehension in elementary school children. In R. Freedle (Ed.), *New directions in discourse processing* (pp. 53-120). Norwood, NJ: Ablex.

Stewart, D., Bennett, D., & Bonkowski, N. (1992). Books to read, books to sign. *Perspectives in Education and Deafness, 10*(3), 4-7.

Stewart, S., & Cegelka, P. (1995). Teaching reading and spelling. In P. Cegelka & W. Berdine (Eds.), *Effective instruction of students with learning difficulties* (pp. 265-302). Boston: Allyn & Bacon.

Swain, M. (1985). Communicative competence: Some roles of comprehensible input and comprehensible output in its development. In S. Gass & C. Madden (Eds.), *Input in second language acquisition* (pp. 235-256). Rowley, MA: Newbury House.

Teale, W. (1984). Reading to young children: Its significance for literacy development. In H. Goelman, A. Oberg, and F. Smith (Eds.), *Awakening to literacy* (pp. 10-130). London: Heinemann.

Topol, D. (1995). *English language acquisition in deaf children.* Final report for the National Institute on Disability and Rehabilitation Research (Grant No. HI 33A80070). Providence, RI: Rhode Island School for the Deaf.

Torgesen, J. (1994). Longitudinal studies of phonological processing and reading. *Journal of Learning Disabilities, 27*(5), 276-286.

Torgesen, J., Morgan, S., & Davis, C. (1992). Effects of two types of phonological awareness training on word learning in kindergarten children. *Journal of Educational Psychological, 84,* 364-370.

Vygotsky, L. (1978). *Mind in society: The development of higher psychological processes* (M. Cole, V. John-Steiner, S. Scribner, & R. Souberman, Trans.). Cambridge, MA: Harvard University Press.

Wandel, J. (1989). *Use of internal speech in reading by hearing and H.I. students in oral, total communication, and cued speech programs.* Unpublished doctoral dissertation, Teachers College, Columbia University, New York City.

Webster, A. (1986). *Deafness, development, and literacy.* New York: Routledge, Chapman & Hall.

Weintraub, L. (1984, November). Once upon a time: Using fairy tales and nursery rhymes to develop pre-reading skills in children. *Perspectives for Teachers of the Hearing Impaired*, 16-19, November.

Wigfield, A., & Asher, S. (1984). Social and motivational influences on reading. In P. Pearson, R. Barr, M. Kamil, and P. Mosenthal (Eds.), *Handbook of research in reading* (pp. 423-452). New York: Longman.

Wiesendunger, K., & Wollenberg, J. (1978). Pre-questioning inhibits third grade reading comprehension. *The Reading Teacher, 31*(8), 892-895.

Wilbur, R., & Goodhart, W. (1985). Comprehension of indefinite pronouns and quantifiers by hearing-impaired children. *Applied Psycholinguistics, 6,* 417-434.

Williams, C. (1994). The language and literacy worlds of three profoundly deaf preschool children. *Reading Research Quarterly, 29*(2), 125-135.

Wilson, K. (1979). *Inference and language processing in hearing and deaf children.* Unpublished doctoral dissertation, Boston University.

Winzer, M. (1985, August). *Encouraging reading through an inactive method: Strategies for hearing impaired children.* Paper presented at the Seventeenth International Congress on the Education of the Deaf, Manchester, England.

Woodcock, R., & Johnson, W. (1989). *Woodcock-Johnson Psychoeducational Battery–Revised.* Allen, TX: DLM Teaching Resources.

Yoshinaga, C., Itano, C., & Snyder, L. (1984). Form and meaning in written language of H. I. children. *The Volta Review, 87*(2), 75-90.

Yurkowski, P., & Ewoldt, C. (1986). A case for the semantic processing of the deaf reader. *American Annals of the Deaf, 131*(3), 243-247.

Chapter 6

Students Reading to Adults and Reading Independently

Day One: Rereading, New Read, and Analyzing

Day Two: Decoding Strategies and Facilitating Meaning

Day Three: Reinforcing Through Word Work and Writing

Day Four: Rereading and Response Activities
  Independent Reading

Resources

Appendix 6-A: Making the Most of a Student
  Reading Session

Appendix 6-B: Narrative Lesson Report

Appendix 6-C: Sight Word Learning

Appendix 6-D: Activities to Extend Reading at
  School or at Home

Appendix 6-E: Literature to Hook Reluctant Readers

Students' reading and writing abilities have been found to reflect their expressive English competence (Horowitz & Samuels, 1987). However, Chall (1983) suggested that by continuing to read and write, students increase language competence. Reading ability can be enhanced when adjustments made in the reading environment optimize the reader's individual skills. Mediation techniques that will help team members create these adjustments are presented in this chapter.

The procedures suggested here are adapted from *Reading Recovery* (RR) (Clay, 1993), a program that uses whole language principles and selective direct instruction procedures (Kelly, 1996) and is designed to *facilitate* and *accelerate* the progress of readers who are not reading on grade level (Clay, 1991a, 1991b). The suggested method is not unlike reciprocal teaching, in which teachers and students take turns leading discussions about text. It includes a repetitive reading strategy, word work, skills facilitated in context, and response or elaboration activities. Introduced in the United States eight years ago, RR is now enthusiastically implemented in more than 40 states (Shanahan & Barr, 1995). (See Center, Wheldall, Freeman, Outhred, & McNaught, 1995a, 1995b; Pinnell, Fried, & Estice, 1990; Pinnell, 1992; and Shanahan & Barr, 1995, for evaluations of the method.)

RR methods supported by research and determined to be effective in promoting proficient readers include practices such as organizing regular reading sessions (for instance, four times a week, for 30–40 minutes a session; Adams, 1994). While many of the practices are being used in both residential and public schools, descriptions or research to verify effectiveness of these procedures with students who are D/HH is scant at this time. Thomas (1997) presented data from applying Reading Recovery procedures to deaf students in Texas over a two-year period. Several researchers (Luetke-Stahlman & Nielsen, 1996; Luetke-Stahlman, Griffiths, & Montgomery, 1998a, 1998b) have reported positive changes in acquisition of English meaning and form variables, as well as positive changes in comprehension of text structure components, after analyzing videotaped retelling samples of a deaf child who had received RR mediation over a two-year period (first and second grades).

This chapter presents four days of student instructional read activities. Team members may already incorporate many of these practices when students who are D/HH read to them. To see to what extent the practices are already used in their programs, team members may wish to take the quiz in Appendix 6–A and discuss the results.

Day One: Rereading, New Read, and Analyzing

One of the main principles of the adapted RR approach is the rereading of level + 1 material. Level + 1 material, as mentioned in Chapter 5, is text that is at the student's instructional reading level—the level slightly more difficult than the student's assessed reading level. Text containing a maximum of five words per every hundred that the student cannot decode independently is considered to be level + 1 text. Series of leveled books can be useful sources of level + 1 material, and new series are continually being published. (See the resource list at the end of this chapter for examples of leveled books and the companies that publish them.)

Day One should begin with the student rereading a level + 1 paragraph, page, or whole text. Although this activity also occurs at the end of the week, it is a good idea to allow the student to demonstrate reading fluency after the natural break from the text that the weekend provides. The reread should take no more than about ten minutes. If the student reads 100 words and fails to decode fewer than five words, the reread is viewed as successful, and material at the next level should be chosen for a "new read." If the student reads the text at less than 95% accuracy, a book of the same level should be selected as a "new read" (see Figure 6–1).

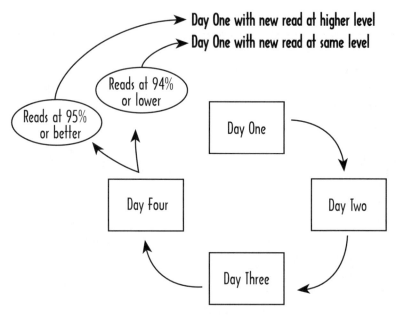

FIGURE 6-1: STUDENT READ PROCESS

The new read might be a whole story or part of it. It might be a chapter of an expository text or only a section of it. The new read should first be introduced; this introduction should take about ten minutes and involve discussion of topics such as the following:

- the meaning of the title or heading
- the relationship of pictures or diagrams to the text
- text structure
- relevant concepts of print (see Figure 6–2)

As part of the introduction, the adult should use any relevant words or phrases that might be unfamiliar to the student.

___ Hold the book like this.	___ Recognize that a sentence can be continued on the next line.
___ Read from the front of the book to the back.	
___ Read left to right.	___ Compare a sentence to a paragraph.
___ At the end of a line, sweep the eyes back to the left side to start a new line.	___ Understand that print tells a story or gives information.
___ Read top to bottom.	___ Identify parts of the book (cover, title, author, illustrator; a page, the first page, the bottom of the page, the last page). *cont.*
___ Compare a letter to a word.	
___ Compare a word to a sentence.	

FIGURE 6-2: CONCEPTS OF PRINT CHECKLIST

FIGURE 6-2, CONT.

___ Identify that a period means to pause.	___ Use the table of contents.
___ Identify that a question mark means a question has been asked.	___ Identify exclamation points.
___ Identify the significance of a capital letter.	___ Use the glossary or dictionary.
	___ Use the index.
___ Identify words emphasized by a different typeface, size, and so forth.	___ Identify Roman numerals.
	___ Compare sizes of headings.
___ Identify italics used for emphasis, stage directions, and so forth.	___ Identify a book that is one of a series.
	___ Understand that words can be hyphenated.
___ Identify quotation marks.	

After the material is introduced, the student reads some or all of the text without interruption or correction, while the adult makes a list of the words or phrases that have been misread. If the student cannot read independently, the adult might write some sentences on sentence strips and practice reading them with the student, reread the book together, or copy pictures from the story or text and ask the student to match them to sentence strips.

Before Day Two activities, the teacher analyzes the words missed by the student on Day One and chooses a few of the most relevant teaching points to emphasize later (for instance, singular versus plural nouns). These words become examples to be used on Days Two and Three as strategies are discussed and practiced. Strategies used by the student to decode and self-correct are noted as well.

> **Study Guide Questions**
>
> 1. *Day One as described has three parts. What examples can you give for each part?*
>
> 2. *How would you practice Day One activities with a peer or a hearing emergent reader? Use the Day One section of the lesson planning sheet in Appendix 6–B.*

Day Two: Decoding Strategies and Facilitating Meaning

The first activity of Day Two involves rereading sentences or paragraphs that contain "new words" that the student was unable to decode the day before. The adult facilitates the correct decoding of these words by modeling a variety of decoding strategies (see Chapter 5). Teaching students strategies to use in decoding unknown words or phrases is a key component of the suggested approach. Phonics, syntactic, visual, and/or orthographic strategies may be used.

- **Phonics strategies:** Sounding out the word is an example of a phonics strategy.
- **Syntactic strategies:** Reading the sentences, skipping unknown words, and then going back and trying again to decode them is an example of a syntactic strategy (also referred to as analysis of content).
- **Visual strategies:** Looking at the pictures and diagrams and going back to another place where the words were used is an example of a visual strategy.
- **Orthographic strategies:** Structural analysis and attention to word families are examples of orthographic strategies. An orthographic activity that may be useful when working with students who are D/HH is provided in Appendix 6–C.

If the student cannot read many words independently, the adult might choose one of the following strategies:

- cut sentence strips into separate word cards
- ask the student to cut sentences into words
- match similar words together and discuss them
- recombine words into the original sentences and compare them to the original text
- replace word cards in a chart and ask the student to pick them out as the adult reads them

Nielsen (1994) suggested that some strategies could be used sequentially, by levels. For example, team members might first try "Level A" strategies to scaffold word recognition skills and then move on to cues that provide the student with less assistance (Levels B, C, D, and E), as shown in Figure 6–3.

Level A: Provide the model.
"That word starts with the /b/ sound." (phonics)
"I saw this word in the title of the story. Here it is." (visual)

Level B: Invite student performance.
"What sound does that word start with?" (visual)
"What is the girl eating?" (meaning)
"Tell me if what I say sounds right: 'The boy are in the house.'
*   Did that sound right"?* (syntactic)
"Find the word rabbit *on this page."* (orthographic)
"Point to the words as you read them." (reinforcing voice-to-
    print match)

Level C: Cue specific elements of a strategy.
"Get your mouth ready." (cue to look at first letter)
"Look at the vowel in that word." (cue to look at vowel)
"Look at the picture." (specific source for meaning)

Level D: Cue specific strategies.
"Did that make sense?" (meaning cue)
"Did that sound right?" (phonics cue)
"Reread that sentence." (syntactic cue)

Level E: Provide general cues.
"What can you try in order to figure that out?"
"What do you do when you are stuck on a word?"
"What are you thinking?" (cue suggesting that self-monitoring
    and taking time to think are valued)

FIGURE 6–3: SCAFFOLDING BY LEVELS

From "Moving from Specific to General Cues," by D. Nielsen, 1994. Unpublished class
handout, University of Kansas, Department of Curriculum and Instruction. Adapted with
permission.

On Day Two, the adult should help the students to define new
words, categorize them, and find synonyms and antonyms for them.
The meaning of sentences, paragraphs, and whole sections of the
text should be discussed interactively; this discussion should be
supported by drawing one or more graphic organizers (word webs,
compare/contrast charts, and so on). Two examples are provided in
Figure 6–4; others appear in the appendix to Chapter 5 and throughout this text.

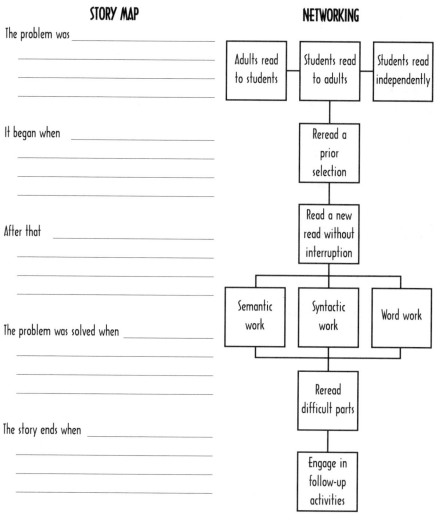

STORY MAP

The problem was _____

_____

_____

It began when _____

_____

_____

After that _____

_____

_____

The problem was solved when _____

_____

_____

The story ends when _____

_____

_____

NETWORKING

| Adults read to students | Students read to adults | Students read independently |

Reread a prior selection

Read a new read without interruption

| Semantic work | Syntactic work | Word work |

Reread difficult parts

Engage in follow-up activities

FIGURE 6–4: GRAPHIC ORGANIZERS TO AID COMPREHENSION

Day Three: Reinforcing Through Word Work and Writing

Study Guide Question
How can you use the lesson plan for Day Two provided in Appendix 6–B?

Word work is the third key component to this reading approach. On Day Three, the adult should manipulate new words to facilitate phonological awareness by using decoding strategies—phonics approach, orthographic approach, or a combination of both. (Some adults might prefer to switch Day Two and Day Three activities.)

Adults should refer to sentences in the text that contain target words, and ask the student to use one of the following strategies.

1. **Sound out a word.**
   - Focus initial assistance on the sounds that appear to be best understood by the student.
   - Assist with the decoding of words that follow the rules before those that do not.
   - Do not avoid words that are irregular and must be memorized.
   - As a last resort, use a multiple-choice question prompt (either with or without speechreading): *"Do you think that word might be* walk, run, *or* hop?*" or *"Do you think it might be* walk, wall, *or* wait?*"*

In using this strategy, team members may want to refer to phonics rules to show patterns of English to students. As is stressed throughout this adapted RR approach, phonics rules should not be taught out of context through workbook pages completed in isolation; they should be taught as students decode difficult words in instructional level materials.

EXAMPLES OF PHONICS RULES

- When the letter *c* is followed by *e, i,* or *y,* its sound is usually /s/ (*city, cent, cycle*).
- When the letter *c* is followed by *a* or *o,* its sound is usually /k/ (*cot, cat, coat, incantation*).
- When *c* and *h* are next to each other, they usually make only one sound, /ch/ (*church, chum, lunch*).

cont.

> - When *s* and *h* are next to each other,
>   they usually make only one sound,
>   /sh/ (*shot, shine, wish*).
> - When a word ends with a vowel-
>   consonant-*e* combination, the vowel
>   sound is usually long (*bake, make,
>   like*).
> - When there are two vowels side by
>   side, the second vowel usually is
>   silent (*coat, mean*).
> - When *y* is the final letter of a word, it
>   usually has the sound /ē/ or /ī/
>   (*candy, my*).
> - Double consonants make only one
>   sound (*fell*).
>
> From *Direct Instruction Reading* (3rd ed.), by D.
> Carnine, J. Silbert, and E. Kameenui, 1997, Upper
> Saddle River, New Jersey: Prentice Hall. Copyright
> 1997 by Prentice Hall. Adapted with permission.

2. **Help the student to distinguish sounds from letters.**
   *"Find a word on this page that starts with b. What sound does
   it say?"*
   *"If I read a word with the /b/ sound in this sentence, can you
   point to the letter?"*

3. **Teach consonant sounds first but introduce vowel
   sounds early, before all consonants are mastered.**

4. **Teach the most common sounds of the letters first.**
   - Continuous sounds: a, e, f, i, m, n, r, s, u, w, z
   - Stops: b, c, d, g, h, j, k, q, t, x

5. **Introduce sound combinations early.**
   Once four or five sounds can be articulated by students,
   ask them to decode CVC (consonant-vowel-consonant)
   words so that discrete skills are given a functional
   application. Continue introducing word structures in
   order of difficulty.

- VC and CVC words (*at, bat*)
- CVCC words that begin with continuous sounds (CS) (*runs, fish*)
- CCVC words beginning with CS (*slap, frog*)
- CCVCC words (*brand, scamp*)
- CCCVC and CCCVCCC words (*split, scratch*)

Specifically teach digraphs, in which consonant pairs make one sound (*ch, sh, th, wh, ng*).

6. **Play Odd One Out, in which three or more words are compared and discussed (for example, *cat, bat, but*).**

7. **Find other words on a page that start or end with the same sound, letter, consonant cluster, and so on.**

8. **Divide words into sounds, letters, syllables.**

9. **Fingerspell words by syllables.**

10. **Segment words.**
    Ms. Gaustad: *"What are the sounds in the word* bike*?"*

    Student: *"/b/ /i/ /k/?"*

    Ms. Gaustad: *"Good job. And what is that word?"*

    Student: *"Bike."*

    Ms. Gaustad: *"Can you find /b/ /i/ /k/ in this paragraph?"*

11. **Blend words.**
    Mr. Conway: *"Somewhere on this page you read yesterday the sounds /b/ /i/ /k/ are found together. Can you find them?"*

    Student: *"Here they are."* (points)

    Mr. Conway: *"And it says . . .?"*

    Student: *"Bike."*

12. Rhyme words.

Ms. Lartz:	*"What word rhymes with* bike*?"*
Student:	*"Hike."*
Ms. Lartz:	*"Let's look at this alphabet strip and see if we can find more words in that family."*
Student:	*"Like, Mike, pike."*
Ms. Lartz:	*"Good work!"*

13. Discuss the compound parts of words and their meanings.

14. Spell words; check their spelling compared to word cards.

15. Make word families.

16. Tell what words contractions comprise.

17. Discuss root words and affixes (see Table 6–1).

Root:	part of a word that gives its derivation or basic meaning
Prefix:	unit at the beginning of a word that changes the meaning of the original word
Suffix:	unit at the end of a word that changes the meaning of the original word
Affix:	general term referring to either a prefix or a suffix

TABLE 6–1: COMMON AFFIXES AND INFLECTED ENDINGS

AFFIX FORMS	MEANING	EXAMPLES
Suffix		
-able	capable of being	agreeable, comfortable
-ance	stage of being	allowance, insurance
-ant	one who	accountant, expectant
-ent	being one who	violent, excellent
-er	relating to, like	harder, older
-ful	full of	joyful, thoughtful
-fy	to make	beautify, magnify
-ish	like	foolish, sheepish
-ist	one who	artist, geologist
-ive	relating to	active, creative
-less	unable to, without	careless, thoughtless
-ly	in a way	honestly, loudly
-ment	state of being	excitement, movement
-ness	state of being	blindness, faithfulness
-ous	full of	mysterious, victorious
-tion	act, state of being	confusion, protection
-ward	turning to	southward, forward
-ible	capable of, worthy	credible, edible
-age	state or act of	advantage, bondage
-ty	quality or state	equality, majesty
-some	like	handsome, lonesome
Prefix		
anti-	against	antiwar, antifreeze
abs-	from	abstain, absent
bi-	two	bicycle, bifocal
co-	with, together with	coworker, coeducation
de-	down, from, away	defrost, desegregate
dis-	opposite	disenchant, disinherit
en-	in, into, make	entrust, engrave
ex-	former, from	exclude, exclaim
im-	not, in	impatient, implant
in-	not, into	incredible, indefensible
inter-	between	interracial, interlude

cont.

TABLE 6–1, CONT.

ir-	not, into	irreversible, irrecoverable
mis-	wrong	misread, misbehave
non-	not	nondrinker, nonvoting
pre-	before	predict, preface
pro-	for, in front of	prolabor, proactivity
re-	back again	rediscover, redirect
semi-	half, partly	semiprofessional, semiannual
sub-	under, less than	subterranean, subtitle
super-	over, above	superhuman, superimposed
trans-	beyond, across	transceiver, transcription
un-	not	unlucky, unhealthy

Common Inflected Endings

-ing	present progressive	running, laughing
-ed	past tense	called, studied
-s	plural	shoes, cats
-'s	possessive	John's, Joyce's
-er	comparative	bigger, stronger
-est	superlative	biggest, strongest

From "Teaching Reading and Spelling," by S. Stewart and P. Cegelka in *Effective Instruction of Students with Learning Difficulties* (p. 282), by P. Cegelka and W. Berdine, 1995, Boston: Allyn & Bacon. Copyright 1995 by Allyn & Bacon. Reprinted with permission.

It is suggested that Day Three end by having each student choose a sentence that contains one or more of the words he or she had difficulty decoding. The teacher dictates the sentence to the student, who writes whatever parts of the sentence he or she can (first and last letters of words, whole words), and the teacher fills in the rest. Together they use the strategies that they have been practicing to determine the letters and write a correct English sentence. The writing of this sentence helps students to make the connection

Study Guide Questions

1. Which of the strategies presented involve phonics and which involve orthographics or structure?

2. How would you teach phonics strategies in context to a student who is hard of hearing?

between writing and reading. Such adult-student experiences also provide team members with opportunities to observe the strategies students are using.

Other word recognition strategies to practice on Day Two or Three include semantic (*"Did that make sense?"*), syntactic (*"What word might fit here?"*), self-correction (*"How did you know that word?"*), cross-checking (*"Is there another way to decide?"*), and self-monitoring strategies (*"What did you notice?"*). Gilbert (1977) also suggested teaching phonological awareness skills through movement experiences. Having students form letters with their bodies or move only when a syllable is accented are two examples from her book.

> **Study Guide Question**
>
> *Can you use the parts of the lesson plan provided in Appendix 6–B to practice Day Three activities?*

Day Four: Rereading and Response Activities

The student should now reread the material from Day One while the adult watches and does not interrupt. The adult again records words or phrases that were not decoded correctly. The Day Four transcription of reading has been called a "running record" (Clay, 1979). If more than five words per hundred (more than 5%) are missed, new material at the same level of difficulty should be read the next week. If the student is able to read three selections with 95% or greater accuracy, the new read should be at the next level. This starts Day One activities over again.

Before moving on from the instructional read of the week, the student should engage in a response activity of some kind:
- giving an oral (signed and/or voice) retell
- reading a written retell to an audience that has not read the material (parents, grandparents, peer) as exemplified in Figure 6–5
- completing a project based on the selection (see suggested activities for extending a reading session in Appendix 6–D)
- dramatizing the materials using English

- responding correctly to comprehension questions that focus on text structure, incorporating novel vocabulary and syntax in the response
- summarizing the text

This letter is an example of a written retell. This retell was supplied by the mother of a nine-year-old deaf girl entering fourth grade. It was written by the mother and daughter together. Ms. Owens is her teacher.

September 11, 1998

Dear Mrs. Owens,

    I read a lot of books this summer and now that we are back in school I want to show you how I can use some of the new vocabulary I learned. Maybe you can use this idea at school. I could learn new vocabulary at school and we could type up a letter to my parents or Grandma Bette that is something like this one.

My Mom typed this outline so I can use new vocabulary from several books. Here goes.

One of the first books I read with Mom was by R. L. Stine. In the story, the author wrote as if I were the main character. At one point in the story, I _____ to a _____ that was two _____ high. It was _____ _____ outside.

       trudged   pitch black   mansion   stories

I could hear some _____ _____ _____ music in the old house that used to belong to a _____. (A professor is a college teacher.) I went in through the _____ and the air smelled _____.

      professor   stale   entryway   rock and roll

cont.

FIGURE 6–5: A WRITTEN RETELL

FIGURE 6-5, CONT.

> The curtains were _____ and the _____ in the living room was old. I found some kids in this club. One girl was named Marcie (almost like me!) and she had a dark _____ of hair.
>
> sofa   faded   mane

The response technique of summarization can be implemented in a variety of ways. Team members might, for example, follow text structure components. For a narrative text, students might be guided by an adult to introduce the main character(s), the setting, and the sequence of events, including the resolution of a problem and conclusion of the story.

Brown and Day (1983) suggested another approach to summarization. Their approach involves a series of rules for summarizing texts: "The first two rules require the deletion of unnecessary material. The third rule, superordination, requires the substitution of a superordinate term for a list of items or actions. The fourth and fifth rules deal with [providing] topic sentences for each paragraph" (p. 509).

Anderson and Hidi (1988) recommended these procedures for teaching students how to summarize:
1. Expect students in the early stages of learning reading to summarize what they've read.
2. Choose short excerpts to be summarized.
3. Begin by summarizing narrative text before other genres.
4. Begin with text that is well-organized, or use students' own work.
5. Initially, allow students to look at the text as they compose their summations.
6. Teach students that a summary includes information that is *important to the author*. Signaling devices that authors use to stress importance include
   a. introductory statements
   b. topic sentences
   c. summary statements
   d. underlining

268

e. italics
f. key phrases
g. repetition
Students should look for these devices in sample text.

Naremore, Densmore, and Harman (1995) recommended the use of a graphic organizer to assist students in summarizing the main idea and supporting details. Figure 6-6 provides a sample of a graphic organizer that is fun and useful for summarizing.

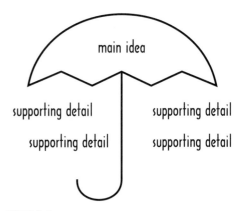

Response activities might also include elaboration activities. Variation in such activities

FIGURE 6-6: GRAPHIC ORGANIZER FOR SUMMARIZING TEXT

can meet individual student needs and affect motivation. Teachers can develop flexibility in their students' abilities to elaborate by asking questions representing different response techniques (analogies, transformations, compare or contrast). Weinstein, Ridley, Dahl, and Weber (1989) suggested using prompts such as the following:

- Have I ever been in a situation where I felt like the main character?
- How could I represent this information in a diagram?
- How could I teach this to my Dad?
- How do I feel about the author's words?
- How does this apply to my life?
- If I lived during this period, how would I feel about my life?
- If I were going to interview the author, what would I ask her?
- What is the main idea of this story?

Naremore et al. (1995) provided the following guidelines for when team members can expect students who are D/HH to include main ideas and details in their summaries (p. 194).

Task	Grade
Main ideas in lists of words	1 and up
Main ideas in sentences	2 and up
Main ideas and details in paragraphs where the main idea is explicitly stated	3 and up
Main ideas and details in paragraphs where the main idea is implicitly stated	4 and up
Main ideas and details in short passages where the main idea is explicit	5 and up
Main ideas and details in short passages where the main idea is implicit	5 and up
Main idea outlines for short passages where the main idea is explicit	6 and up
Main idea outlines for short passages where the main idea is implicit	6 and up
Main ideas in long passages (such as entire chapters in a textbook)	7 and up

Independent Reading

Study Guide Question
Can you use the lesson plan report found in Appendix 6–B as you facilitate a "student-read-to-adult" session? Discuss the challenging parts of the lesson with a peer.

Students should be encouraged to read daily at their independent reading level. By definition, students are able to read proficiently materials at this level without adult mediation. Independent-level materials are those that are at a student's assessed reading level. Reading independently with success can bolster self-esteem. Again, leveled books previously read with an adult could be used. Many publishers indicate the grade level of paperbacks on the back cover to assist in choosing appropriate independent reading materials. Parents can also find books in the library or local bookstores that are at the student's assessed reading level.

   Independent read books = Books at student's assessed reading level

Worthy (1996) noted that "when students have strong interests in what they read, they can frequently transcend their so-called reading level" (p. 205). She provided a helpful list of books that will "hook" reluctant readers and keep them reading. The list is provided in Appendix 6–E.

Students often enjoy series books and Worthy (1996) suggested a number of them on her list (Appendix 6–E). Mackey (1990) speculated that the popularity of series books is due to the familiarity students feel toward the characters (their personalities, relationships to one another, and so on) and toward the events in the stories. The English language and content grow more familiar with the reading of each book in the series. Series books allow students who are D/HH to behave like experienced readers. Students can also enter a bookstore or library and locate the books in their favorite series, make independent choices, and decide when they have outgrown the series. Greenlee, Monson, and Taylor (1996) found that students reported a large collection of series books at the local public library but only a few at school libraries. Both Greenlee et al. (1996) and Worthy contend that students will read independently if allowed to choose what they read, including series books. Students enjoy literature of a higher quality but sometimes need guidance in finding such literature, whereas series books are more easily identifiable.

Independent reading time can occur at school ("SSR time" or Silent Sustained Reading periods) but can also be organized by parents at home. For example, one parent asks her deaf children to be in their pajamas with teeth brushed by 8:00 p.m. and expects to find them in bed reading from 8 p.m. to 9:00 p.m. She reports that these third and fifth graders really enjoy this quiet time with their books.

> **Study Guide Question**
>
> *Interview an administrator, a teacher of the deaf, a general education teacher, and a parent. How much independent reading time do they plan for students who are D/HH?*

Summary

Activities to assist in the organizing of weekly student reading sessions are provided in this chapter. With practice and evaluation, team members can become skilled at including the suggested activities in daily lessons so that students who are D/HH become more proficient readers.

Activities

1. Take the quiz in Appendix 6–A. Give three more ways to incorporate some of the activities discussed in this chapter into reading sessions when students who are D/HH read to adults.

2. Use the lesson plan report form provided in Appendix 6–B for a week, and discuss the strengths and weaknesses with a peer.

3. Add to the list of activities for parents in Appendix 6–C; have parents discuss their impressions of these activities.

4. Ask teachers which of the following recommended pictorial dictionaries they prefer:
   Guralnik, D. (1983). *New World Dictionary for Readers.* New York: Simon and Schuster.
   Levey, J. (1990). *Macmillan First Dictionary.* New York: Macmillan.
   Macmillan Visual Dictionary (1992). New York: Macmillan.
   Vienna, F. (1979). *Children's Dictionary: An American Heritage Dictionary.* Boston: Houghton Mifflin.
   Wittels, H. & Greisman, J. (1985). *A First Thesaurus.* New York: Golden Books.

Resources for Leveled Books for Young Readers

Hello Reader
Scholastic
730 Broadway
New York, NY 10003

Rigby
P.O. Box 797
Crystal Lake, IL 60039-0797
800-822-8661

STEP Into Reading
Random House
201 E. 50th St.
New York, NY 10022

I Can Read Books
HarperCollins
10 E. 53rd St.
New York, NY 10022-5299

School Zone
School Zone Publishing
P. O. Box 777
Grand Haven, MI 49417

Wright Group
19201 120th Ave, NE
Bothell, WA 08011

High Interest/Low Read Resources

Globe Fearon
4350 Equity Drive
P.O. Box 2649
Columbus, OH 43216

New Readers Press
Dept. 597
P.O. Box 888
Syracuse, NY 13210-0888

Phoenix Learning Resources
2349 Chaffee Drive
St. Louis, MO 63146

Steck-Vaughn
P.O. Box 26015
Austin, TX 78755

Appendix 6-A

Making the Most of a Student Reading Session: How Do You Rate?

"Student read to adult" is an activity during which a student (or small group of students) reads to an adult by speaking, cueing, and/or signing the printed text. The adult might be a teacher, parent, librarian, or any interested adult. Recent research has demonstrated that while many teachers of the deaf facilitate reading sessions with their students, they are not always including important components (Bilson, Hayes, & Luetke-Stahlman, 1996). The research supporting the need for these components or essential practices is provided by Luetke-Stahlman, Hayes, and Nielsen (1996). To see if you (as well as parents and others in your program) are including the essential aspects of student-read sessions, you are invited to take this quiz. Keep track of your responses and check them against the information provided at the end of the quiz. Good luck!

1. When choosing an "appropriate" book or story, I might make my selection because the content (a) uses a particular story structure; (b) calls attention to a unit theme; (c) includes a specific vocabulary word or phrase that was experienced in another story; (d) has beautiful pictures; (e) is of interest to the student; (f) all except "e"; (g) all of the above.

2. Students should always be reading (a) selections that include English grammar and vocabulary that is slightly more difficult than what they themselves express; (b) "instructional level" selections; (c) both "a" and "b."

3. I schedule student-read sessions (a) as often as I can; (b) twice a week; (c) three times a week; (d) four or five times a week.

4. I begin the student-read session by (a) asking the student to reread material from the previous session; (b) reading some of the selection to the student; (c) allowing the student to read without interruption; (d) introducing a new selection (see #5 below); (e) all of the above.

5. I introduce a new selection for the student-read if the student reads some familiar material (a) perfectly; (b) 95% correctly; (c) 90% correctly; (d) less than 90% correctly.

cont.

6. During the introduction the student and I also (a) discuss the title or headings; (b) make predictions; (c) discuss the author or illustrator; (d) use novel or technical vocabulary in our interactive dialogues; (e) discuss relevant concepts of print; (f) cover the print and look instead at the pictures or diagrams; (g) link text to life; (h) all of the above; (i) all but "e."

7. Once the student has started reading, I should be (a) reading some of the selection to the student; (b) allowing the student to read without interruption.

8. As the student reads, I model that I enjoy reading and value the experience (a) often with each story or text; (b) sometimes; (c) rarely.

9. I have the student read the selection again (a) once or twice in a week; (b) three times in a week; (c) when we have time; (d) rarely.

10. If I do have the student read a second time, I (a) don't stop to talk much and possibly risk losing the story line; (b) discuss the selection with the student at the end of the reading; (c) engage the student before, during, and after in an interactive dialogue about the selection.

11. If I do have the student read a narrative a second time, I usually discuss (a) the main characters; (b) primarily the main characters, setting, and conclusion of the story; (c) all of the story structure elements.

12. If I do have the student read a second time and if he or she mispronounces a word (in speech, cues, or signs), I might stop at the next logical place (end of paragraph, end of page, and so on) and facilitate decoding by (a) signing, fingerspelling, or cueing the word; (b) calling attention to pictures or parts of the word; (c) providing a synonym for the word.

13. I (a) often; (b) sometimes; (c) rarely suggest that the student reread a sentence that contains a word he or she has mispronounced.

14. If the student doesn't hear sound at all, I might look at one or more words from those I recorded during the first student-read and help the student to (a) define it; (b) give me one or more synonyms; (c) fingerspell it; (d) engage in structural analysis of the word (finding the root word, covering parts of a compound word, discussing affixes and inflections, and so on); (e) sound it out; (f) all of the above except "e"; (g) all of the above during the third reading.

cont.

15. If the student has some hearing ability, I look at my list (see #14) and ask him or her to (a) blend; (b) segment; (c) rhyme; (d) discuss word families; (e) all of the above during the third reading.

16. I (a) often; (b) sometimes; (c) rarely ask about a concept of print.

17. I (a) often; (b) sometimes; (c) rarely ask the student to give an oral response (in speech, cues, or signs) or a written response.

18. I (a) often; (b) sometimes; (c) rarely have students act out all or part of the story, send the story or a shortened version home, and/or have the student draw a picture or diagram about some part of the text.

Answers: One Point for Each Correct Response

1. (g) all of the above. Criteria used to make a selection are currently being researched and usually include all of these factors to some degree.

2. (c) both "a" and "b"   Texts should be chosen that are within the student's "zone of proximal development"—challenging but not frustrating to comprehend (Vygotsky, 1978). Reading assessments can be conducted so that the student's level of English comprehension is known. Then, based on this information, texts should be chosen that are written at a slightly more difficult grammatical and semantic level than is understood by the student (level + 1). This level is the same as the instructional level.

3. (d) Students should read on their instructional level at least four times a week, if not more often.

4. (a) At the start of each daily session, students should be asked to reread a whole story, page, or paragraph of text that they have read previously at 95% accuracy.

5. (a) or (b) This criterion is based on the Reading Recovery model. Although it has not been empirically studied in deaf education, it is highly recommended.

6. (h) Adults should always take the time to introduce the story and link it to the student's life, helping students to make text-to-life connections. Adults can do this by activating thinking about the title of the text, explaining the historical period in which a story occurs, discussing the

cont.

material as fact or fiction, and discussing predictions about context. Naming the author or illustrator, using novel vocabulary in discussions, discussing concepts of print, and talking through the material while looking at pictures, diagrams, and so on, are also important introduction activities.

7. (b) The student should read without interruption as the adult notes words that are misread and the page numbers on which they occur. Strategies used when self-correction occurs should be noted if possible. And yes, it is hard to write and at the same time watch a student sign/read!

8. (a) Books and stories modeled by adults as those particularly enjoyed are the same materials that students want to read and discuss. School staff and parents can increase the enjoyment of a read aloud by using a language or system that is easily understood by the student and by choosing stories for which the child has the required background knowledge or interest.

9. (c) Rereading text is highly recommended by researchers and educators and depends on what is being read. The student should be asked to read approximately 100 words of what was read previously at least three times in a week. Parents and older students or siblings can also be asked to listen to the student reread the text.

10. (c) Adults need to mediate the story, making it a meaning-making experience. Analytical conversation, which causes the student to compare or contrast, make judgments, and so on, should occur through an interactive dialogue using questions, strategy talk, and making predictions. As the story unfolds, relevant ideas should be emphasized and irrelevant predictions discarded. Plenty of open-ended questions should be asked, focused on keeping the student from attending to relatively unimportant story details. The atmosphere should be one that encourages the student's risk-taking in using English structures, discussing the text with regard to his or her own life, and responding cognitively (summarizing, providing a new title, and so on).

11. (c) The adult and student should discuss all of the story structure elements—character, setting, problem, solution.

12. (a) Novel or challenging vocabulary should be signed, cued, or fingerspelled and not avoided. Instead of only preteaching vocabulary that

cont.

is important to text comprehension, adults can discuss words and phrases in context when they introduce the story, again during the reading of the story, and once again after the story has been read.

If the students understand English signing, then signs and markers can be used to further discuss the form and meaning of the word or phrase. If the students use ASL, then the adult can facilitate discussion that compares and contrasts the meaning of the English word(s) and the ASL equivalent(s).

Paul and Quigley (1994) suggested that special attention be given to text that includes pronouns (including *this* and *that*, and making sure the children can identify the word or words they represent), variations of verbs (*break, breaking, broke, broken*), the meaning of clauses, the shades of meaning that modals represent (*can, could, might*), and inferences.

13. (a) When students are asked to reread sentences, paragraphs, or pages, they are the beneficiaries of multiple exposures to specific grammar, vocabulary, and complex story structure. Hickman (1981) noted that repeated readings affect the depth of student responses, their ability to make more complicated predictions, and their literacy achievement.

14. (f) or (g) The order of these essential practices is not important, but planning lessons so that they are included will facilitate reading proficiency.

15. (e) If students have some hearing ability, adults might call attention to some initial and final sounds, rhyming patterns, the blending of sounds to form words, and the names of sounds as compared to the names of letters. Adults might also facilitate the student's knowledge of words that cannot be sounded out easily (such as *night*) and spelling similarities (*back* compared to *black*).

16. (a) Students should be asked to use fingerspelling or signs to label concepts of print used in a story. These might include basic concepts such as the direction of the print or what an exclamation point is, as well as more sophisticated terms such as *chapter* and *subheading*. See Andrew and Akamatsu (1993) for more detail.

17. (a) or (b) Retelling the story is a very important activity and should not be overlooked.

cont.

18. (a) Adults should provide a variety of verbal responses (retell or paraphrase, journal) and nonverbal responses (art, mime) to the read aloud. They can have the student retell the story using puppets; role play the story; or use graphic organizers such as story maps, networking, and word webs, so that the story elements are clarified and understood as important components of every story. Retell activities can deepen the students' comprehension of the story and increase their ability to discuss the form and meaning of the text. Older students might be asked to decide on a new title, develop test questions, or invent a new ending.

Tallying Your Score

Count up your points. How did you do? Can you set some professional goals for improvement?

15–18 points
Congratulations! Your students are effectively reading to adults at home and at school. Keep them at it.

11–14 points
Your students have made a good start in the reading program you are providing, but there is room for improvement. They are including many of the essential components when they read to school staff or parents, but you need to facilitate the inclusion of more of the suggested practices.

0–10 points
Perhaps the information provided in this chapter will help you to modify the school reading program so that students can improve their reading sessions with adults.

Appendix 6-B

Narrative Lesson Report*

Day One

STUDENT _____

DATE _____

LEVEL _____

TEACHER _____

LESSON _____

WEEK _____

1. FAMILIAR REREAD of a page, story, or several stories.
(Independent Level ____)

Description/Title(s) _____

Word Recognition: P F G   Fluency: P F G   Cueing: M S V
(P=poor; F=fair; G=good)

Comments: Student's Strategy Talk: M S V
(M = meaning, including picture   S = syntax of sentence
V = visual aspects of words; phonics decoding, sight words)

Running Record:

In every 100 words, student is missing 5 words or fewer ____ (yes) Are
mistakes made in a meaningful way? ____ (Do errors make sense? ____
Is the student self-correcting? ____)

cont.

*Unpublished report form prepared by B. Luetke-Stahlman, D. Nielsen, & P. Hayes, 1995. University of Kansas Medical Center, Kansas City.

2. NEW MATERIAL

New book _____ Level _____

Focus of this lesson _____

Introduction:

value _____ enjoyment _____ predictions _____

Link: history _____ culture _____ child's life _____

past stories _____

Cover: title _____ author _____ illustrator _____ headings _____

Story structure: characters _____ setting _____

problem _____ events _____ conclusion _____ pictures _____

graphics _____

Concepts of print and books: period _____ comma _____

quotation marks _____ exclamation _____ headings _____

first/last sentence _____ table of contents _____ paragraph _____

index _____

3. FIRST READ

New vocabulary (misread by the student):

Day Two

DECODING STRATEGIES

1. Discussed strategies for decoding unknown words

Phonetic strategies:

Syntactic strategies:

Visual strategies:

Orthographic strategies:

Combinations:

cont.

2. Discussed
    figurative English ＿＿＿ multiple meanings ＿＿＿
    verb particle (come on, come over) ＿＿＿ inferences ＿＿＿
    vocabulary ＿＿＿

3. Discussed

    Definitions of: ＿＿＿＿＿＿＿＿＿＿＿＿＿＿＿＿＿＿＿＿＿＿＿＿＿＿

    Antonyms of: ＿＿＿＿＿＿＿＿＿＿＿＿＿＿＿＿＿＿＿＿＿＿＿＿＿＿

    Synonyms of: ＿＿＿＿＿＿＿＿＿＿＿＿＿＿＿＿＿＿＿＿＿＿＿＿＿＿

    Explanations of: ＿＿＿＿＿＿＿＿＿＿＿＿＿＿＿＿＿＿＿＿＿＿＿＿

4. Discussed grammar
    Anaphoric relationships within conjoined sentences (Sally went home and she slept.): ＿＿＿＿＿＿
    Verb inflections (*breaks, breaking, broke, broken*): ＿＿＿＿＿＿
    Indefinite pronouns (*this, that*): ＿＿＿＿＿＿
    Relative clauses: ＿＿＿＿＿＿
    Modals (*can, will, should*): ＿＿＿＿＿＿
    Syntactic parsing (by clauses; by noun/verb phrases; by noun/verb/object; and so on): ＿＿＿＿＿＿

MEANING FACILITATION

5. Discussed story structure
    Characters: ＿＿＿ Setting: ＿＿＿ Problem/goals: ＿＿＿
    Conclusion/resolution: ＿＿＿

6. Asked comprehension questions (who, what, when, where, why, how related to the key episodes of the story):

cont.

Day Three

PHONOLOGICAL AWARENESS

1. Phonics approaches
    __ Sound it out
    __ Sounds versus letters
    __ Introduce sound combinations
    __ Tell me a word that starts/ends like _____
    __ Oddity tasks (odd one out: *boy, bird, plane, ball*) ____
    Rhyming ___ Initial consonants ____ Mixed sets ____

    __ Find other words on the page that start or end with the same
    letter _____
    __ Divide words into syllables ____
    __ Segment ("In the word *boat*, how many sounds do you
    hear?") ____
    Adult says word, student moves markers. ____
    Student says and segments. ____
    Given a word, student writes letters in boxes. ____
    __ Blend (*"Listen to these sounds. What word do they make?"*) ____
    __ Rhyme words ____

2. Orthographic approaches
    __ Discuss compound words
    __ Spell words
    __ Discuss word families
    __ Inflection work
    __ Root words and affixes
    __ Contractions

Student's strengths: _____

Areas of need: _____

(Priority need) Focus for next lesson: _____

Appendix 6-C

Sight Word Learning: An Orthographic Strategy

Gaskins, Ehri, Cress, O'Hara, and Donnelly (1997) described the phases that children go through in learning to read sign words. As they discussed, students use cues to remember sight words and move from a prealphabetic phase to full and consolidated alphabetic phases as illustrated in the figure.

Phases of Sight Word Learning

Prealphabetic phase
Remembering a distinctive, purely *visual* cue
Example: tall posts for double *l*s

yellow

Partial alphabetic phase
Remembering limited matches between
salient letter sounds
Example: matches between *K* and *N* only

KitteN
↓   ↓
K it n

Full alphabetic phase
Remembering matches between *all* letters
and sounds
Example: 4 letter units matched to 4 sound units

C L O C K
↓ ↓ ↓ ↓
k l o k

Consolidated alphabetic phase
Remembering matches between multiletter
units and syllabic units
Example: matching onset and rime units

CRATE
↓   ↓
kr at

From "Procedures for Word Learning: Making Discoveries about Words," by I. Gaskins, L. Ehri, C. Cress, C. O'Hara, & K. Donnelly, 1997, *The Reading Teacher, 50* (4), pp. 312-327. Copyright 1997 by the International Reading Association. Adapted with permission.

Appendix 6-D

Activities to Extend Reading at School or at Home*

1. Read the story and be mindful of its content. Talk about related content when opportunities arise at school, home, or out in the community.

2. Upon request by a teacher, gather the materials that might be needed to tell the story at school. For example, for one particular story, a third grade teacher asked a parent to supply a fake, potted, tall tree; three Chinese dolls; a cardboard wolf; a basket; and some thin rope. Parents' willingness to hunt up items allows the teacher time to concentrate on other aspects of reading the story and gives the parents the satisfaction of assisting.

3. Upon request by a teacher, collect pictures needed to augment a story. For example, for one story a parent was asked to photocopy scale pictures of a mouse, a mole, a chipmunk, a fox, a donkey, and a horse. These were glued on a strip of paper sequenced by size. This size comparison was used to help students comprehend the setting of the story. These strips were later made into bookmarks.

4. Adults can rent videos or secure them from The National Captioning Institute (1447 E. Main Street, Spartanburg, SC 29307), and provide opportunities for students to watch them. Research suggests that multiple exposure to the same stories benefits students. If captioned versions cannot be found, show the uncaptioned version. This global exposure to the story will still be helpful as students read the tale with a better visual understanding.

5. Adults can buy single copies of the stories that are bound in the basal text or check them out from the public library. This allows students the opportunity to reread the story at home and share it with others. It also clarifies that the story is really a book in and of itself.

6. Provide a quiet time and a comfortable spot for reading on a daily basis. Sit near the student and read independently, too.

cont.

*From "Literacy . . . the most important challenge: Checklist," by B. Luetke-Stahlman, C. Griffiths, and D. Stryker, 1997, *Perspectives in Education and Deafness, 15* (4) pp. 10-11. Copyright 1997. Adapted courtesy of *Perspectives in Education and Deafness*, Pre-College National Mission Programs, Gallaudet University.

7. Provide experiences mentioned in stories. For example, perhaps it is important to know where particular countries are in relationship to each other. In *How My Parents Learned to Eat* by Iva Friedman (Macmillan/McGraw-Hill, 1993), for example, knowing how the British hold a fork compared to how Americans hold a fork is the key to comprehending the final episode.

8. Challenge yourself to be able to do one or two activities with "Some Signing Involved." See below.

Literacy Activities—Some Signing Involved

1. Go to the library or bookstore for books on topics related to the story currently being read. These could be other narratives or expository pieces. For example, a book about teeth, an illustration of a bicuspid, or a tool book illustrating a winch would be helpful additions to reading the story, *Doctor De Soto* by William Steig (Farrar, Strauss & Giroux, 1982). Discuss these materials with the student.

2. Make a concept book and add to it as stories are read. For example, on a page with the heading "Material," the words *gauze* and *flannel* from *Doctor De Soto* could be defined. Real swatches could be displayed on the page as well.

3. Invite over another child or a parent to read the current story together. Everyone can help everyone else sign the reading. Serve cookies and socialize afterwards.

4. Invite or hire a deaf adult to read the story with you and your student. Videotape sessions so that they can be used as sign practice tapes.

5. Ask adults at school to videotape the current story for you and use it as a practice tape. Watch it alone as well as with the student. Have the student sign along with the video.

6. If a sign exists for a difficult vocabulary word, paste the description of the sign opposite the word on a flash card. Practice signing and defining the word together.

7. Act out or mime the characters. All family members can participate at dinnertime by pretending to be the characters in a particular story.

cont.

8. Challenge yourself to be able to do one or two activities requiring "Advanced Signing" (see below).

Literacy Activities—Advanced Signing Involved

1. Read each story to the student before, during, and/or after it is read at school. Do not be shy in acknowledging your need to refer to sign dictionaries for specific vocabulary; elicit help from the student in this process. It is also helpful for the student to see you using special resources and asking for help.

2. Discuss the theme, moral, or main idea of the story. Compare these ideas to past stories, real experiences in the student's life, or real experiences in your life.

3. Discuss the characters, problem, events, and conclusion in the story. Identify these parts of the story structure, elaborate on each, and assist the student in retelling them to you.

4. Have the student retell the story. The student can independently retell the story on video, in writing, or in pictures, or you can assist in the retelling. This can be done by alternating contributions. Your modeling of how to retell certain components of each story can provide the student with an example of what he or she might say or sign next (or in the next story).

5. Reverse interpret as the student tells the story to an audience that has never heard the tale. Enlist the cooperation of a grandparent, a neighbor, or younger siblings and peers to be an authentic audience. Ask audience members to make specific, realistic comments after the retelling. (*My favorite part was ___. The word ___ was new to me. Help me make the sign for ___. I'd like to read that story myself.*)

Appendix 6-E

Literature to Hook Reluctant Readers*

Repetitive texts

Pattern books
Aardema, V. (1981). *Bringing the rain to Kapiti Plain*. Jefferson City, MO: Scholastic.
Komaiko, L. (1988). *Earl's too cool for me*. New York: Harper & Row.
Zemach, H. (1969). *The judge*. Toronto, ON: Collins.

Poetry and verse
Adoff, A. (1982). *All the colors of the race*. New York: Beech Tree Books.
Adoff, A. (1995). *Street music: City poems*. New York: Harper Collins.
Agard, J., & Nichols, G. (Eds.) (1994). *A Caribbean dozen: Poems from Caribbean poets*. Cambridge MA: Candlewick.
Bruchac, J., & London, J. (1992). *Thirteen moons on turtle's back: A Native American year of moons*. New York: Philomel.
Carlsen, L. (Ed.) (1994). *Cool salsa: Bilingual poems on growing up Latino in the United States*. New York: Holt.
Cole, W. (Ed.). (1981). *Poem Stew*. New York: Harper Trophy.
Feelings, T. (Ed.) (1990). *Soul looks back in wonder*. New York: Dial.
Giovanni, N. (1993). *Ego tripping and other poems for young people*. New York: Lawrence Hill.
Linthwaite, I. (Ed.) (1990). *Ain't I a woman? A book of women's poetry from around the world*. New York: Wings.
Prelutsky, J. (1980). *Rolling Harvey down the hill*. New York: Mulberry.
Prelutsky, J. (1984). *The new kid on the block*. New York: Greenwillow.
Rylant, C. (1994). *Something permanent*. New York: Harcourt Brace.
Silverstein, S. (1974). *Where the sidewalk ends*. New York: Harper & Row.
Silverstein, S. (1981). *A light in the attic*. New York: Harper & Row.
Tripp, W. (Ed.) (1973). *A great big ugly man came up and tied his horse to me: A book of nonsense verse*. Boston: Little, Brown.
Viorst, J. (1981). *If I were in charge of the world*. New York: Aladdin.

Jump rope and street rhymes
Cole, J. (Ed.) (1989). *Anna banana: 101 jump-rope rhymes*. New York: Scholastic.
Cole, J., & Calmenson, S. (Eds.) (1990). *Miss Mary Mack, and other children's street rhymes*. New York: Beech Tree Books. *cont.*

---

*From "A Matter of Interest: Literature that Hooks Reluctant Readers and Keeps Them Reading," by J. Worthy, 1996, *The Reading Teacher*, 50(3), pp. 204-212. Copyright 1996 by the International Reading Association. Adapted with permission.

Yolen, J. (Ed.) (1992). *Street rhymes around the world*. Honesdale, PA: Boyds Mills Press.

Performance texts

Speeches
Berry, J. (Ed.) (1995). *Classic poems to read aloud*. New York: Kingfisher.
McKissack, P.C. & McKissack, F. (1992). *Sojourner Truth: Ain't I a woman?* New York: Scholastic.
Stevens, L. (1978). *Cesar Chavez: A mini-play*. Stockton, CA: Relevant Instructional Materials.
Walker, R.J. (Ed.) (1992). *The rhetoric of struggle: Public address by African American women*. New York: Garland.

Books and poems for readers theater
Cole, B. (1987). *Prince Cinders*. New York: G. P. Putnam's Sons.
Cuyler, M. (1991). *That's good! That's bad!* New York: Holt.
Fleischman, P. (1988). *Joyful noise: Poems for two voices*. New York: Harper & Row.
Hooks, W. H. (1989). *The three little pigs and the fox*. New York: Macmillan.
Martin, B., & Archambault, J. (1985). *The ghost-eye tree*. New York: Holt.
Martin, B., & Archambault, J. (1987). *Knots on a counting rope*. New York: Holt.
Raschka, C. (1993). *Yo! Yes?* New York: Scholastic.
Scieska, J. (1991). *The frog prince, continued*. New York: Viking.
Trivizas, E. (1993). *The three little wolves and the big bad pig*. New York: Margaret K. McElderry.

Popular texts

Cartoon collections and comics
The adventures of TinTin by Herge. Boston: Little, Brown.
Archie. Mamaroneck, NY: Archie Comics.
Asterix by R. Goscinny & A. Uderzo. Paris: Dargaud.
Batman. New York: D. C. Comics
Calvin and Hobbes by B. Watterson. Kansas City, MO: Andrews & McMeel.
Garfield by J. Davis. New York: Ballantine Books.
Spiderman. New York: Marvel Comics.
Superman. New York: D. C. Comics.
X-men. New York: Marvel Comics.

Series books
The baby sitters club by A. M. Martin. New York: Scholastic.
The Bailey School kids by D. Dadey & M. T. Jones. New York: Scholastic.
The boxcar children by G. C. Warner. New York: Scholastic.

cont.

Cam Jansen by D. Adler. New York: Puffin.
Choose your own adventure by S. Saunders. New York: Bantam Skylark.
The Culpepper adventures ("Dunc") by G. Paulsen. New York: Dell.
Goosebumps by R. L. Stine. New York: Scholastic.
The Hardy boys by F. W. Dixon. New York: Grosset.
Nancy Drew by C. Keene. New York: Grosset.
Nate the great by M. W. Sharmat. New York: Dell Yearling.
The time warp trio by J. Scieska. New York: Puffin.

Magazines
Cracked, Ebony, Gamepro, Hot Rod, Jet, People, Road and Track, Seventeen, Sports Illustrated, Zoobooks.

Sophisticated picture books
Allard, H. (1974). *The Stupids step out*. New York: Trumpet.
Emberley, M. (1990). *Ruby*. Boston: Little, Brown.
Garland, S. (1993). *The lotus seed*. San Diego, CA: Harcourt Brace Jovanovich.
Hooks, W. H. (1990). *The ballad of Belle Dorcas*. New York: Knopf.
Innocenti, R. (1985). *Rose Blanche*. New York: Stewart, Tabori, & Chang.
Locker, T. (1987). *The boy who held back the sea*. New York: Dial.
Maruki, T. (1980). *Hiroshima no pika*. New York: Lothrop, Lee & Shepard.
Pilkey, D. (1993). *Dogzilla*. New York: Harcourt Brace.
Scieska, J. (1989). *The true story of the three little pigs by A. Wolf*. New York: Viking.
Scieska, J. (1992). *The stinky cheese man and other fairly stupid tales*. New York: Viking.
Steig, W. (1988). *Spinky sulks*. New York: Trumpet.
Steig, W. (1990). *Shrek*. New York: Trumpet.
Van Allsburg, C. (1981). *Jumanji*. New York: Scholastic.
Van Allsburg, C. (1991). *The wretched stone*. Boston: Houghton Mifflin.
Wegman, W. (1993). *Cinderella*. New York: Hyperion.
Yorinks, A. (1990). *Ugh*. New York: Michael di Capua.

Nonfiction books
Bird, L. with B. Ryan (1989). *Drive: The story of my life*. New York: Doubleday.
Boyd, B., & Garrett, R. (1989). *Hoops: Behind the scenes with the Boston Celtics*. Waltham, MA: Little, Brown.
Hollander, P., & Hollander, Z. (1990). *Bo knows Bo: The autobiography of a ballplayer*. New York: Doubleday.
Lake, E. D. (1995). *Low rider*. Minneapolis, MN: Capstone.
Lee, S., & Vuscema, J. (1978). *How to draw comics the Marvel way*. New York: Simon and Schuster.

cont.

Lovett, S. (1992). *Extremely weird animals series*. Santa Fe, NM: John Muir.
Parker, S. (1992). *Inside the whale and other animals*. New York: Doubleday.
Parsons, A. (1990). *Eyewitness Juniors animals series*. New York: Alfred A. Knopf.
Sabin, L. (1992). *Roberto Clemente: Young baseball hero*. New York: Troll.

Authors who appeal to reluctant readers
Christopher, M. (1992). *Return of the home run kid*. Waltham, MA: Little, Brown.
Colville, B. (1990). *My teacher is an alien*. New York: Minstrel.
Dahl, R. (1980). *The Twits*. New York: Puffin.
Dahl, R. (1982). *The BFG*. New York: Trumpet.
Jacques, B. (1991). *Seven strange and ghostly tales*. New York: Avon.
Manes, S. (1991). *Make four million dollars by next Thursday*. New York: Bantam Skylark.
Pinkwater, D. M. (1977). *Fat men from space*. New York: Dell.
Rockwell, T. (1973). *How to eat fried worms*. New York: Dell.
Schwartz, A. (1991). *Scary stories 3: More tales to chill your bones*. New York: Harper Collins.

Adult books and authors who appeal to adolescent reluctant readers
Angelou, M. (1969). *I know why the caged bird sings*. New York: Random House.
Anthony, P., & Kornwise, R. (1989). *Through the ice*. New York: Simon and Schuster.
Asprin, R. (1983). *Hit or myth*. Norfolk, VA: Conning.
Cisneros, S. (1994). *The house on Mango Street*. New York: Knopf.
Chrichton, M. (1980). *Congo*. New York: Dell.
King, S. (1981). *Cujo*. New York: Viking Press.
Rivera, T. (1992). *This migrant earth*. (R. Hinojosa, Trans.) Houston: Arte Publico (original work published 1970).

References

Adams, M. (1994). *Beginning to read: Thinking and learning about print.* Cambridge, MA: MIT Press.

Anderson, V., & Hidi, S. (1988, December). Teaching students to summarize. *Educational Leadership,* 26-28.

Andrew, J., & Akamatsu, C. (1993). Building blocks for literacy: Getting the signs right. *Perspectives, 11*(3).

Bilson, M., Hayes, P., & Luetke-Stahlman, B. (December, 1996). Reading aloud with children who are deaf and hard of hearing. A survey of teachers working in state schools for the deaf. *Canadian Association of Educators of the Deaf and Hard of Hearing Journal, 22*(2/3), 56-71.

Brown, A., & Day, J. (1983). Macrorules for summarizing texts: The development of expertise. *Journal of Verbal Learning and Verbal Behavior, 22,* 1-14.

Carnine, D., Silbert, J., & Kameenui, E. (1990). *Direct Instruction Reading* (3rd ed.). Upper Saddle River, NJ: Prentice Hall.

Center, Y., Wheldall, K., Freeman, L., Outhred, L., & McNaught, M. (1995a). An evaluation of Reading Recovery. *Reading Research Quarterly, 30*(2), 240-263.

Center, Y., Wheldall, K., Freeman, L., Outhred, L., & McNaught, M. (1995b). Response to Rasinski. *Reading Research Quarterly, 30*(2), 272-275.

Chall, J. (1983). *Stages of reading development.* New York: McGraw-Hill.

Clay, M. (1979). *The early detection of reading difficulties.* Portsmouth, NH: Heinemann.

Clay, M. (1991a). Syntactic awareness and reading recovery: A response to Tunmer. *New Zealand Journal of Educational Studies, 22,* 35-58.

Clay, M. (1991b). Introducing a new storybook to young readers. *The Reading Teacher, 45,* 264-273.

Clay, M. (1993). *Reading recovery: A guideline for teachers in training.* Portsmouth, NH: Heinemann.

Gaskins, I., Ehri, L., Cress, C., O'Hara, C., & Donnelly, K. (1997). Procedures for word learning: Making discoveries about words. *The Reading Teacher, 50*(4), 321-327.

Gilbert, A. (1977). *Teaching the three Rs through movement experiences.* Minneapolis: Burgess.

Greenlee, A., Monson, D., & Taylor, B. (1996). The lure of series books: Does it affect appreciation for recommended literature? *The Reading Teacher, 50*(3), 216-225.

Hickman, J. (1981). A new perspective on response to literature: Research in an elementary school setting. *Research in the Teaching of English, 15*, 343-354.

Horowitz, R., & Samuels, J. (1987). *Comprehending oral and written language.* San Diego, CA: Academic Press.

Kelly, L. (1996). The interaction of syntactic competence and vocabulary during reading by deaf students. *Journal of Deaf Studies and Deaf Education, 1*(1), 75-90.

Luetke-Stahlman, B., Griffiths, C., & Montgomery, N. (1998a). Development of text structure knowledge as assessed by signed and spoken retellings of a deaf student. *American Annals of the Deaf, 143*(4), 337-346.

Luetke-Stahlman, B., Griffiths, C., & Montgomery, N. (1998b, accepted). A deaf child's language acquisition verified through text retelling. *American Annals of the Deaf.*

Luetke-Stahlman, B., Griffiths, C., & Stryker, D. (1997). Literacy . . . the most important challenge: Checklist. *Perspectives in Education and Deafness, 15*(4), 10-11.

Luetke-Stahlman, B., Hayes, L., & Nielsen, D. (1996). Essential practices as adults read to meet the needs of deaf and hard of hearing students. *American Annals of the Deaf, 141*(4), 309-320.

Luetke-Stahlman, B., & Nielsen, D. (1996). *A deaf child learns to read.* Unpublished manuscript, University of Kansas Medical Center, Kansas City.

Luetke-Stahlman, B., Nielsen, D., & Hayes, P. (1995). *Narrative lesson plan report.* Unpublished manuscript, University of Kansas Medical Center, Kansas City.

Mackey, M. (1990). Filling the gaps: The baby-sitters club, the series book, and the learning reader. *Language Arts, 67*, 484-489.

Naremore, R., Densmore, A., & Harman, D. (1995). *Language intervention with school-aged children: Conversation, narrative, and text.* San Diego, CA: Singular.

Nielsen, D. (1994). *Moving from specific to general cues.* Unpublished class handout. University of Kansas, Lawrence.

Paul, P., & Quigley, S. (1994). *Language and deafness* (2nd ed.). San Diego, CA: Singular.

Pinnell, G. (1992). Reading recovery swift, effective in reversing reading failure, MacArthur study finds. *The Running Record, 4,* 1-3.

Pinnell, G., Fried, M., & Estice, R. (1990). Reading recovery: Learning how to make a difference. *The Reading Teacher, 43,* 282-295.

Shanahan, T., & Barr, R. (1995). Reading recovery: An independent evaluation of the effects of an early instructional intervention for at risk learners. *Reading Research Quarterly, 30*(4), 958-996.

Stewart, C., & Cegelka, P. (1995). Teaching reading and spelling. In P. Cegelka & W. Berdine, *Effective instruction of students with learning difficulties,* (pp. 265-299). Boston: Allyn & Bacon.

Thomas, C. (1997). *Adapting reading recovery strategies for small groups of emergent readers.* Paper presented at the Literacy and Deafness Conference, Ft. Worth, Texas, July, 1997.

Vygotsky, L. (1978). *Mind in society: The development of higher psychological processes.* Cambridge, MA: Harvard University Press.

Weinstein, C., Ridley, D., Dahl, T., & Weber, S. (1989). Helping students develop strategies for effective learning. *Educational Leadership, 46*(4), 17-19.

Worthy, J. (1996). A matter of interest: Literature that hooks reluctant readers and keeps them reading. *The Reading Teacher, 50*(3), 204-212.

Chapter 7

Assessing and Facilitating Writing

Writing Assessment

Beginning Writers

Process Writing

Reading about Writing

Using Computers

Resources

Appendix: Six Trait Rubric

Writing abilities are necessary for a wide range of communication needs. In fact, Bruner (1966) regarded writing as the ultimate tool for thinking! At school, writing activities typically include response journals passed back and forth between teacher and student, retells of narrative and expository materials, reports, short stories, poems, and so forth. Unfortunately, students who are D/HH traditionally have not developed age-appropriate writing skills. One reason may be that teachers of the deaf have not felt confident about ways to help students become better writers. Also, early writing instruction for students who are D/HH targeted sentence level constructions (Wilbur, 1977): Examples include the Wing Symbols (Wing, 1887) and the Fitzgerald Key (Fitzgerald, 1949). It is now realized that segments of text larger than sentences should be facilitated as well.

Success with writing activities correlates to students' reading abilities. In addition, the ability to use speech has been shown to be an advantage in being able to write well (Polloway & Smith, 1992). The information provided in this chapter can assist team members in the assessment and facilitation of students' writing abilities and in the integration of writing with other literacy skills.

Writing Assessment

As with other assessments discussed in this text, instruments to evaluate writing should be based on the questions of team members. A parent may want assurance that the child's ability to write a letter or a creative story is similar to that of hearing peers. The speech-language pathologist may wonder if the student can make reasonable guesses about how to write the initial sounds of the phonemes he or she can pronounce. Teachers may be concerned that a student cannot construct a paragraph about what has been learned in social studies or science. Team members may ask, "What strategies can be used to facilitate the writing abilities of students who are D/HH?" Motivated by questions such as these, team members can plan a comprehensive formal and informal battery of *question-directed writing assessments* to evaluate students' writing.

Formal Assessment

Formal methods of writing assessment typically require students who are D/HH to analyze another person's writing sample and to respond to multiple-choice test questions. Heefner (1993) noted that examples of formal measures are provided in the *Stanford Achievement Test* (SAT) (Psychological Corporation, 1989), *The Test of Written Language* (TOWL) (Hammill & Larsen, 1983), the *Iowa Tests of Basic Skills* (ITBS) (Cantor, 1986), and the Written Language Cluster of Part Two of the *Woodcock-Johnson Psychoeducational Battery* (Woodcock & Johnson, 1977). Taylor (1997) recommended the *Test of Written Expression* (TOWE) (McGhee, Bryant, Laren, & Rivera, 1995). In addition, the *Test of Early Written Language* (TEWL) (Hresko, 1988) may be helpful when assessing emergent writing abilities.

> **Study Guide Question**
>
> *What formal writing assessment has been used with a student who is D/HH whom you know? Interview parents and teachers about the usefulness of the assessment and share what you learn.*

Informal Assessment

To use informal assessment, a representative writing sample (or samples) must first be collected. Students may or may not be given a specific time limit in which to write the sample. The sample can be analyzed using any of the following:

1. T-unit analysis: measuring the degree to which students use more complex sentences by counting grammatically complete segments, called terminable units or T-units (as used by Klecan-Aker and Blondeau, 1990)
2. error analysis
3. checklists
4. holistic or analytical scoring

Bourne (1994) suggested a sequence for the informal assessment of early drawing/writing performance. That sequence is shown in Figure 7–1.

PERFORMANCE						
Picture Only	Picture & Text	Imbalance (Pictorial)	Complementary	Imbalance (Textual)	General to Specific	Text Only
■ picture unaided by text	■ redundant ■ text duplicates picture	■ picture is more specific and informative than text	■ both picture and text supply information	■ text is more specific and informative than picture	■ text is more specific and informative than picture	■ text carries the meaning ■ no accompanying picture

FIGURE 7-1: AN OVERVIEW OF EARLY DRAWING/WRITING

Holistic Scoring

Holistic scoring is a method by which a single overall score is subjectively given to a written sample. The scoring may consider several different aspects of writing, such as organization, cohesion, voice, ideas, mechanics, and so on (Heefner, 1993), but only one score is granted. Holistic scoring may enable team members to determine whether a student is falling below proficiency, but the method does not provide information about students' strengths and weaknesses that can be used for instructional purposes (Luetke-Stahlman & Luckner, 1991). If teachers find that holistic scoring does not meet their needs, analytical scoring should be considered.

Analytical Scoring

Analytical scoring of a written sample (the trait method) gives a separate score for each predetermined trait or characteristic of writing. "Diederich, the pioneer of the trait method, devised his original analytical writing scale to include ideas (the message), organization (order and flow), wording (the vocabulary and correct usage), and flavor (voice or personal style)" (Heefner, 1993, p. 11). The Six Trait Analytical Writing Assessment Model (Northwest Regional Educational Laboratory, 1995) is a popular example of the analytical scoring procedure. The traits assessed in this model are ideas and content, organization, voice, word choice, sentence fluency, and conventions. A rubric for this model appears in Appendix 7–A.

Scoring systems for traits differ. Often, the traits are provided with suggested scores for "beginner," "improving," and "proficient" levels of ability. The Six Trait method (Appendix 7–A) uses a 1, 3, 5 system for allocating points in which:

- 1 represents beginning development
- 3 represents taking control and gaining a sense of purpose
- 5 represents a strong sense of control that has direction and purpose

To collect the written sample, students are usually asked to choose between two or more prompt options (a series of pictures or slides, a starter sentence, a paragraph that suggests a writing topic, and so on) and to write a sample based on the prompt. Then trained raters evaluate the sample and assign it a score for each of the six separate traits.

The Six Trait method has been used at elementary, middle, and high school levels (Duncan & Neuberger, 1987; Slater, 1994; Poggio, Glasnapp, Nielsen, Barry, & Sundbye, 1995). Several states have adopted the procedure as a teaching tool, as well as for local and state assessment. Because of the popularity of this method, Duncan and Neuberger were able to identify these advantages of analytical scoring:

- Assessment results are clear to various audiences.
- Students understand what qualities are important in good writing.
- Beginning writers establish an orderly, systematic plan for editing and revising their writing.
- Teachers design writing instruction based on the qualities they wish to see demonstrated.
- Team members and students understand how student writing is evaluated.
- Consistency is provided in the way teachers rate student writing.
- Technical vocabulary is used that provides educators, students, and parents with terms to use in talking about writing and writing instruction.

The Six Trait assessment checklist in Figure 7–2 is a tool for team members who are evaluating the writing skills of students who are D/HH.

1. **Ideas and Content**
   Writing is ___ interesting, ___ well-focused, ___ precise, ___ clear.

2. **Organization**
   The passage has ___ an introduction, ___ effective transitions, ___ a strong conclusion, ___ appropriate use of details.

3. **Voice**
   It is written ___ honestly, ___ expressively, ___ in a manner that creates interest.

4. **Word Choice**
   Writer uses ___ precise vocabulary, ___ strong verbs, ___ figures of speech, ___ effective imagery.

5. **Sentence Fluency**
   Sentences are ___ coherent, ___ grammatically correct, ___ easy to read aloud.

6. **Conventions**
   Passage is written with correct ___ spelling, ___ punctuation, ___ grammar ___ capitalization, ___ paragraphing.

FIGURE 7–2: SIX TRAIT ASSESSMENT CHECKLIST

Significant findings have resulted from the use of analytical scoring in research with students who are D/HH. Gormley and Sarachan-Deily (1987), for example, used an analytical scoring system to report information concerning the similarities and differences between the papers of good and poor writers who were D/HH. Heefner (1993) used analytical scoring to measure six traits of writing by deaf and hard-of-hearing residential students. Her work included 206 students, ages 8 to 21, and four years of scores. Her results showed that, although students who were D/HH scored lower on average than their hearing peers, their improvement over the years was greater on average than their hearing peers'. Heefner also found validity for the trait method when means were summed across the traits and correlated with the students' means on the *Stanford Achievement Test for Hearing Impaired Students* (SAT–HI) (Gallaudet University, 1983) reading component. She deduced that the process writing approach (explained later in this chapter) used at the school where she did her research contributed greatly to the outcome of general improvement in student writing ability.

Beginning Writers

Study Guide Question

Can you score a written sample using the Six Trait method? Work with a peer and discuss the strengths and weaknesses of this approach.

Many children begin to write by drawing. For writing to emerge, team members should provide a time and place for art activities, provide materials, and value any attempts to communicate through drawing, scribbling, or writing. At some point, scribbles become letters; drawing becomes writing. Team members can help the process along by providing written labels on pictures for students and modeling writing. Team members might work alongside children, saying and signing things such as *"I think I'll make the letter* o.*"*

The language experience approach for reading (Stauffer, 1980) is an effective way to introduce students who are D/HH to writing. In this approach students work as a group to dictate a story about a specific experience. An adult then writes student contributions in correct English on large chart paper. Afterwards the adult and students take turns reading the story to each other. Finally, each student copies the story and takes it home to share. Clay (1975) noted that students begin to generate their own writing by first tracing, copying, and inventing symbols as they copy stories such as those generated through the language experience approach. Other reading approaches, such as *Reading Recovery* (Clay, 1993), include writing and spelling activities as well. Beginning readers can be helped through these approaches to write a single sentence using words that they had difficulty reading in a particular story.

Collective writing is another way to give beginning writers confidence and support. Collective writing occurs when students work together in cooperative groups to produce a single piece of work. Team members ask students to write on any topic, or require that they write on a given topic and use specific vocabulary words, such as those studied in reading, social studies, or science. Students take turns making suggestions for sentences and recording their peers' contributions. This approach allows students to receive immediate feedback on ideas, grammar, vocabulary, and punctuation. When a first draft is finished, one student reads the composition aloud to the others, and students respond and suggest revisions.

Purposeful writing, such as creating needed lists or labels, can also motivate students who have just begun to write. Students can be encouraged, for example, to list foods needed at home and supplies used at school. Adults can help students create labels for their belongings or for the location of certain materials. Emergent writers can also be asked to label graphic organizers. Adults should assure children that correct spelling is not necessary to communicate a functional message and that pictures or a combination of pictures and words is acceptable. Students can be shown how to photocopy their drawings so that they can include them when they are writing to other students, to relatives, or to authors. Letters to friends or notes of thanks or apology at school are other forms of purposeful writing. Teachers can model purposeful writing by leaving notes on students' desks about their work or behavior. To share thoughts with parents about school events, children can be helped to label drawings completed at school or fill in assignment notebooks. Students should be encouraged to copy the words that adults write for them and to create small personal dictionaries in which they write and can look up needed words.

When students hesitate to write because of difficulties with grammar, adults can support their learning by providing them with a paragraph in which they fill in words (the words may or may not be separately provided). This is also a good way to practice spelling. Sentence starters and story frames can also be used to assist emergent writers in learning grammar. A sentence pattern (The ___ I'm wearing is ___) can later be altered in a minor way (I'm wearing a ___ ___). These aids support the acquisition of grammar that may be unknown to students who are D/HH.

Adults can also help emergent writers by brainstorming ideas with them and recording responses in a notebook or on the blackboard. A teacher might list several characters from a story that has been read and then ask students to describe them. The teacher can list the descriptive phrases students suggest as well as actions that occurred in the story or places that the characters visited. These lists allow students access to many of the words they will need to communicate their own ideas in writing.

Process Writing

Study Guide Question
What are some other ways to help emergent writers begin to draw, scribble, and write? Share three ideas with your peers.

There is agreement in contemporary literature (Heefner, 1993) that students who are D/HH can benefit from a process approach to writing. Such an approach involves four stages: planning, writing, conferencing and revising, and publishing (see Figure 7–3). The following activities comprise the team member's role in a process approach:

- have students choose topics and set goals
- have students establish a purpose for writing
- with students, determine the audience for the writing
- provide instruction and support during each writing stage
- demonstrate and model each writing stage
- hold brief writing conferences at each writing stage
- have students evaluate their own progress
- teach grammar and mechanics in context at the editing stage
- encourage dialogue and collaboration among students
- encourage peer critiques
- provide opportunities for writing across the curriculum
- informally assess ongoing writing projects
- evaluate student-selected portfolios
- focus evaluation on particular behaviors for individual writing projects

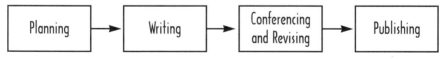

FIGURE 7–3: A PROCESS APPROACH TO WRITING

The Planning Stage

During the planning stage, students brainstorm topics to write about, identify an audience, and establish a plan for writing. Research by Oliver (1995) documented the importance of students' choosing topics that are relevant to their lives. Luetke-Stahlman (1998) discussed the factor of relevance with regard to providing an environment that is optimal for language acquisition. Many of the factors she described can be applied to the writing process. For example, she suggested that adults ask open-ended questions about student experiences and ideas to help them collect their thoughts:

> Ms. Montgomery: Have you found an idea that you want to write about? How is the writing going? Have you solved the problem we talked about before? What part of your writing do you want to discuss today?

Often a booklet of ideas is used to keep a list of topics students have thought about and may later want to expand.

To develop cognitive or academic skills, team members might suggest that students who are D/HH write about material they have recently read. Noyce and Christie (1989) made the following suggestions for writing about recently read material:
- write a preface to the story, describing what happened before the story began
- write a sequel to the story, continuing the plot
- write an alternative ending to the story
- write a parallel story from another point of view
- write a parallel story in another setting
- compare or contrast two characters or events in the story

Planning writing includes being clear about its purpose and, thereby, its type. Heefner (1993) clarified that students who are D/HH might be assigned at least four types of writing during their academic years.
- **Narrative writing** tells a real or imaginary story. Its text structure includes all the elements of story structure: characters, setting, episode, conclusion, and so forth.

- **Expository writing** explains concepts about social studies, history, math, or other subjects. The text structure of expository writing can be compare and contrast, classify, and so on.
- **Descriptive writing** creates a picture using rich, detailed vocabulary that enhances a visual or other sensory image.
- **Persuasive writing** presents supporting information to attempt to convince the reader of a particular opinion.

A graphic organizer such as the one provided in Figure 7–4 can help students systematically plan their writing. An example of an organizer for a five-paragraph narrative piece appears in Figure 7–5.

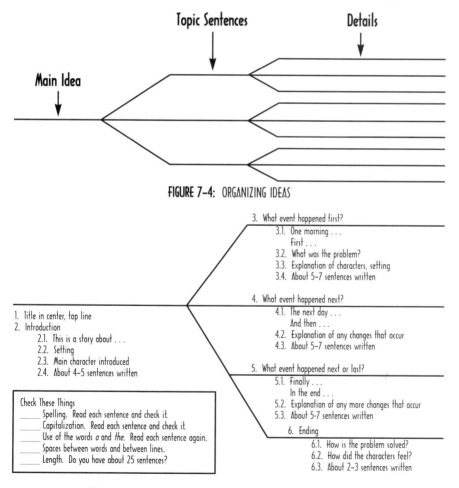

FIGURE 7–4: ORGANIZING IDEAS

FIGURE 7–5: STRUCTURE FOR WRITTEN NARRATIVE RETELL WITH MEDIATION

The Writing Stage

Study Guide Question
How can you help a student plan to write? Read a professional article or book chapter on this topic and share three ideas with a peer.

During the writing stage, students draft their written piece by following their plan. A first draft is completed during this stage (McAnally, Rose, & Quigley, 1994). It may be written by hand, but many students who are D/HH enjoy word processing on computers. During this stage adults can assist by focusing on producing ideas rather than on mechanics (Luetke-Stahlman & Luckner, 1991).

Phenix (1990) suggested that adults can facilitate writing content, organization, and style by asking questions such as the following:

Questions about Writing*

Content
- What are you writing about?
- What is the most important thing you want me to learn from this paragraph?
- I don't understand what you are saying here. Can you explain it in a different way?
- I'm surprised you didn't write more about this. I know it's a subject you know a lot about.
- Is there anything you need to know more about?
- Is there anything you would like help with?

Organization
- You seem to have things a little mixed up here. What do you think should come first?
- I'm not sure this is the best order for your information. What do you think?
- Do you think it might be clearer if you divided this up into sections?
- You haven't organized this into paragraphs yet. Do you know how to do that?
- Have you thought about putting this information into a list rather than a paragraph?

*From *Teaching Writing*, by J. Phenix, 1990, Markham, Ontario: Pembroke Publishers. Copyright 1990 by Pembroke Publishers. Adapted with permission.

- What do you think you ought to do next?
- Is there anything you would like help with?

Style
- You seem to be using this word over and over again. Can you think of any other words you could use instead?
- Did you consider writing this as a diary, letter, or play? Do you think it might be effective that way?
- You haven't used any dialogue. Was there any special reason for this?
- Is there anything you need help with?

Narrative or story writing is one of the first types of writing done by most children. The text structure of a story includes a main character, a setting, a problem faced or action performed by the main character, the resolution of the problem, and a conclusion. Archer and Gleason (1995) suggested guiding the student's narrative writing process with questions and ideas such as these:

- Explain this graphic organizer (picture stimulus item).
- Write about each of these:
    Who is the main character?
    Where does the story take place?
    What does the main character do?
    What happens when he or she does it?
    How does the story end? How does the main character
      feel?
- What are your story part ideas for each of these parts?

For more advanced writers who are writing a persuasive piece (essay), La Paz and Graham (1997) suggested incorporating one strategy (DARE) within another (STOP), as in Figure 7–6. Their strategy involves using cue cards to aid the writing process.

Planning Strategy: **STOP**	Instructions for Each Planning Step
1. **S**uspend judgment	Consider each side before taking a position. Brainstorm ideas for and against the topic. When you can't think of more ideas, use these cue cards: (a) Did I list ideas for each side? If not, do this now. (b) Can I think of anything else? Try to write more ideas. (c) Another point I haven't considered yet is . . . .
2. **T**ake a side	Read your ideas. Decide which side you believe in, or which side can be used to make the strongest argument. Place a "+" on the side that shows your position.
3. **O**rganize ideas	Choose ideas that are strong, and decide how to organize them for writing. To help you do this, use these cue cards: (a) Put a star next to the ideas you want to use. Choose at least ___ idea(s).* (b) Choose at least ___ argument(s)* to refute. (c) Number your ideas in the order you will use them.
4. **P**lan more as you write	Continue to plan as you write. Use all four essay parts (use a DARE cue card to jog your memory): **D**evelop your topic sentence. **A**dd supporting ideas. **R**eject possible arguments for the other side. **E**nd with a conclusion.

*Note: In the third step, "Organize ideas," goals to choose the number of supporting ideas and arguments are adjusted for each writer based on initial writing ability. Remind students that their primary goal is to be convincing, so that they may include more (or even fewer) items as they write.

FIGURE 7–6: THE ESSAY PLANNING STRATEGY

From "Strategy Instruction in Planning: Effects on the Writing Performance and Behavior of Students with Learning Difficulties," by S. La Paz and S. Graham, 1997, *Exceptional Children, 63*(2), pp. 167-186. Copyright 1997 by the Council for Exceptional Children. Adapted with permission.

The Conferencing and Revising Stage

The best writing is not written but *rewritten* (Willis, 1977). During the revising stage, students polish, clarify, augment, and change their composition. At this point, the adult and student work cooperatively to understand the meaning of the writing. The adult may use mediation strategies (as discussed in Chapter 1) and may also decide at this time to identify a particular skill to be improved without marking or without extensively marking on the student's paper.

Daiute and Kruidenier (1985) found that students' written work improved when they were simply asked to reread it! Hacker, Plumb, Butterfield, Quathamer, and Heineken (1994) studied several ways to help students revise their writing. They found that students might be able to identify an error but would not necessarily know how to correct it. They also found that allowing more time with the student's draft, specifying that a grammatical error was made (as opposed to a semantic error), and rehearsing expressive language use required in the written piece could help students successfully revise their work.

Students might be encouraged to check their writing using the CaPS learning strategy (Levy & Rosenberg, 1961):

C = Have I *capitalized* the first word and proper nouns?
a = Have I made *any messy errors* in handwriting, margins, and so on?
P = Have I used *punctuation*—commas, periods, and semicolons—carefully?
S = Are words *spelled* correctly? Can I sound them out or use the dictionary?

The lowercase *a* in the "CaPS" mnemonic device is associated with the word *errors*. This sound-symbol mnemonic may not be helpful for all students who are D/HH.

Facilitating Correction

Hayward and LeBuffe (1985) contend that self-correction is a better approach to revision than the alternative of having teachers mark student papers. They recommend that editing symbols be used to prompt the student's self-correction. Table 7–1 shows editing codes that team members can write in the margin on the lines where a revision is suggested.

TABLE 7–1: EDITING CODES FOR SELF-CORRECTION

Code	Meaning	Interpretation	Example
sp	Spelling	A word in this line is spelled incorrectly.	The gril sat down.
C	Capitalization	A capital letter is needed in this line.	She and i are friends.
lc	Lowercase	A word in this line has an incorrect capital letter that should be changed to lowercase.	The Man chased the dog.
p	Punctuation	There is an error in punctuation in this line (to clarify, specify the punctuation needed).	John said, Stop that!
#	Number (singular or plural)	A word in this line is singular when it should be plural, or vice versa.	These car were stolen.
ill	Illegible	Something on this line is illegible. I can't read it.	Do you like ppoue?
vt	Verb tense	A verb in this line is in the wrong tense.	Tom was lost and cries.
V	Verb error	A verb in this line is in the wrong form.	She is go to college.
pro	Pronoun error	There is a wrong pronoun on this line.	The boy ate him supper.

From "Self-Correction: A Positive Method for Improving Writing Skills," by L. Hayward and J. LeBuffe, 1985, *Teaching Exceptional Children, 18*(1), pp. 68-73. Copyright 1985 by the Council for Exceptional Children. Adapted with permission.

Students who are D/HH can review their own work to identify and revise areas of concern. The adult role is to praise students for locating errors and revising. Only one editing code or symbol should be introduced and explained at a time.

Conferences

Conferencing discussions can serve as "cogni-calisthenics" for building the skills needed for writing (Rubin, 1987, p. 59). Peers may be able to use standard symbols when they conference about written work.

A SAMPLING OF STANDARD EDITING SYMBOLS

Symbol	Meaning	Example
————	Delete something	The ball ~~bounced and~~ bounced.
∧	Insert something	The ball bounced ∧ᵃⁿᵈ bounced.
≡	Capitalize	the ball bounced.
¶	New paragraph	¶Today was the beginning . . . .

Adult-Student Conferences. Various team members can be trained to conference with students who are D/HH. This is not a job for a teacher assistant or volunteer. Knudson (1989) found that when adults modeled writing techniques with students, students' writing improved. The language strategies of self talk, parallel talk, and inform talk described by Luetke-Stahlman (1998) could be adapted to model writing strategies. Englert, Raphael, Anderson, Anthony, and Stevens (1991) found that adult self talk, also called "think alouds," was a facilitation technique that helped students improve their writing. Skill instruction should use students' writing and include "brief, targeted instruction" (Willis, 1997, p. 6).

Phenix (1990) gave many examples of when adult-student conferences might occur, as well as what the content might be. She suggested sticking to one section and choosing only one or two subjects for discussion. What is chosen to work on depends on the stage of the writing and the writer's experience. Phenix's suggested questions were presented earlier in this chapter; her strategies by writing stage are presented below:

Writing Strategies
---

1. Draft (before and during early-draft writing)
Topic
- Help the student select a topic, if necessary.
- Encourage the student to talk about the topic.
- Show an interest in what the student is writing about.
- Help the student clarify intentions. (Discuss purpose and possible audience.)

Focusing
- Help the student to narrow down the topic. Rather than "Japan," for example, select "Sumo Wrestling" or "How Pearl Divers Work."
- Find out what the writer is really interested in.
- Help the writer stay on topic. Draw attention to irrelevant material. (*"I'm not sure what this part has to do with your main topic."*)

Expanding
- Help the writer to recall information or generate ideas. (*"Where else did you go on your trip?" "What other disasters might your characters experience?"*)
- Ask questions. (*"What did you do when it started to rain?" "Do you really think people would behave that way?"*)
- Share your own experience. (*"Did I ever tell you about the time I . . . "*)
- Suggest resources. (*"Maria knows a lot about stamps. Have you talked to her?"*)

2. Process (after first draft)
- Help with revision.
- Focus the writer on the process of writing. (*"What do you think you should do next?"*)
- Discuss possible ways to organize the writing.
- Teach revision shortcuts, such as arrows indicating where material is to be moved, omission marks, cut-and-paste.

3. **Evaluate (after some revision has been done)**
   - Review purpose and audience.
   - Help decide whether the writing is finished, needs more revision, needs more research.
   - Together, decide whether the piece is to be shared, displayed, published, and so on.
   - Encourage the writer to reflect on the writing. (*"What made it difficult?" "How does it compare with other pieces you have written?"*)

4. **Edit (before writing a final draft)**
   - Give instruction on a particular skill.
   - Help the writer identify and correct spelling errors.
   - Help the writer check punctuation and other print conventions.
   - Help the writer prepare pieces for publication or display.

From *Teaching Writing* (pp. 28-29), by J. Phenix, 1990, Markham, Ontario: Pembroke Publishers. Copyright 1990 by Pembroke Publishers. Adapted with permission.

Peer Conferences. Writing improves when students have a real audience. Students might read aloud to an audience of other students or switch papers on an individual basis. Members of the audience respond by making comments or asking questions about parts they did not understand, "showing an interest, being positive, seeking clarification, offering more information on the topic, suggesting solutions to problems, or helping with proofreading" (Phenix, 1990, p. 32).

> **Study Guide Question**
> *Can you make a student response sheet using Phenix's conferencing ideas?*

Students might also use a peer conference summary sheet (see Figure 7–7) for brief periods of directed instruction. Such sheets can be taken with them for a reminder as they prepare their revision.

> Name:_____ Date:_____
> Topic:_____
>
> Conference Partner:_____
>
> 1. What is my story/project about?
> 2. What do you like best about it?
> 3. Did I say anything confusing? Did you have any questions?
> 4. Do I need to add more details? Where?
>   _____ beginning _____ middle _____ ending
>   _____ characters _____ setting
> 5. What other suggestions would you make?

FIGURE 7–7: PEER CONFERENCE SUMMARY

The Publishing Stage

Although not every piece of work will be published, the publishing stage should conclude the writing process at least some of the time. After students choose which of their pieces they would like to share, publishing can occur in many different ways, including making a book, reading the work to the class, or making the work available for others to read (McAnally, Rose, Quigley, 1994).

Six Trait Rubrics Used in Process Writing

The Six Trait assessment method explained earlier in this chapter is sometimes used to facilitate process writing. However, Knudson (1989) advised against this. She found that improvement in writing samples was not evidenced when students in elementary and middle school grades were presented with scales, questions, or criteria to guide writing. She suggested that this was because students were presented with too much information in too short a time period. "Either students need more models before being introduced to questions/scales/criteria, or they need more time to write without models" (p. 94).

Dialogue Journals and Learning Logs ———————

A method that may prove to be successful with some students who are D/HH involves the use of dialogue journals and learning logs (Feathers, 1993). Using this approach, a student writes daily (or often) for 10–15 minutes in a notebook specified for this activity. The topic of the writing could be in response to a specific question or activity or could be free choice. Journals allow students to take ownership in their writing and to reflect on a novel being read, a science experiment, a social studies topic, their personal experiences, their interest in other writers, and so forth. Requiring the use of specific words and phrases from studied topics might facilitate cognitive academic language proficiency.

Reading about Writing

A list of trade books about young people who write was compiled by Noyce and Christie (1989). These books might inspire writers when used as adult reads or instructional text.

Books about Young People Who Write

For Third Graders
Cleary, B. (1984). *The Ramona Quimby Diary*. New York: Morrow.
Hess, L. (1982). *Diary of a Rabbit*. New York: Scribner.
For Fourth Graders
Hahn, M. (1984). *Daphne's Book*. New York: Clarion.
Klein, R. (1984). *Penny Pollard's Letters*. New York: Merrimack.
For Older Students
Blos, J. (1979). *A Gathering of Days*. New York: Scribner.
Cleary, B. (1983). *Dear Mr. Henshaw*. New York: Yearling.

Noyce and Christie (1989) also list books by complex English patterns. Their lists, categorized by "if clauses," "that clauses," "when clauses," "where clauses," and "who clauses," might be useful to team members.

Using Computers

Graham, Harris, MacArthur, and Schwarts (1991) suggested that "the combination of word processing, a process approach to writing, and strategy instruction provided a viable mechanism for improving the writing of participating students with learning disabilities" (p. 108). Computers can provide an alternative to handwritten work for students who are D/HH as well. Graham et al. believed that word processing and desktop publishing software appear to have the ingredients that can stimulate both student use and understanding. Graphics, spellcheck, and grammar checks, as well as text body clues should enhance writing and assist students in printing a piece of work that looks polished.

Software programs made commercially available include the following titles; grade levels are indicated for each title. Publishers' addresses are provided in the resource list at the end of this chapter.

Software on Writing

Mavis Deacon Teaches Typing. Personalized practice based on error analysis. The Learning Company.

Sentence Starters (K–4). Supports writers by giving them an assortment of sentence starters. Children can also select graphics to produce unique storybooks. Cambridge Developmental Laboratory.

The Amazing Writing Machine (K–8). Invites students to express their ideas in story, letter, journal essay, or poem. Page layouts and graphics are provided. Educational Resources.

Read, Write, and Type (1–2). An early literacy program that allows students to apply phonics and typing skills and to combine sounds to make words, sentences, and stories. The Learning Company.

Storybook Weaver Deluxe (1–6). Provides graphics and music when students create their own original stories. The Learning Company.

Write On Plus: Elementary (3–6). Integrates writing and literature. Engaging activities motivate students to edit, combine sentences, and practice punctuation, as well as prewrite, draft, revise, and edit their responses to classic stories. Educational Resources.

The Process of Writing (3–6). Allows student to write short essays, book reports, posters, and poems. Children learn prewriting and drafting techniques, sentence and para graph structure, revising, and editing skills. Sunburst.

Easy Book Deluxe (3–8). Includes a spell-checker, thesaurus, text-to-speech option, and editing and formatting tools to provide support as students create stories. Sunburst.

Writing about Books (3–8). An interactive literacy program designed to assist students in writing about preselected books. Illustrations, worksheets, and quotations can be inserted into students' writing. Educational Resources.

Student Report Writer (3 and up). An interactive writing program that includes 50 templates for a variety of school subject reports. The Learning Company.

My Own Stories (4–10). Inspires students to create stories by providing 48 backgrounds/foregrounds, 162 people, 54 buildings, 90 interior items, 45 items from nature, 135 vehicles and objects, 12 borders, 15 fonts, and 42 sound effects. Cambridge Developmental Laboratory.

Visual Planner (4–12). Can be used by adults and students to organize text in a graphic way. Students can create concept maps, story webs, Venn diagrams, and flow charts. Sunburst.

Writing Skills (6–9). Provides students with structured practice of sentence development, structured paragraphs, and the development of essays. Children can rewrite and proof as they assume the role of editor. Sunburst.

> **Study Guide Question**
>
> *How is computer software used to assist students you know with their writing? Share your description with peers and comment on at least one improvement you would like attempted in your school.*

Summary

This chapter has focused on question-driven assessment, formal and informal assessment, and the facilitation of writing across the curriculum. Specific checklists and strategies to assist students in composing and editing their written work have been presented. The aim of the strategies is to move students from dependence to independence in writing. The adult's role as a mediator has also been stressed as an essential component of the writing program.

Activities

1. Interview a teacher who works with students who are D/HH. What questions or concerns about facilitating writing with these students does the teacher have?

2. Conduct a formal or informal assessment of the writing abilities of a student who is D/HH.

3. Use the Six Trait Writing Assessment Model (Appendix 7–A) to determine several writing objectives for a student. Discuss them with a teacher.

4. Describe and exemplify the four principal writing stages.

5. Complete several stages of the writing process with a student who is D/HH. Evaluate your mediation and conferencing skills and share your ideas with a peer.

Resources for Facilitating Writing

Books

Bridges, L. (1997). *Writing as a Way of Knowing.* York, ME: Stenhouse.

Gillie, J., Ingle, S., & Mumford, H. (1997). *Read to Write: An Integrated Course for Non-Native Speakers of English.* New York: McGraw-Hill.

Peyton, J., & Reed, L. (1990). *Dialogue Journal Writing with Normative English Speakers: A Handbook for Teachers.* Alexandria, VA: TESOL.

Software

Cambridge Developmental Laboratory
86 W. Street
Waltham, MA 02154
1-800-637-0047

Educational Resources
P.O. Box 1900
Elgin, IL 60121-1900
1-800-624-2926

Learning Services
P.O. Box 10636
Eugene, OR 97440
1-800-877-3278

Sunburst
101 Castleton Street
P.O. Box 40
Pleasantville, NY 10570
1-800-321-7511

320

Appendix 7-A

Six Trait Rubric*

With this six trait rubric for assessing writing, points are allocated using a 5, 3, 1 point system:
- 5 = a strong sense of control with direction and purpose
- 3 = taking control and gaining a sense of purpose
- 1 = beginning development

Ideas and Content

5 *This paper is clear and focused. It holds the reader's attention. Relevant anecdotes and details enrich the central theme or story line.*
- Ideas are fresh and original.
- The writer seems to be writing from knowledge or experience and shows insight: an understanding of life and a knack for picking out what is significant.
- Relevant, telling, quality details give the reader important information that goes beyond the obvious or predictable.
- The writer develops the topic in an enlightening, purposeful way that makes a point or tells a story.
- Every piece adds something to the whole.

3 *The writer is beginning to define the topic, even though development is still basic or general.*
- It is pretty easy to see where the writer is headed, though more information is needed to "fill in the blanks."
- The writer seems to be drawing on knowledge or experience, but has difficulty going from general observations to specifics.
- Ideas are reasonably clear, though they may not be detailed, personalized, accurate, or expanded enough to show in-depth understanding or a strong sense of purpose.
- Support is attempted, but doesn't go far enough yet in fleshing out the main point or storyline.
- Details often blend the original with the predictable.

1 *As yet, the paper has no clear sense of purpose or central theme. To extract meaning from the text, the reader must make inferences based on sketchy details. The writing reflects more than one of these problems:*

cont.

*From *Student Friendly Guide to Writing with Traits*, by the Northwest Regional Educational Laboratory, 1995, Portland: Northwest Regional Educational Laboratory. Originally developed by teachers from the Beaverton, Oregon, School District. Copyright 1995 by the Northwest Regional Educational Laboratory. Adapted with permission.

- The writer is still in search of a topic, or has not begun to define the topic in a meaningful, personal way.
- Information is very limited or unclear.
- The text may be repetitious, or may read like a collection of disconnected, random thoughts.
- Everything seems as important as everything else; the reader has a hard time sifting out what's critical.

Organization

5 *The organization enhances and showcases the central idea or storyline. The order, structure, or presentation of information is compelling and moves the reader through the text.*
- Details seem to fit where they're placed; sequencing is logical and effective.
- An inviting introduction draws the reader in; a satisfying conclusion leaves the reader with a sense of resolution.
- Pacing is well controlled; the writer knows when to slow down and elaborate, and when to pick up the pace and move on.
- Thoughtful transitions clearly show how ideas connect.
- Organization flows so smoothly that the reader hardly thinks about it.

3 *The organizational structure is strong enough to move the reader through the text without undue confusion.*
- The paper has a recognizable introduction and conclusion. The introduction may not create a strong sense of anticipation; the conclusion may not tie up all loose ends.
- Sequencing is usually logical, but may sometimes be so predictable that the structure takes attention away from the content.
- Pacing is fairly well controlled, though the writer sometimes spurts ahead too quickly or spends too much time on details that do not matter.
- Transitions often work well; at other times, connections between ideas are fuzzy.
- The organization sometimes supports the main point or storyline; at other times, the reader feels an urge to slip in a transition or move things around.

1 *The writing lacks a clear sense of direction. Ideas, details, or events seem strung together in a loose or random fashion; there is no identifiable internal structure. The writing reflects more than one of these problems:*
- Sequencing needs work.
- There is no real lead to set up what follows, no real conclusion to wrap things up.

cont.

- Pacing feels awkward; the writer slows to a crawl when the reader wants to get on with it, and vice versa.
- Connections between ideas are confusing or missing.
- Problems with organization make it hard for the reader to get a grip on the main point or storyline.

Voice

5 *The writer speaks directly to the reader in a way that is individual, compelling, and engaging. Clearly, the writer is involved in the text, is sensitive to the needs of an audience, and is writing to be read.*
- The reader feels a strong interaction with the writer, sensing the person behind the words.
- The tone and voice give flavor to the message and seem appropriate for the purpose and audience.
- Narrative writing seems honest, appealing, and written from the heart.
- Expository or persuasive writing reflects a strong commitment to the topic, and brings the topic to life by showing why the reader should care or want to know more.

3 *The writer seems sincere, but not fully engaged or involved. The result is pleasant or even personable, but not compelling.*
- The writing communicates in an earnest, pleasing manner. Moments here and there surprise, amuse, or move the reader.
- Voice may emerge strongly on occasion, then retreat behind general, dispassionate language.
- The writing hides as much of the writer as it reveals.
- The writer seems aware of an audience, but often weighs words carefully or discards personal insights in favor of safe generalities.

1 *The writer seems indifferent, uninvolved, or distanced from the topic and/or the audience. As a result, the writing is lifeless or mechanical; depending on the topic, it may be overly technical or jargonistic. The paper reflects more than one of the following problems:*
- It is hard to sense the writer behind the words. The writer does not seem to reach out to an audience or to anticipate their interests and questions.
- The writer speaks in a kind of monotone that flattens all potential highs or lows of the message.
- The writing may communicate on a functional level, but it does not move or involve the reader.
- The writer does not seem sufficiently at home with the topic to take risks, share personal insights, or make the topic/story personal and real for the reader.

cont.

Word Choice

5 *Words convey the intended message in a precise, interesting, and natural way. The words are powerful and engaging.*

- Words are specific and accurate; it is easy to understand just what the writer means.
- The language is natural and never overdone; words and phrasing are highly individual and effective.
- Lively verbs energize the writing. Precise nouns and modifiers create pictures in the reader's mind.
- Striking words and phrases often catch the reader's eye—and linger in the reader's mind.
- Clichés and jargon are used sparingly, only for effect.

3 *The language is functional, even if it lacks punch. It is easy to figure out the writer's meaning on a general level.*

- Words are almost always correct and adequate; they simply lack flair.
- Familiar words and phrases communicate but rarely capture the reader's imagination. Still, the paper may have one or two fine moments.
- Attempts at colorful language come close to the mark, but sometimes seem overdone.
- Energetic verbs or picturesque phrases liven things up now and then; the reader longs for more.

1 *The writer struggles with a limited vocabulary, searching for words to convey meaning. The writing reflects more than one of these problems:*

- Language is so vague (e.g., *It was a fun time, She was neat, It was nice, We did lots of stuff*) that only the most general message comes through.
- Persistent redundancy distracts the reader.
- Jargon or clichés distract or mislead.
- Words are used incorrectly, sometimes making the message hard to decipher.
- Problems with language leave the reader wondering what the writer is trying to say.

Sentence Fluency

5 *The writing has an easy flow and rhythm when reading aloud. Sentences are well built, with strong and varied structure that invites expressive oral reading.*

- Sentences are constructed in a way that helps make meaning clear.

cont.

- Purposeful and varied sentence beginnings show how each sentence relates to and builds upon the one before it.
- The writing has cadence, as if the writer has thought about the sound of the words as well as the meaning.
- Sentences vary in length as well as structure.
- Fragments, if used, add style.
- Dialogue, if used, sounds natural.

3 *The text hums along with a steady beat, but tends to be more pleasant or businesslike than musical, more mechanical than fluid.*

- Sentences may not seem artfully crafted or musical, but they are usually grammatical. They hang together. They get the job done.
- There is at least some variation in sentence length and structure. Sentence beginnings are NOT all alike.
- The reader sometimes has to hunt for clues (e.g., connecting words and phrases like *however, therefore, naturally, after a while, on the other hand, to be specific, for example, next, first of all, later, but as it turned out, although, etc.*) that show how sentences interrelate.
- Parts of the text invite expressive oral reading; others may be stiff, awkward, choppy, or gangly.

1 *The reader has to practice quite a bit in order to give this paper a fair interpretive reading. The writing reflects more than one of the following problems:*

- Sentences are choppy, incomplete, rambling, or awkward; they need work.
- Phrasing does not sound natural, the way someone might speak. The reader must sometimes pause or read over to get the meaning.
- Many sentences begin in the same manner and may follow the same patterns (e.g., subject-verb-object) in a monotonous way.
- Endless connectives (*and, and so, but then, because, and then,* etc.) create a massive jumble of language in which clear sentence beginnings and endings get swallowed up.

Conventions

5 *The writer demonstrates a good grasp of standard writing conventions (e.g., grammar, capitalization, punctuation, usage, spelling, paragraphing) and uses conventions effectively to enhance readability. Errors tend to be so few and so minor that the reader can easily overlook them unless hunting for them specifically.*

- Paragraphing tends to be sound and to reinforce the organizational structure.

cont.

- Grammar and usage are correct and contribute to clarity and style.
- Punctuation is accurate and guides the reader through the text.
- Spelling is generally correct, even on more difficult words.
- The writer may manipulate conventions—especially grammar and spelling—for stylistic effect.
- GRADES 7 AND UP ONLY: The writing is sufficiently long and complex to allow the writer to show skill in using a wide range of conventions.
- Only light editing would be required to polish the text for publication.

3 *The writer shows reasonable control over a limited range of standard writing conventions. Conventions are sometimes handled well and enhance readability; at other times, errors are distracting and impair readability.*

- Paragraphing is attempted, but paragraphs sometimes run together or begin in the wrong places.
- Problems with grammar or usage are not serious enough to distort meaning.
- Terminal (end-of-sentence) punctuation is usually correct; internal punctuation (commas, apostrophes, semicolons, dashes, colons, parentheses) is sometimes missing or wrong.
- Spelling is usually correct or reasonably phonetic on common words.
- Moderate editing would be required to polish the text for publication.

1 *Errors in spelling, punctuation, usage and grammar, capitalization, and/or paragraphing repeatedly distract the reader and make the text difficult to read. The writing reflects more than one of these problems:*

- Paragraphing is missing, irregular, or so frequent that it has no relationship to the organizational structure of the text.
- Errors in grammar or usage are very noticeable, and may affect meaning.
- Punctuation (including terminal punctuation) is often missing or incorrect.
- Spelling errors are frequent, even on common words.
- The reader must read once to decode, then again for meaning.
- Extensive editing would be required to polish the text for publication.

References

Archer, A., & Gleason, M. (1995). Skills for school success. In P. Cegelka & W. Berdine (Eds.), *Effective instruction of students with learning difficulties* (pp. 227-264). Boston: Allyn & Bacon.

Bourne, J. (1994). *An overview of early drawing performance.* Unpublished manuscript, University of Kansas Medical Center, Kansas City.

Bruner, J. (1966). *Toward a theory of instruction.* Cambridge, MA: Harvard University Press.

Cantor, N. (1986). *The reliability and validity of the Iowa Test of Basic Skills writing supplement.* Unpublished master's thesis, University of Iowa, Iowa City.

Clay, M. (1975). *What did I write.* Portsmouth, NH: Heinemann Books.

Clay, M. (1993). *Reading recovery: A guidebook for teachers in training.* Portsmouth, NH: Heinemann.

Daiute, C., & Kruidenier, J. (1985). A self-questioning strategy to increase young writers' revising processes. *Research in Teaching of English, 15*(10), 5-22.

Duncan, V., & Neuberger, W. (1987). *Results and analysis of the 1987 Oregon statewide writing assessment.* Salem, OR: Oregon Department of Education.

Englert, C., Raphael, T., Anderson, L., Anthony, H., & Stevens, D. (1991). Making strategies and self-talk visible: Writing instruction in regular and special education classrooms. *American Educational Research Journal, 28*(2), 337-372.

Feathers, K. (1993). *Info text: Reading and learning.* Scarborough, Ontario: Pippin.

Fitzgerald, E. (1949). *Straight language for the deaf.* Washington, DC: Alexander Graham Bell Association for the Deaf.

Gallaudet University (1983). *Stanford Achievement Test for Hearing Impaired Students.* Washington, DC: Gallaudet University. (Available from the Center for Assessment and Demographic Studies, Gallaudet University; 800 Florida Avenue, NE; Washington, DC 20002–3695)

Gormley, K., & Sarachan-Deily, A. (1987). Evaluating hearing-impaired students' writing: A practical approach. *The Volta Review, 89*(3), 157-166.

Graham, S., Harris, K., MacArthur, C., & Schwarts, S. (1991). Writing and writing instruction for students with learning disabilities: Review of a research program. *Learning Disability Quarterly, 14*, 89-114.

Hacker, D., Plumb, E., Butterfield, E., Quathamer, D., & Heineken, E. (1994). Text revision: Detection and correction of errors. *Journal of Educational Psychology, 86*(1), 65-78.

Hammill, D., & Larsen, S. (1983). *Test of Written Language.* Austin, TX: Pro-Ed.

Hayward, L., & LeBuffe, J. (1985, Fall). Self-correction: A positive method for improving writing skills. *Teaching Exceptional Children 18*(1), 68-73.

Heefner, D. (1993). *Assessing written narratives of deaf students with the six trait analytical scale.* Unpublished master's thesis, University of Kansas Medical Center, Kansas City.

Hresko, W. (1988). *Test of Early Written Language.* Austin, TX: Pro-Ed.

Klecan-Aker, J., & Blondeau, R. (1990). An examination of the written stories of H.I. school-age children. *The Volta Review, 92*(6), 275-282.

Knudson, R. (1989). Effects of instructional strategies on children's informational writing. *Journal of Educational Research, 83*(2), 93-96.

La Paz, S., & Graham, S. (1997). Strategy instruction in planning: Effects on the writing performance and behavior of students with learning difficulties. *Exceptional Children, 63*(2), 167-186.

Levy, N., & Rosenberg, M. (1961). Strategies for improving the written expression of students with learning disabilities. *LD Forum, 16*(1), 27-30.

Luetke-Stahlman, B. (1998). *Language issues in deaf education.* Hillsboro, OR: Butte Publications.

Luetke-Stahlman, B., & Luckner, J. (1991). *Effectively educating students with hearing impairments.* New York: Longman.

McAnally, P., Rose, S., & Quigley, S. (1994). *Language learning practices with deaf children* (2nd ed.). Austin, TX: Pro-Ed.

McGhee, R., Bryant, B., Laren, S., & Rivera, D. (1995). *Test of Written Expression.* Austin, TX: Pro-Ed.

Mercer, C. (1997). *Students with learning disabilities.* Columbus, OH: Merrill.

Northwest Regional Educational Laboratory (1995). *Student friendly guide to writing with traits.* Portland: Northwest Regional Educational Laboratory.

Noyce, R., & Christie, J. (1989). *Integrating reading and writing instruction in grades K-8.* Boston: Allyn & Bacon.

Oliver, E. (1995). The writing quality of seventh, ninth, and eleventh graders, and college freshmen: Does rhetorical specification in writing prompts make a difference? *Research in the Teaching of English, 29,* 422-450.

Phenix, J. (1990). *Teaching writing: The nuts and bolts of running a day-to-day writing program.* Markham, Ontario: Pembroke.

Poggio, J., Glasnapp, D., Nielsen, D., Barry, A., & Sundbye, N. (1995). *Overview of the Kansas assessment programs.* Lawrence, KS: Center for Educational Testing and Evaluation, School of Education, University of Kansas.

Polloway, E., & Smith, T. (1992). *Language instruction for students with disabilities* (2nd ed.). Denver: Love.

Psychological Corporation (1989). *Stanford Achievement Test* (8th ed.). San Antonio, TX: Harcourt Brace.

Rubin, D. (1987). Divergence and convergence between oral and written communication. In K. Butler (Ed.), *Best Practices I: The classroom as an assessment arena* (pp. 56-73). Gaithersburg, MD: Aspen.

Slater, S. (1994). *1994 Oregon statewide assessment press briefing packet.* Salem, OR: Oregon Department of Education.

Stauffer, R. (1980). *The language experience approach to the teaching of reading.* New York: Harper.

Taylor, R. (1997). *Assessment of exceptional students: Educational and psychological procedures.* Boston: Allyn & Bacon.

Wilbur, R. (1977). An explanation of deaf children's difficulty with certain syntactic structures. *The Volta Review, 79,* 85-92.

Willis, S. (1997). *Teaching young writers: Feedback and coaching help students hone skills.* Alexandria, VA: Association for Supervision and Curriculum Development.

Wing, G. (1887). The theory and practice of grammatical methods. *American Annals of the Deaf, 32,* 84-89.

Woodcock, R., & Johnson, M. (1977). *Woodcock-Johnson Psychoeducational Battery.* Allen, TX: DLM.

Chapter 8

Assessing and Facilitating Spelling

Spelling Assessment

Three Spelling Approaches

Phonological Awareness and Students Who Are D/HH

Spelling Facilitation

Appendix 8-A: Basic Sight Vocabulary List

Appendix 8-B: Spelling and Phonics Monitoring Form

"For centuries, adults spelled as well as they could using the Roman alphabet as they struggled to write English. They invented spellings as they wrote. Standard spelling is a fairly recent notion, growing from the 1755 dictionary of Samuel Johnson. . . . Two spelling tasks have emerged in the 1990s: learning strategies of spelling and learning how to spell individual words" (McCracken & McCracken, 1995, p. 113).

Given the history of spelling, it is not surprising that educators are currently faced with at least three different approaches to facilitating the development of spelling skills in students. Whatever methodology is chosen, team members should be mindful that recent research (e.g., Perfetti, Rieben, & Fayol, 1997) has confirmed that spelling proficiency requires both (a) an understanding of the relationship between the spoken sounds of English and how those sounds are represented when written and (b) the ability to read a large number of whole words. With these requirements in mind, spelling assessment and facilitation strategies are explained in this chapter. The chapter includes weekly lesson plans to assist team members who wish to facilitate spelling and to integrate reading, writing, and spelling activities.

Spelling Assessment

The assessment of spelling should be driven by relevant questions and can be achieved through both formal and informal techniques. Using a combination of both kinds of tools is recommended in preparation for team meetings regarding the literacy skills of students who are D/HH. Instruments described by Mercer (1997) and Polloway and Smith (1992) include the following:

Formal Spelling Assessment Instruments
Diagnostic Spelling Potential Test (Arena, 1981)
Gates-Russell Spelling Diagnostic Test (Gates & Russell, 1937)
Test of Written Spelling–2 (Larsen & Hammill, 1986)
Peabody Individual Achievement Test–Revised (Dunn & Markwardt, 1989)
Wide Range Achievement Test–3 (Wilkinson, 1993)

Informal Spelling Assessment Tools
Dictated tests
Informal spelling inventories
Curriculum-based assessment
Spelling error analysis
Cloze procedure
Interviews and questionnaires to obtain information
from a student perspective
Observation

Three Spelling Approaches

Study Guide Question
What do teachers in your area use to assess spelling ability when students are D/HH? Compare your findings with those of a peer.

To spell proficiently, students require a knowledge of the spelling system in English and opportunities to read and study many words. At the present time, spelling practices combine three approaches. These approaches have been synthesized from the literature for discussion here.

One Word at a Time. One approach teaches spelling one word at a time and uses spelling lists determined by word frequency alone (Morris, Blanton, Blanton, & Penny, 1995). Lists of the words most frequently used in conversation and reading are available in many language arts texts and can be used by team members interested in working with this word-by-word approach. A sample list is provided in Appendix 8–A.

Orthographic Patterns. A second approach to facilitating spelling achievement promotes the formal study of approximately 3000 words taught during second through eighth grades. Spelling textbooks which present orthographic patterns (spelling rules) are used, and students are asked to pay attention to chosen patterns. Words for study do not originate from students' actual writing needs. This approach includes repeated teaching of small steps of material, guided practice, and often the use of cooperative learning. Fulk and Stormont-Spurgin (1995) emphasized the importance of providing direct instruction of spelling rules but advocated spending short periods of time doing so.

Strategies and Generalizations. In a third approach to facilitating spelling achievement, adults determine each student's spelling level and monitor the difference between the student's ability to demonstrate knowledge of how to spell and his or her actual use of spelling conventions when writing. Inherent in this approach is the recognition that the student needs a "spelling base" in much the same way that he or she needs a language base (Morris et al., 1995). Invernizzi, Abouzeid, and Gill (1994) described basic elements of this approach:

- assessment of the student's present level of orthographic awareness
- design of a systematic study of word features that match the student's developmental knowledge, including knowledge of spelling rules
- use of text that the student has read or written as a context for studying spelling

Implementation of this approach includes

- comparing and contrasting words so the student can examine them (for example, comparing regular and irregular past tense verb spellings)
- categorizing words so the student can manipulate them (for example, sorting out past tense verb spellings that sound like /t/, those that sound like /d/, and those that are irregular)
- discussing the spelling of words and spelling rules so the student's attention is directed toward word patterns (*What is the most common spelling of past tense verbs in English?*)
- providing adult supervision (for instance, confirming student observations)

The result of this approach is that students learn spelling strategies and generalizations that extend beyond learning how to spell individual words (see also Zutell, 1996).

Proponents of the spelling strategies approach advocate that students learn and apply phonological coding: That is, when students hear, say, or kinesthetically feel a sound, they write a letter or letter sequence (see Figure 8–1).

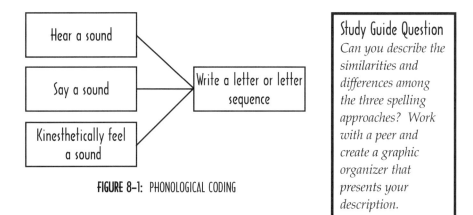

FIGURE 8-1: PHONOLOGICAL CODING

Study Guide Question
Can you describe the similarities and differences among the three spelling approaches? Work with a peer and create a graphic organizer that presents your description.

Phonological Awareness and Students Who Are D/HH

Marschark (1993) commented that the "central issue . . . seems to be how deaf children, especially those who are severely to profoundly deaf, can make use of phonological coding in the absence of hearing" (p. 209). Hung, Tzeng, and Warren (1981) found that some students who are D/HH do use sound-to-spelling correspondences (see Figure 8–2). This appears to be true both for students who sign and for students who use only oral communication (Hanson, 1989; Marschark; Tzeng, 1993; Gibbs, 1989). Use of Cued Speech or visual phonics may be required (Luetke-Stahlman, 1998).

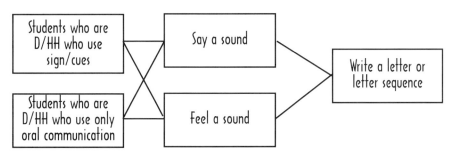

FIGURE 8-2: STUDENTS WHO ARE D/HH USE PHONOLOGICAL CODING

Marschark (1993) noted that "variability in the use of phonological coding doesn't seem to be directly tied to degree of hearing loss, at least among students with more severe losses" (p. 209). Also, Hanson, Shankweiler, and Fischer (1983) found no connection between hearing status and the ability of college students to spell words with regular spelling patterns.

Because strong phonological awareness is so closely linked to literacy, Luetke-Stahlman and Luckner (1991) suggested that professionals work with students who are D/HH for at least 6 to 12 months to facilitate phonological coding. Work by Becker (1993) supported this idea, finding that students who are D/HH may be capable of acquiring and applying phonics skills. Students with assistive listening devices may be able to learn phonics skills over time, given training. A checklist for monitoring the teaching of phonics to first, second, and third graders is provided in Appendix 8–B.

In summarizing the work of Leybaert, Content, and Alegria (1987), Marschark (1993) suggested that phonological awareness can be trained using a combination of
- grapheme-to-sound awareness
- spelling-to-speaking articulation awareness
- speechreading ability
- fingerspelling awareness
- writing

None of these methods, he emphasized, is adequate in and of itself. In a spelling approach promoting the uses of structured lessons, Oldrieve (1997) concurred with using a combination of these methods.

> **Study Guide Question**
> *What are the phonological awareness abilities of students you know who are D/HH? Ask a teacher of the deaf or a speech-language pathologist to assist you in describing the students' abilities.*

Spelling Facilitation

Logically, students who are D/HH would benefit from thoughtful facilitation of spelling. Currently, however, most of these students' present level of orthographic awareness is unassessed, and they are not taught spelling strategies. The result is that there is little transfer from weekly spelling tests to spelling in students' writing. Willis (1995) conducted an informal study of professionals involved with the education of students who are D/HH in seven school districts in one major city. These professionals reported that students were often able to spell weekly word lists correctly, but spelled poorly in "authentic writing" assignments (writing that is functional or about real-life contexts).

☛   **Correct weekly**   ≠   **Correct spelling in**
               spelling   **authentic writing**

The practice of simply telling students how to spell a word when they ask for help as they write needs to be reevaluated. Students can be provided with individual dictionaries where words are added as requested, but thereafter words should be independently located by the student. To choose the best spelling method(s) to use with a particular student, adults may need to consider the three approaches to spelling reviewed earlier in this chapter. In addition, they may need to *identify the desired outcomes* of spelling achievement. To do so, and to choose the best mediation strategies, team members may find the Cummins Model of Language Proficiency (Cummins, 1984) useful.

As explained in earlier chapters, the upper right-hand quadrant of the Cummins model characterizes the demands of the general education classroom or real life. Consideration of the other quadrants assists in understanding the degree of language proficiency and the linguistic skills required by specific learning tasks, such as spelling. An example adapting the model for spelling mediation appears in Figure 8–3.

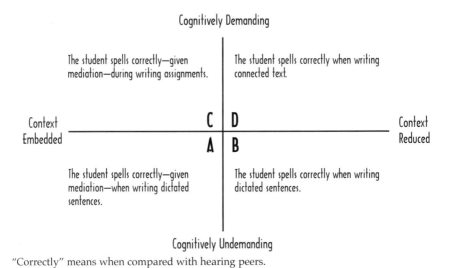

Cognitively Demanding

The student spells correctly—given mediation—during writing assignments. | The student spells correctly when writing connected text.

Context Embedded

C | **D**

A | **B**

Context Reduced

The student spells correctly—given mediation—when writing dictated sentences. | The student spells correctly when writing dictated sentences.

Cognitively Undemanding

"Correctly" means when compared with hearing peers.

FIGURE 8-3: THE CUMMINS MODEL ADAPTED FOR SPELLING

Consideration of spelling mediation activities in terms of the Cummins model can assist team members in developing an organizational plan for spelling instruction for students who are D/HH. Adults will be aware of the desired outcomes specified in the upper right-hand quadrant and can focus on the characteristics of the other quadrants to develop and sequence appropriate mediation activities.

Examples of spelling mediation include the following. Other mediation strategies are discussed in Chapter 1.

> **Study Guide Question**
> *Can you write 3–5 spelling objectives based on the spelling assessment of a hypothetical student and using the Cummins model?*

Examples of Spelling Mediation Activities

1. Teachers identify each student's zone of proximal development (Vygotsky, 1962, 1978) between word features that are correctly represented and those that are omitted (Invernizzi et al., 1994). This is the student's "instructional spelling level."

2. As promoted by Allred (1977), Dolch (1943), Henderson (1990), and Horn (1960), students practice spelling at their assessed instructional level (or level + 1, as described in Chapters 5

and 6; Krashen, 1982). This practice might occur individually or in small groups. When practicing in groups, students work with others of their same ability level, allowing them to retain a greater number of correctly spelled words (Morris et al., 1995).

3. Students receive immediate feedback when they misspell words. Immediate feedback can be provided by word-processing software that includes spellchecker, by working with peers at the board, and by peers' helping each other self-correct. Pronunciation, speechreading of target words, and fingerspelling letters as they are signed also provide feedback.

4. Students sort words from a given list into contrasting categories. The words are later copied into a notebook (Invernizzi et al.).

5. Students locate words from specific word families in materials they are reading and writing that fit the word family (*ick, ock; fact, factory*). They classify these words in columns (Invernizzi et al.).

6. Students are helped to observe words that are difficult to spell or word families with irregular forms. Students are helped to make hypotheses about the variance involved. Each student copies the words into a notebook, grouping them in columns by orthographic patterns (Invernizzi et al.).

7. Adults help students to be aware of how spellings can have different sounds. For example, the suffix *-ed* can have three different pronunciations: *batted*, /ed/; *jumped*, /t/; or *played*, /d/. When students are inconsistent in their spelling of such words, it is a clue that they are ready for word attack work (see Invernizzi et al.).

8. Weekly spelling lists of 10–20 words are compiled, consisting of words that students need for creative writing, high frequency words, and words that fit a particular word sort or rule pattern. These words are discussed daily, 4–5 words at a time, so that all words are practiced before the weekly quiz. Miller (1995) advocated flow lists rather than

fixed lists. Using a flow list, words are dropped from the list as they are mastered, and new words are added.

9. Students are given a pretest so that target words for study are identified (Morris et al.). Fulk and Stormont Spurgin (1995) labeled this same concept "test-teach-test" (p.16).

10. Students demonstrate accountability. They are given retention tests every six weeks to encourage them to remember the spellings of words learned previously (Morris et al.). Praise and reinforcement are lavished on students who demonstrate that the correct spelling of words has been remembered.

> **Study Guide Question**
>
> *Use the spelling mediation activities listed in this chapter to create an instructional plan for one of your students who is D/HH. What is the plan and what is the outcome of the lesson (incorporate information from this chapter)?*

To make spelling assessment and mediation materials more useful to team members, Ganske (1993) organized work by Henderson's (1990) four levels of spelling ability: the letter-name stage, within-word pattern stage, syllable-juncture stage, and derivational constancy stage. Ganske particularly promoted assessment to determine each student's level of spelling ability so that the appropriate instructional spelling level, such as level + 1, can be identified. In addition she described an approach in which Henderson's spelling stages were used to assign students to spelling groups. Students with similar abilities could then work cooperatively to use spelling in authentic writing activities.

Getting Ready for Spelling Facilitation

Team members need to prepare for spelling facilitation in several ways. First, they need to have some important tools:

- a list (or lists) of high-frequency words required for an individual student's written work
- a list of words that are difficult to learn to spell and must therefore be learned by rote
- a list of basic spelling rules (these can be found in many

standard grammar texts—see Figure 8–4 for a sampling of spelling rules)

■ knowledge of each student's spelling level

1. When the sound is /k/, use *ck* at the end of a one-syllable word immediately after a short vowel sound: *black, fleck, trick, lock, stuck.*

2. When the sound is /ch/, use *tch* at the end of a one-syllable word immediately after a short vowel sound: *match, stretch, ditch, scotch, hutch.* Exceptions are *such, much,* and *rich.*

3. When the sound is /j/, use *dge* at the end of a one-syllable word immediately after a short vowel sound: *badge, ledge, bridge, lodge, nudge.*

4. In a one-syllable word that ends in one consonant after one vowel, double the final consonant before adding a suffix that begins with a vowel:
run + ing = running, thin + est = thinnest, but *glad + ly = gladly.*

5. When a word ends in a silent *e*, drop the *e* before adding a suffix that begins with a vowel: *give + ing = giving, love + able = lovable,* but *safe + ly = safely.*

6. When a word ends in *y* after a consonant, change the *y* to *i* before adding any suffix, except one that begins with *i*: *copy + ed = copied, copy + es = copies, copy + ing = copying.*

FIGURE 8–4: A SAMPLING OF BASIC SPELLING RULES

After these materials are assembled, adults need to organize the week so that activities based on the three approaches to spelling are used, and both direct instruction and induction are incorporated into lesson plans. The weekly plan in Figure 8–5 provides an example of how team members can ensure that essential spelling practices as well as effective teaching strategies are included in weekly lessons.

Study Guide Question

How does a teacher in your area prepare for spelling facilitation? Interview a teacher of the deaf and determine how his or her preparation is similar to or different from the techniques described here.

Monday

- Adults provide students with a list of 10–20 words to study. Some of these words are high frequency, some are hard to spell, and some are of the pattern the students need to study (Henderson, 1990).
- Adults pretest to determine which words the students cannot spell correctly.
- Adults guide a word sort on the board and assist students individually to determine relevant spelling patterns.
- Students practice spelling words at home.

Tuesday

- Students practice word sorts and spelling the words on the weekly list by being given short, relevant sentences that incorporate other school content.
- Adults ask students to write words, checking that students can
  - (a) name the first letter, final letter, then medial letter(s)
  - (b) write the upper- and lowercase variant of the first letter
  - (c) name the sounds the first letter, final letter, and medial letters represent
  - (d) describe the way the first, final, and medial letters sound/feel
- The teacher keeps track of each student's ability to succeed with letter combinations in each position (initial, medial, final) and continually introduces letters that are appropriate for each student.
- Students practice spelling words at home.

Wednesday

- Students work cooperatively to sort the spelling words without a model and to search their reading and writing materials for other words that fit the target pattern(s).
- When writing, teachers model rule application, word sort application, and so forth. Opportunities include writing lessons, "think alouds," and writing on the board.
- Students practice word sorts and spelling words at home.

Thursday

- As a practice test, adults dictate sentences that include spelling words and school subject content (McCracken & McCracken, 1995).
- Teachers check for correct spelling patterns rather than misspelled whole words and praise students for partial spelling success.
- Students practice word sorts and spelling words at home.

cont.

FIGURE 8–5: A WEEKLY SPELLING ACTIVITY PLAN

FIGURE 8–5, CONT.

> **Friday**
> - Students take the weekly spelling test and demonstrate that they can spell at least some of the target words correctly in their own writing.
> - Students identify 3–5 misspelled words from their independent writing and include them in the following week's spelling list.
> - Teachers complete a check point accountability grid for each student (see, for example, Mercer & Mercer, 1989).

Finally, team members might plan to intertwine spelling activities with reading and writing activities as shown in Figure 8–6 (specific reading and writing activities are discussed in Chapters 5, 6, and 7). As systematic spelling instruction occurs, adults should design checklists or save examples of student's original work to demonstrate and document the progress that is made.

Basal* Read Aloud	Instructional Read	Response Work	Spelling
Monday (Day 1) ■ Focus on purpose. ■ Introduce book (characters, setting, problem, solution). ■ Explain vocabulary and grammar. ■ Have students paraphrase definitions.	■ Reread part of an old story. ■ Introduce leveled text. ■ Discuss author, illustrator, title; make predictions, etc. ■ Introduce concepts of print. ■ Tell story to students using pictures or graphics and new words.	■ Share weekend writing. Use the following: – special chair – rubric for scoring – peer responses (*I like the way . . . ; My favorite part was . . . ; I learned ____ from your story; The word ___ was new to me*).	■ Provide words. ■ Pretest. ■ Present guided sentences.
Tuesday (Day 2) ■ Read text. ■ Make life-to-text, text-to-school studies linkages. ■ Present graphic organizer.	■ Students read text. ■ Adults record misread words but do not tell words to or correct student.		■ Practice spelling in context. ■ Write and sort words. *cont.*

*Could be any text used in a subject area

FIGURE 8–6: INTEGRATING SPELLING, READING, AND WRITING ACTIVITIES

342

FIGURE 8-6, CONT.

Wednesday (Day 3)			
■ Introduce concepts of print based on needs. ■ Continue reading. ■ Ask comprehension questions, using novel vocabulary and grammar.	■ Present semantic work. ■ Present phonics work. ■ Present structure analysis work. ■ Spell new words and needed vocabulary. ■ Practice letter/sound(feel) writing.		■ Re-sort words. ■ Model the rule with words from school subjects.
Thursday (Day 4) ■ Continue reading. ■ Present derivations of words (e.g., *unlike, unusual, unused*). ■ Use blending or segmenting. ■ Identify word patterns. ■ Practice spelling key words.	■ Continue Day 3 discussion. ■ Have students read rest of story or text, or reread if it was completed previously.		■ Dictate spelling words. ■ Monitor student progress.
Friday (Day 5) ■ Videotape oral retell of basal or instructional read.	■ Discuss and apply rules. ■ Keep list of rules taught.	■ Have students write retell using a graphic organizer. ■ Hold a mini-conference. ■ Color-code edit: red = punctuation; green = misspelling; blue = capitalization	■ Spell text in context. ■ Identify authentically misspelled words. ■ Measure accountability.
Weekend ■ Rewrite final story to share with others.			

Activities That Help or Hinder the Learning of Spelling—

Phenix (1990) published summary lists of activities that help and activities that hinder the facilitation of spelling. These lists have been enhanced with suggestions from Perfetti et al. (1997):

How to Help the Learning of Spelling

- Create genuine needs for standard spelling. Publish and display student's writing (letters to relatives, creative pieces and so on).
- Teach students when, where, and why spelling matters.
- Remind students that spelling is a thinking activity, not just a remembering activity.
- Encourage any attempt students make to spell.
- Help students move to their next stage of developmental spelling.
- Provide information about words when students need it but do not tell them the correct spelling of words.
- Point out interesting facts about links between words, word origins, and so on.
- Help students link words into word families that have the same spelling pattern.
- Facilitate spelling by grouping words that share a spelling pattern.
- Show the students how their knowledge of spelling is growing by charting progress.
- Assess spelling proficiency in real writing contexts and at final-draft stage rather than earlier.
- Encourage board and computer games and puzzles that involve words and spelling.
- Teach self-editing or proofreading for specific items, such as plural endings.
- Teach students about the function of spelling patterns. For example, an -er ending often indicates a person who does something (baker, teacher, and so on).
- Give regular, explicit instruction in spelling concepts, the patterns of words, and the construction of words.

- Inform parents about your spelling program and help them understand how their children are learning to spell.
- Link reading, writing, and spelling throughout the day.

How to Hinder the Learning of Spelling

- Expect to see accurate spelling at early stages in learning.
- Make spelling a major priority in your writing program.
- Teach students that all words have to be memorized.
- Expect students to look up all their spelling errors in a dictionary.
- Require corrected spelling in every piece of writing the students do.
- Teach spelling by using lists of words that do not share a spelling pattern or generalization. (This makes memorization the only strategy for learning words.)
- Measure spelling proficiency by test scores.
- Draw conclusions about spelling ability by evaluating first-draft writing.
- Focus on students' weaknesses.
- Send home lists of words to be memorized.

From *Teaching Writing* (pp. 91-92), by J. Phenix, 1990, Markham, Ontario: Pembroke Publishers. Copyright 1990 by Pembroke Publishers. Adapted with permission.

Study Guide Question

Do older students and team members agree with Phenix's ideas about helping or hindering spelling facilitation? Interview an older (high school) student who is D/HH or a teacher of the deaf and share her or his opinions with a peer.

Summary

A review of the literature pertaining to spelling reveals at least three basic approaches to helping students become independent spellers. Readers are urged to assess the spelling abilities of students and combine the approaches suggested in this chapter. They are encouraged to compile weekly spelling lists that include

- high-frequency words
- words that are difficult to spell
- words that the student needs for writing
- words that reflect the student's current spelling level

Much of the information provided in this chapter promotes students' applying spelling strategies to genuine literacy work and being accountable for their own spelling achievement.

Activities

1. Interview teachers working in a program that serves students who are D/HH. Ask how spelling is facilitated in the program and how requirements or materials might be modified for particular students. Ask the opinion of these professionals with regard to the integration of the spelling activities described in this chapter.

2. Facilitate a spelling lesson using the lesson plan provided in this chapter.

3. Read two current research articles on spelling instruction from journals outside the field of deaf education.

Appendix 8-A

Basic Sight Vocabulary List: The 200 Most Frequently Used Words*

1	the	33	you	65	some
2	of	34	were	66	could
3	and	35	her	67	time
4	to	36	all	68	these
5	a	37	she	69	two
6	in	38	there	70	may
7	that	39	would	71	then
8	is	40	their	72	do
9	was	41	we	73	first
10	he	42	him	74	any
11	for	43	been	75	my
12	it	44	has	76	now
13	with	45	when	77	such
14	as	46	who	78	like
15	his	47	will	79	our
16	on	48	more	80	over
17	be	49	no	81	man
18	at	50	if	82	me
19	by	51	out	83	even
20	I	52	so	84	most
21	this	53	said	85	made
22	had	54	what	86	after
23	not	55	up	87	also
24	are	56	its	88	did
25	but	57	about	89	many
26	from	58	into	90	before
27	of	59	than	91	must
28	have	60	them	92	through
29	an	61	can	93	back
30	they	62	only	94	years
31	which	63	other	95	where
32	one	64	new	96	much *cont.*

97	your	134	while	171	once
98	may	135	last	172	general
99	well	136	might	173	high
100	down	137	us	174	upon
101	should	138	great	175	school
102	because	139	old	176	every
103	each	140	year	177	don't
104	just	141	off	178	does
105	those	142	come	179	got
106	people	143	since	180	united
107	Mr.	144	against	181	left
108	how	145	go	182	number
109	too	146	came	183	course
110	little	147	night	184	war
111	state	148	used	185	until
112	good	149	take	186	always
113	very	150	three	187	away
114	make	151	states	188	something
115	would	152	himself	189	fact
116	still	153	few	190	through
117	own	154	house	191	water
118	see	155	use	192	less
119	men	156	during	193	public
120	work	157	without	194	put
121	long	158	again	195	thing
122	get	159	place	196	almost
123	here	160	American	197	hand
124	between	161	around	198	enough
125	both	162	however	199	far
126	life	163	home	200	look
127	being	164	small		
128	under	165	found		
129	never	166	Mrs.		
130	day	167	thought		
131	same	168	went		
132	another	169	say		
133	know	170	part		

Appendix 8-B

Spelling and Phonics Monitoring Form*

Suggested Teaching Order for Phonics Adult points/cues, student says the sound	
Grade One	**Date Learned**
Introducing *m*	
Introducing *s*	
Practicing *m* and *s*	
Introducing *f*	
Practicing *m, s,* and *f*	
Introducing *b*	
Practicing *m, s, f,* and *b*	
Introducing *t*	
Practicing *m, s, f, b,* and *t*	
Introducing *c*	
Practicing *m, s, f, b, t,* and *c*	
Reviewing what has been taught so far	
Teaching short vowels	
Introducing short *a*	
Teaching short *a* in medial position	
Spelling whole words after teaching short *a*	
Introducing *r*	
Practicing *m, s, f, b, t, c,* and *r*	
Introducing *l*	
Practicing *m, s, f, b, t, c, r,* and *l*	
Practicing short *a* with *m, s, f, b, t, c, r,* and *l*	
Introducing *p*	
Practicing *m, s, f, b, t, c, r, l,* and *p*	
Reviewing what has been taught so far	
Introducing short *o*	
Introducing *d*	
Practicing *d* with short *a* and short *o*	*cont.*

*From *Spelling Through Phonics*, 2nd ed., by M. McCracken and R. McCracken, 1996, Winnipeg, Manitoba, Canada: Peguis Publishers. Copyright 1996 by Peguis Publishers. Adapted with permission.

Grade One, cont.	Date Learned
Introducing *g*	
Practicing *g* with short *a* and short *o*	
Reviewing what has been taught so far	
Writing sentences	
Introducing *n*	
Practicing *n* with short *a* and short *o*	
Introducing *w*	
Introducing short *i*	
Practicing short *i*	
Reviewing what has been taught so far	
Introducing *h*	
Practicing *h* with all known consonants and vowels	
Introducing *j*	
Introducing *k*	
Introducing *v*	
Practicing *w, j, k,* and *v* with short *a, i,* and *o*	
Introducing short *u*	
Practicing short *u* in medial position	
Reviewing what has been taught so far	
Introducing *y*	
Introducing *qu*	
Introducing *z*	
Introducing *x*	
Introducing short *e*	
Reviewing consonant sounds, sequencing of sounds, and short vowels	
Spelling two-syllable words	
Practicing two-syllable words	
Practicing three- and four-syllable words	
Adding the endings *-s, -ing, -y,* and *-er*	
Adding *-s* to words that require no other change	
Adding *-ing* to words that require no other change	
Using *-y* on the end of words	
Using *-er* on the end of words	*cont.*

Grade One, cont.	Date Learned
Introducing *ch* in initial and final position	
Introducing *sh* in initial and final position	
Introducing *th* in initial and final position	
Practicing *ch, sh,* and *th*	
Introducing long vowels	
Long *a*	
Long e	
Long *i*	
Long *o*	
Long *u*	

Grade Two	Date Learned
Reviewing short vowels with what has been taught so far	
Short *a*	
Short *e*	
Short *i*	
Short *o*	
Short *u*	
Reviewing one- and two-syllable words and the word endings *-er, -ed, -ing, -y, -es,* and *-s* with the short vowels	
Short *a*	
Short *e*	
Short *i*	
Short *o*	
Short *u*	
Teaching words with short vowels followed by *r*	
er	
ar	
or	
ir	
ur	
Dictating sentences	
Reviewing simple two-syllable words	*cont.*

Grade Two, cont.	Date Learned
Reviewing two-syllable words with *er*	
Teaching common spelling patterns	
ck	
ic	
le	
g representing /j/	
ge representing /j/	
dge representing /j/	
Teaching double consonant words	
ll	
ss	
ff	
Teaching double consonant words with -*er*	
Teaching the *ng* spelling patterns	
ang	
ing	
ong	
ung	
Teaching vowel sound patterns	
The patterns of *oi* and *oy*	
The pattern of *ow* as in *now*	
The pattern of *ow* as in *snow*	
The pattern of *ou* as in *out*	
The pattern of *ous* to sound /us/	
Reviewing what has been taught so far	
Teaching long vowels	
Teaching long *a* vowel patterns	
ai spelling long /a/	
a-e spelling long /a/	
ay spelling long /a/	
Teaching long *e* vowel patterns	
e-e spelling long /e/	
ee spelling long /e/	
ea spelling long /e/	
ie spelling long /e/	*cont.*

Grade Two, cont.	Date Learned
Teaching long *i* vowel patterns	
i-e spelling long /i/	
igh spelling long /i/	
ie spelling long /i/	
Teaching long *o* vowel patterns	
o-e spelling long /o/	
oa spelling long /o/	
ow spelling long /o/	
o followed by *ld* spelling long /o/	
o followed by *lt* spelling long /o/	
Teaching long *u* vowel patterns	
u-e spelling long /u/ or /oo/	

Grade Three	Date Learned
Reviewing the spelling learned so far	
Phonetic words	
Words with *er*	
Words with *y*	
Words with *ing*	
Words with *er* for "good spellers"	
Words with *ic*	
Adding -*ed*	
Doubling the consonant before adding -*ed*	
Teaching changing *y* to *i* and adding -*es* or -*ed*	
Teaching the *oo* spelling patterns	
oo as in *look*	
oo as in *toot*	
Teaching the double *ll* patterns	
all	
ull	
ill	
ell	
Teaching the use of -*tion* to spell /shun/	*cont.*

Grade Three, cont.	Date Learned
Teaching prefixes and suffixes	
-able	
be-	
re-	
dis-	
auto-	
un-	
uni-	
bi-	
tri-	
sub-	
super-	

References

Allred, R. (1977). *Spelling applications of research findings.* Washington, DC: National Education Association.

Arena, J. (1981). *Diagnostic Spelling Potential Test.* Novato, CA: Academic Therapy.

Becker, K. (1993). *Increasing the accuracy of reading decoding skills exhibited by hearing-impaired students with the use of a sound/letter unit instructional approach.* Nova University. (ERIC Document Reproduction Service No. 367 070)

Cummins, J. (1984). *Bilingualism and special education: Issues in assessment and pedagogy.* San Diego, CA: College-Hill Press.

Dolch, E. (1943). *Better spelling.* Champaign, IL: Garrard.

Dunn, L., & Markwardt, F. (1989). *Peabody Individual Achievement Test–Revised.* Circle Pines, MN: American Guidance Service.

Fulk, B., & Stormont-Spurgin, M. (1995). Fourteen spelling strategies for students with learning disabilities. *Intervention in School and Clinic, 31,* 16-20.

Ganske, K. (1993). *Developmental spelling analysis: A qualitative measure for assessment and instructional planning.* Barboursville, VA: Author.

Gates, A. & Russell, D. (1937). *Gates-Russell Spelling Diagnostic Test.* New York: Columbia University Press.

Gibbs, K. (1989). Individual differences in cognitive skills related to reading ability in the deaf. *American Annals of the Deaf, 134,* 214-218.

Hanson, V. (1989). Phonology and reading: Evidence from profoundly deaf readers. In D. Shankweiler & I. Liberman (Eds.), *Phonology and reading disability: Solving the reading puzzle* (pp. 69-89). Ann Arbor, MI: University of Michigan Press.

Hanson, V., Shankweiler, D., & Fischer, F. (1983). Determinants of spelling ability in deaf and hearing adults: Access to linguistic structure. *Cognition, 14,* 323-344.

Henderson, E. (1990). *Teaching spelling* (2nd ed.). Boston: Houghton Mifflin.

Horn, E. (1960). Spelling. In C. Harris (Ed.), *Encyclopedia of educational research* (3rd ed.) (pp. 1337-1354). New York: Macmillan.

Hung, D., Tzeng, O., & Warren, D. (1981). A chronometric study of sentence processing in deaf children. *Cognitive Psychology, 13*, 583-610.

Invernizzi, M., Abouzeid, M., & Gill, J. (1994). Using students' invented spelling as a guide for spelling instruction that emphasizes word study. *The Elementary School Journal, 95*(2), 155-167.

Johnson, D. (1971). The Dolch list reexamined. *The Reading Teacher, 24*(5), 455-456.

Krashen, S. (1982). Accounting for child-adult differences in second language rate and attainment. In S. Krashen (Ed.). *Child-adult differences in second language acquisition*, (pp. 202-226). Cambridge, MA: Newbury House.

Larsen, S. & Hammill, D. (1986). *Test of Written Spelling–2*. Austin, TX: Pro-Ed.

Leybaert, J., Content, A., & Alegria, J. (1987). *The development of written word processing: The case of deaf children*. Workshop presentation, ISPL Congress, University of Kassel.

Luetke-Stahlman, B. (1998). *Language issues in deaf education*. Hillsboro, OR: Butte Publications.

Luetke-Stahlman, B., & Luckner, J. (1991). *Effectively educating students with hearing impairments*. New York: Longman.

Marschark, M. (1993). *Psychological development of deaf children*. New York: Oxford University Press.

McCracken, M., & McCracken, R. (1995). *Reading, writing and language: A practical guide for primary teachers*. Winnipeg, Manitoba, Canada: Peguis.

McCracken, M., & McCracken, R. (1996). *Spelling through phonics*. Winnipeg, Manitoba, Canada: Peguis.

Mercer, C. (1997). *Students with learning disabilities*. Columbus, OH: Merrill.

Mercer, C., & Mercer, A. (1989). *Teaching students with learning problems* (3rd ed.). Columbus, OH: Merrill.

Miller, L. (1995). Spelling and handwriting. In J. Choate (Ed.), *Curriculum-based assessment and programming*. Boston: Allyn & Bacon.

Morris, D., Blanton, L., Blanton, W., & Penny, J. (1995). Teaching low-achieving spellers at their instructional level. *The Elementary School Journal, 96*(2), 163-176.

Oldrieve, R. (1997, March/April). Success with reading and spelling. *Teaching Exceptional Children*, 57-61.

Perfetti, C., Rieben, L., & Fayol, M. (1997). *Learning to spell: Research, theory, and practice across languages.* Mahwah, NJ: Lawrence Erlbaum.

Phenix, J. (1990). *Teaching writing.* Markham, Ontario, Canada: Pembroke Publishing.

Polloway, E., & Smith, T. (1992). *Language instruction for students with disabilities* (2nd ed.). Denver: Love.

Tzeng, S. (1993). *Speech recoding, short-term memory, and reading ability in immature readers with severe to profound hearing impairment.* Unpublished doctoral dissertation, Ohio State University, Columbus.

Vygotsky, L. (1962). *Thought and language* (E. Hanfonann & G. Vakar, Trans.). Cambridge, MA: MIT Press.

Vygotsky, L. (1978). *Mind and society: The development of higher psychological processes* (M. Cole, V. John Steiner, S. Schribner, & E. Souberman, Eds. and Trans.). Cambridge, MA: MIT Press.

Wilkinson, G. (1993). *Wide Range Achievement Test–3.* Wilmington, DE: Jastak Associates.

Willis, T. (1995). *Spelling and deafness.* Unpublished manuscript, University of Kansas Medical Center, Kansas City.

Zutell, J. (1996). The directed spelling thinking activity (DSTA): Providing an effective balance in word study instruction. *The Reading Teacher, 50*(2), 98-108.

Chapter 9

Math and Language

Math Assessment

Cognition and Math

Semantics and Math

Syntax and Math

Teaching about Time and Money

Word Problems

Math Facilitation Tips

Resources

Appendix: Ten-Step Word Problem Worksheet

"To fully participate in life, students must become competent in the language and reasoning of mathematics" (Maryland State Department of Education Mathematics Framework Task Force, 1987). Students who are deaf or hard of hearing "must be taught how to interpret and express mathematical concepts not only in American Sign Language (ASL) but in spoken and written English as well" (Schroeder & Strosnider, 1997, p. 13). In a mathematical environment, students must be able to read texts, understand the linguistic interactions of the teacher and peer group, participate in discussions, and complete assignments correctly. These tasks require ASL and/or English linguistic comprehension and expression, as well as the ability to do reading and writing activities in decontextualized situations (Coelho, 1982).

In this chapter, assessment and facilitation ideas are described that will enable team members to assist students who are D/HH specifically in the acquisition of math language abilities. The cognitive academic language skills required in math as well as other subject areas are then summarized in Chapter 10 (see Figure 10–1).

Math Assessment

Motivated by questions concerning a student's math skills, team members might choose a combination of formal and informal math assessment tools. As with other subject areas, standardized tools are also useful for math assessment to compare students who are D/HH to hearing peers, document progress over a year's time, and ensure that specific skills have been mastered.

Two recommended formal math assessments are the *Key Math–Revised* (Connolly, 1988) and *the Woodcock-Johnson Psychoeducational Battery–Revised (Woodcock & Johnson, 1989)*. McCoy (1995) reported that the standardized math assessments most commonly administered are the *Iowa Test of Basic Skills* (Hieronymus, Hoover, & Lindquist, 1986), the *Metropolitan Achievement Tests* (Comprehension and Basic Skills subtests)

(Prescott, Barlow, Hogan, & Farr, 1984), and the *Stanford Achievement Test* (SAT) (The Psychological Corporation, 1989). Recommended is the version of the SAT normed on students who are D/HH available from Gallaudet University: the *Stanford Achievement Test for Hearing Impaired Students* (SAT–HI) (Gallaudet University, 1983).

Criterion-referenced information is available from the *Diagnostic Mathematics Inventory/Mathematics Systems* (Gessell, 1983) and the *Stanford Diagnostic Mathematics Test* (SDMT) (Beathy, Madden, Gardner, & Karlsen, 1985). These tests assess an individual student's strengths and weaknesses in math skills.

Informal math assessment tools allow team members to evaluate whether a student is gaining curriculum competencies. They also provide insight into the student's ability to use math in real-life situations. Recent trends suggest that teachers assess the *process* students use to arrive at answers. This assessment can be done informally by observing and interviewing, analyzing worksheet samples, or accumulating samples in a portfolio. McLoughlin and Lewis (1994) suggested that such portfolios include the following:

- quizzes and tests
- assignments
- interview results
- standardized test results
- projects
- checklists of progress
- self-assessments
- curriculum-based assessments
- task analysis hierarchy

Task analysis involves a hierarchy of math skills. Such skills can be found listed in materials developed for students with learning disabilities or mild cognitive impairments (see, for example, Mercer & Mercer, 1993).

Cognition and Math

Math comprehension is dependent on the integration of language and mathematical skills. Crandall (1987) stated that, unlike natural interpersonal language, mathematical language lacks redundancy. Problems are often decontextualized and difficult; on the Cummins model they would be charted in the upper right-hand quadrant (Crandall; Cummins, 1984). In order to successfully meet problem-solving challenges in math, students must be able to apply background knowledge, previous mathematical applications, and mathematical thinking (Crandall; see Figure 9–1).

Problem solving has been identified as the most important math skill by the National Council for Teachers of Mathematics (NCTM) (1989). McCoy (1995) explained that recent concern about students' ability to problem solve stemmed from

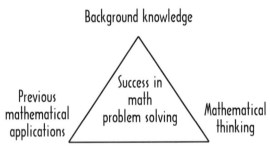

FIGURE 9–1: PROBLEM-SOLVING COMPONENTS IN MATH

a number of sources, including the National Assessment of Educational Progress (NAEP), whose members worried that students could not choose correct math operations in context. "Students knew *how* to add and subtract, but not *when*" (Hodgkinson, 1979, p. 161).

Mathematical thinking incorporates a wide range of cognitive functions (Chamot & O'Malley, 1994):

- Seek information
- Inform
- Compare
- Order
- Classify
- Analyze
- Infer
- Justify and persuade
- Solve problems
- Synthesize
- Evaluate

Chamot and O'Malley also noted that students of mathematics need language to perform these cognitive functions. For example, seeking information requires the language to explore and inquire; informing requires the language to identify and report; comparing requires the language to describe similarities and differences; and so forth.

These cognitive functions and language abilities can be ordered hierarchically to form the vertical axis when team members apply the Cummins model to mathematics. Where each cognitive function or language ability is placed on a vertical axis depends on individual student abilities. The primary value of using the Cummins model in this way is to task analyze in order to determine which skills the student uses presently and which might be facilitated next.

> **Study Guide Question**
>
> *What language is required for cognitive functions? For each of the cognitive functions listed, describe how language is used and give at least one specific example. For example, to seek information uses language to explore and inquire; specifically, a student might use "who" and "what" questions to perform this function.*

Semantics and Math

Semantic knowledge of math terms and mathematical phrases should be assessed so that needs can be identified and objectives written as required. In math, many familiar English words are used in novel ways (*table, altogether, rounded*), and many specialized terms must be learned (*addend, quotient, square root, multiplication, least common denominator, divisor, coefficient*). When two or more mathematical concepts are combined to form a new concept, the semantic demands of the task are compounded (*least common multiple, negative exponent*, and *a quarter of the ___*; Crandall, 1987). English terms with verb particles, such as *divided by* or *divided into*, can cause confusion (Crandall, Dale, Rhodes, & Spanos, 1985).

Students of mathematics also often need to be able to infer meaning from statements and questions, using their ability to determine the referents of key words (Crandall, 1987). For example, problems involving English phrases such as *the number* or *a number* require such inferencing (*Five times the number 6 is three more than 9 times a number*). Also, adults are often inconsistent and do not always use a single term to refer to a math operation. For example, they might use *less*, *take away*, and *minus* all to refer to subtraction (Polloway & Patton, 1993).

 ## Students with Cognitive Academic Language Proficiency (CALP) in math are better able to achieve.

Students who can communicate using the technical language of math in decontextualized situations are better able to construct and share their understanding than students who never learned or were never given linguistic access to specialized English terms and phrasing (Trafron & Claus, 1994). Garnett (1989) found that students who could not understand or use English math vocabulary were not proficient problem-solvers, could not communicate mathematically, and did not have confidence in their mathematical ability. For this reason, adults need to fingerspell (and expect comprehension of fingerspelled terms), write, or borrow sign system signs for key math terms (see Figure 9–2).

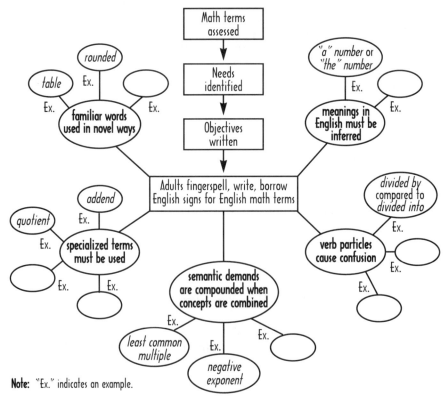

Note: "Ex." indicates an example.

FIGURE 9-2: KEY MATH VOCABULARY REQUIRES FACILITATION

Syntax and Math

English syntactic structures distinctive to mathematics need to be understood by (and sometimes modified for) students who are D/HH if they are to acquire skill in math. For example, because math is the study of relationships, comparative English syntactic structures are an essential and recurring part of the language used (Knight & Hargis, 1977). Students who are D/HH need to understand these structures. Chamot and O'Malley (1994) listed comparative English grammatical structures that occur in mathematical problems including

- *as ___ as* (*Sam is as tall as Roberto*)
- *-er than* (*Kent is a year older than Barb.*)
- *greater/less than* (*Six is greater than four. Name all the numbers that are less than eight.*)
- *times as much* (*Mary Pat earns two times as much as Lynn.*)

Study Guide Questions

1. *Can you list several examples of difficulties that students who are D/HH might experience in comprehending math problems?*

2. *In what ways do you think requiring a student to maintain a "math dictionary" might be helpful?*

3. *How would you complete Figure 9–2? Fill in examples where they are missing in this concept web.*

Word order is also important—and can be confusing—in mathematical phrases. The order of words in math can at times signify a meaning which is counter-intuitive. For example, the numbers in the expression *two divided into eight* must be transposed to write the synonymous mathematical expression *8 ÷ 2* (Crandall, 1987). Team members need to facilitate students' comprehension of the special significance of word order in mathematics.

 In mathematical utterances, learners must rely on the semantics inferred and not interpret the surface English structure or syntax as they would standard text (Kessler, Quinn, & Hayes, 1985).

Logical connectors such as *if . . . then, if and only if, because, that is, for example, such that, but, consequently,* and *either . . . or* are all difficult for students who are not native speakers of English (Kessler, Quinn, & Hayes, 1985). Consider the following math problem adapted from Crandall (1987). This problem would be very difficult for many students who are D/HH:

> If Breeze can word process one page in 20 minutes, how long will it take her to type two pages?

Yet, if the syntax is modified, the problem can often be successfully solved by students who are D/HH:

> Breeze word processed one page in 20 minutes. How much time will it take her to type two pages?

Teaching about Time and Money

Methods used in the general education curriculum to help students tell time and use money are appropriate for students who are D/HH. (Resources for related teaching materials and software are listed at the end of this chapter.) In addition, real-life application of these skills is a necessity. Having a clock in the classroom and a wristwatch worn by the student are both helpful for learning real-life skills. Parents are particularly essential team members when it comes to students' practicing real-life applications: For instance, parents can have students routinely make small purchases and tell time for authentic purposes.

FUNCTIONAL TIME ACTIVITIES

School	Home
Discuss when classes start, when special classes and recess occur, when it's time for speech or computer lab, and so forth.	Use a vibrating alarm so that the student gets up at a particular time; request "lights off" at night at a particular time; ask student to be ready to go "in five minutes"; and encourage independence.

Word Problems*

Students who are D/HH historically have had difficulty solving word problems in English. This is, of course, because their emerging math skills usually interface with their English acquisition needs and reading skills. Team members are encouraged to mediate word problem activities and to focus on the underlying *meaning* of each problem to solve it. The optimal input factors discussed by Luetke-Stahlman (1998) should be revisited when organizing math strategies. Everyone should work hard to incorporate genuine English word problems into students' lives at home and school. Recommended resources for word problems are listed at the end of this chapter.

Procedure for Solving Word Problems

"Word problems . . . can be described in terms of different networks of concepts and relationships underlying the problem" (De Corte & Verschaffel, 1991, pp. 118-119). A crucial step in solving word problems is to construct an internal representation of their conceptual networks. De Corte and Verschaffel suggested a five-stage "competent problem-solving model of elementary arithmetic word problems" (p. 118) that emphasizes a semantic approach to the task. This model has been adapted and expanded into the ten-step procedure presented below and is arranged and included as a worksheet in Appendix 9–A.

Ten-Step Word Problem Procedure

---

1. **Rewrite word problems so that they are relevant to the student's life.**
   Hannah, you know that Mrs. Tombs will give your class a pop party with a movie when the class has earned 100 marbles in her jar, right?

---

*Material incorporated in this section from "Some Factors Influencing the Solution of Addition and Subtraction Word Problems," by E. De Corte and L. Verschaffel, 1991, in K. Durkin and B. Shire (Eds.), *Language in Mathematical Education: Research and Practice*, Buckingham, U.K.: Open University Press. Copyright 1991 by Open University Press. Adapted with permission.

(Student responds.) *About how many marbles do you think she has in there now?* (Student gives a number. It is unimportant whether it is the actual number or not.) *So about how many more marbles does Mrs.Tombs need before your class gets the party?*

2. **Ask the student to draw a representation of the problem.**

3. **Compare the accuracy of the drawing (Step 2) with your own perception of a visualization.** Make changes together as needed to obtain at least one representation of the problem. Do not enable the student by *telling* information or moving the drawing to your part of the work space.

4. **Help the student to explain verbally (in speech, signs, cues) how to solve the problem.** The description should include an appropriate formal math operation or an informal counting strategy.

5. **Repeat and clarify what the student has expressed, making a visual list of steps if needed.**

6. **Have the student write the problem sentence.** For example: *83 + ? = 100.*

7. **Have the student execute the mathematical action or operation.**

8. **Have the student replace the unknown element in Step 6 and verbally express the solution by paraphrasing the original word problem.**
   Mrs. Tombs has 83 marbles, and we need 100 for a pop party can be paraphrased: *If Mrs. Tombs has 83 marbles and we earn 17 more, we will have 100 marbles and can have a pop party.*

9. **Have the student verify the information in Step 8 by solving the word problem another way or by drawing a new picture and checking for errors.**

10. **Ask the student to decide whether he or she could solve a similar word problem.**

Study Guide Question
How could you redesign the word problem worksheet provided in Appendix 9–A so that it can be used as a data collection tool?

Task Characteristics of Word Problems

De Corte and Verschaffel (1991) conducted a series of word problem studies with hearing first and second graders and suggested that task characteristics include three elements:
1. the semantic intent of the information

2. the clarity of this semantic intent in the wording of the problem

3. the order of presentation of the known information stated in the problem

Two additional characteristics have been added here:
4. the range of numbers used in the problem

5. the extent to which a systematic procedure (such as the one suggested above) is routinely used

Each of these characteristics is discussed below.

The Semantic Intent and Its Clarity

Three semantic categories in simple addition and subtraction word problems are discussed in De Corte and Verschaffel (1991):
1. **Change problems** are those in which an event changes the value of a quantity: *Xavier had 3 marbles; Cheng gave him 5 more marbles; how many marbles does Xavier have now?*

2. **Compare problems** are those that compare two amounts and involve the difference between them: *Xavier has 3 marbles; Cheng has 5 more marbles than Xavier; how many marbles does Cheng have?*

3. **Combine problems** involve static situations concerning two amounts considered either separately or in combination: *Xavier has 3 marbles; Cheng has 5 marbles; how many marbles do they have altogether?*

De Corte and Verschaffel found that combine problems are easier than change problems for young students.

These three semantic categories can be further subdivided, depending on the identity of the unknown quantity and the characteristics of the event or relationship described. For example, both of these problems are change problems, but the answers and the events described differ:

1. *Xavier had some marbles; then Cheng gave him 5 more marbles; now Xavier has 8 marbles; how many marbles did Xavier have in the beginning?*

2. *Xavier had 8 marbles; then he gave some marbles to Cheng; now Xavier has 3 marbles; how many marbles did he give to Cheng?*

Riley, Greeno, and Heller (as cited in De Corte & Verschaffel, 1991) identified fourteen types of simple addition and subtraction problems—six types of change problems, two types of combine problems, and six types of compare problems.

Pauwels (as cited in De Corte & Verschaffel, 1991) conducted a study illustrating that although some of the fourteen problem types can be solved using the same mathematical operation, the differences in their characteristics create semantic differences. These semantic differences make some problems harder to solve than others. In addition, some problem representations are more easily expressed by a mathematical operation than are others, and this can affect the rate at which these types of problems are understood by students who are D/HH (see Figure 9–3).

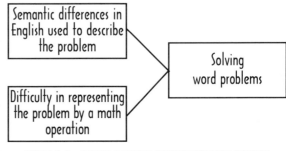

FIGURE 9–3: FACTORS AFFECTING THE UNDERSTANDING OF WORD PROBLEMS

Carpenter (1985) demonstrated that clarifying the wording in story problems significantly assisted young students in solving them. In the study, rewriting complex English sentences into successive simple sentences and changing verb tenses influenced student success. Hudson (1983) found that beginning the question part of the problem description with a question word (*How many more birds than worms are there?*) is more helpful than a conversational or indirect approach (*If each bird catches a worm, how many worms will be left?*).

The Order of Presentation

The sequence in which numbers are presented in a text can influence a student's ability to solve the problem correctly. De Corte and Verschaffel (1987) studied this characteristic systematically with first graders. They found that students are more successful when the first number in an addition problem is the smaller one. They also found that the order of numbers is influential in subtraction word problems. For example, *If 2 puppies hop out of a bed that holds 6 puppies, how many are left?* is more difficult than *There are 6 puppies in a bed and 2 hop out. How many are left?*

The Range of Numbers Used

Because comprehending the semantic underpinnings of a word problem may be difficult for students who are D/HH, mathematical operations should initially be those that are familiar and easy to solve. For example, when a student has demonstrated the ability to solve several types of problems using the numbers 0–9, identically structured word problems with numbers 10–19 can be used. The following number groupings can be helpful to team members attempting to write appropriate IEP objectives:

> **Study Guide Question**
> *How could you use the information from De Corte and Verschaffel (1991) to task analyze the difficulties a student who is D/HH might be having in solving word problems? Discuss the advantages and disadvantages of rewording problems so that the semantic intent is explicit, and consider rewording as a step in your task analysis.*

> **Study Guide Question**
> *How would you illustrate the information about order of presentation with your own examples?*

0–9	50–99	1,000–1,999
10–19	100–119	2,000–2,999
20–29	120–149	3,000–9,999
30–39	150–199	10,000–99,999
40–49	200–999	100,000–999,999

> **Study Guide Question**
> *Using three different sets of number groupings, how would you write three objectives for a student you know who is D/HH?*

The Use of a Systematic Procedure

Students who are D/HH can benefit from teaching procedures in which each student's abilities are assessed, appropriate objectives are written, and lessons are taught in an organized manner. The concept of input + 1 or level + 1 is as relevant to math and to word problems as it is to other linguistic and academic areas. Using the word problem worksheet provided in Appendix 9–A or another organizational device will help ensure that each   student is working with team members at level + 1, the level slightly above his or her independent level.

Math Facilitation Tips

> **Study Guide Question**
> *Discuss the information provided from De Corte and Verschaffel (1991). How can it be used to ensure level + 1 for word problems?*

To begin a math facilitation plan for a student who is D/HH, team members should clarify the desired outcomes of a particular math course for the student:

- What specific curricular competencies are to be demonstrated as learned by the student?
- What are the reading, speaking, and writing requirements for demonstrating these competencies? Can they be modified? (Refer and add to Figure 10–1 in Chapter 10.)
- What are the technical vocabulary English requirements of the subject?
- What are the cognitive skills required of the student?

The following activities (adapted from Crandall, 1987) can also help ensure mathematical achievement:

- Teach problem-solving and self-monitoring strategies.
- Include students in setting goals.

- Teach relationships and rules.
- Facilitate improvement in English language proficiency and reading ability.
- Make sure that textbooks and computer programs match students' needs (see resource list at the end of this chapter).
- Teach students to think mathematically at a cognitive and metacognitive level.
- Teach students to be both patient and persistent.
- Use interactive math activities that incorporate students' real-life experiences.
- Provide positive experiences: Use overt feedback and keep the affective filter low (for example, make sure that students are comfortable taking risks and enjoy the learning process).

Students who are not achieving in math classes at the same rate as their peers will require the assistance of a team member to mediate instruction in the general education math class. In addition to the supports and services discussed in Chapter 1 and listed in Appendix 1–A, team members might need to adapt instruction for math (and other school subjects) in public schools as follows:

Mediations for Math and Other School Subjects

1. Make sure that the student can see the interpreter, the teacher, and the board.
2. Make sure that the teacher provides constant time for interpreting and does not expect the student to use his or her eyes for two purposes simultaneously (watching the interpreter and tracking an explanation at the board).
3. Repeat what has been said more slowly.
4. Provide English or ASL sentence starters to help the student express ideas.
5. Use self talk, parallel talk, inform talk to practice mathematical language (see Luetke-Stahlman, 1998).
6. Cue or fingerspell important (key) words and write them on the board or display them using an overhead projector; the student should be responsible for learning, using, and if possible, pronouncing/cueing each word.
7. Define key English math vocabulary and clarify characteristics that distinguish closely related or opposite terms.

8. Make math problems visually clear; use space, directionality, eye-gaze, and so on, to clarify the English being used.
9. Facilitate or monitor peer communication and participation of students who are D/HH in pairs or small groups.
10. Encourage text-to-life, life-to-text connections.
11. Provide direct feedback about the appropriateness of the student's ideas, comments, and so forth.
12. Ensure that assistive listening devices are working.
13. Provide a place on each worksheet for the student to indicate the math process that will be used, as well as space to show computation work.
14. Make sure that students (if capable) can pronounce and fingerspell key words.

These considerations could be charted on the left side of a Cummins model to supply context as team members task analyze a particular student's abilities and promote independence.

> **Study Guide Question**
> *What mediation activities would you and your peers add to the list provided?*

A Second Language Approach to Facilitating Skills in Mathematics

Since math comprehension is dependent on the integration of linguistic as well as mathematical skills, application of hearing bilingual research and practice should be considered. The information presented below restates that provided earlier in this chapter, serving as a reminder of the similarities among the needs of all students who have not developed proficient cognitive academic language skills and are attempting age-appropriate work in school subject areas.

Cuevas (1984), a hearing bilingual educator, developed an approach to mathematics that would apply to working with students who are D/HH. The approach consisted of two strands: one focusing on mathematics content and the other emphasizing related English language skills. The *content strand* involves

- use of preventive strategies (review and reinforcement of prerequisite skills)
- analysis of what concepts or skills need to be taught

- diagnosis (task analysis of the strategies being used by the student and how the lesson might be organized so that new skills can be learned)
- design of a lesson plan (activities targeted at the student's level, involving manipulatives and using effective teaching practices)

The *language strand* involves
- analysis of the English language required
- diagnosis of the student's comprehension of the cognitive, meaning, and form skills required
- discussion of the mathematics content in ASL (if that is the student's dominant language) and practice using the English necessary to comprehend the target mathematical concept

Strategy Instruction

Whether a student who is D/HH is solving a computation problem or a word problem, use of strategy can improve performance (Bezuk & Cegelka, 1995). One example of a math strategy appears in Figure 9–4. Others can be found in books and journal articles for professionals working with students who have learning disabilities. Team members will need to evaluate whether the English used to describe a strategy or the complexity of the strategy make it inappropriate for use with a student who is D/HH.

Study Guide Question
Read a current journal article on the topic of teaching math to hearing bilingual students. How is it relevant to deaf education?

1. Visibly read or sign the problem

2. Paraphrase
    Give the important information
    Visibly repeat the question that is being asked
    Ask yourself, *"What is asked? What am I looking for?"*

3. Visualize
    Draw a diagram of the problem

4. State the problem
    Say/Sign: *"I have . . . I want to find . . . . "*

5. Hypothesize/Predict
    "If I . . . then . . . . "

6. Estimate
    Round the numbers in the problem
    Estimate an answer

7. Calculate the answer
    Write a label for what the number represents (e.g., *3 marbles*)
    Circle the answer

8. Self-check your work
    Check every step, beginning at the beginning
    Check your calculations to make sure you correctly added,
    subtracted, etc.

9. Decide whether your answer makes sense when compared to the
    estimating you did (#6)

10. Highlight your answer (e.g., circle it again)

FIGURE 9–4: ACTIVITIES IN A VERBAL (SPOKEN OR SIGNED) MATH PROBLEM-SOLVING STRATEGY

From "The Effect of Cognitive Strategy Training on Verbal Math Problem Solving Performance of Learning Disabled Adolescents," by M. Montague and C. Bos, 1986, *Journal of Learning Disabilities, 19*(1), pp. 26-33. Copyright 1986 by Pro-Ed, Inc. Adapted and reprinted with permission.

Summary

In this chapter, the integration of cognition, mathematics, and language skills was explored. Team members responding to questions raised with regard to the math and language abilities of students who are D/HH should assess appropriately, write objectives as needed, and facilitate learning in a systematic way using the principles of effective teaching and mediated learning. Math mediation strategies, worksheets, and resource lists were provided in this chapter, and reading in the areas of learning disabilities and hearing bilingual studies was suggested.

Activities

1. Assess the needs of a student who is D/HH in an area of mathematics.

2. Facilitate a student's ability to comprehend word problems.

3. Critically evaluate the commercial word problem materials that are available.

4. Using the work of De Corte and Verschaffel (1991), discuss with colleagues how you might organize a word problem workbook.

Resources for Math Materials

Butte Publications, Inc.
P.O. Box 1328
Hillsboro, OR 97123-1328
1-800-330-9791
Distributor of materials on math (time, money, word problems) specifically for students who are D/HH

Pro-Ed
8700 Shoal Creek Blvd.
Austin, TX 78757-6897
512-451-3246
Materials about telling time and counting money, originally published by Dormac (which sold products specifically for use with students who are D/HH)

Attainment Company
P. O. Box 930160
Verona, WI 53593-0160
Software for time and money activities

Also see companies listed in Chapter 10.

Recommended Word Problems Curricula*

How to Solve Story Problems (1987) by R. D'Apice
Weekly Reader Skill Books
4343 Equity Drive
Columbus, OH 43228

Understanding Math Story Problems by M. McGlothlin
Pro-Ed
8700 Shoal Creek
Austin, TX 78757
1-800-897-3202
Three workbooks focusing on the English terms used in math word problems: Book 1 for students who read at a second-grade level; Book 2 for third-grade level;

*Suggested by teachers of the deaf in the Kansas City area

Book 3 for fourth-grade or higher level. Problems are controlled for vocabulary, sentence length, and complexity according to reading level. Each workbook contains a pretest to identify students who are unable to perform the required calculations. These workbooks could be incorporated into the word problem procedure described in this chapter.

Recommended Math Software**

Preschool
Thinking Things Collection 1 (Edmark)

Elementary
Math Blaster (Davidson)
Math Workshop (Broderbund)
Thinking Things Collections (Edmark)
Treasure Math Storm (The Learning Company)
Math Rabbit (The Learning Company)
Math Munchers Deluxe (MECC)
Coin Critters (Nordic)
Graph Club (Tom Snyder)

Middle School
The Cruncher (The Learning Company)
Number Munchers (MECC)

High School
Algeblaster 3 (Davidson)
Math Ace (Sanctuary Words)

All software available from publishers (indicated in parentheses) or from the following distributor:

Learning Services
3895 E. 19th Ave.
Eugene, OR 97403
1-800-877-9378

**Top choices in software suggested by Kent Luetke-Stahlman, middle school technology coordinator and parent of two deaf daughters (15540 S. Downing; Olathe, KS 66062)

378

Appendix 9-A

Ten-Step Word Problem Worksheet*

Name_____ Date_____

1. Write the relevant word problem:

2. Student draws the problem.

3. Make changes as needed to Step 2.

4. Student verbally explains the math operation required.

5. Adult lists the steps suggested by the student if needed.

6. Student writes the math problem sentence:

7. Student solves the math problem sentence (Step 6) in this work space:

8. Student rewrites the math problem sentence in Step 6 and includes the problem solution (Step 7), then verbally expresses the solution to the problem by paraphrasing the original word problem.

9. Student verifies the solution by solving the problem another way or drawing it.

10. Student decides whether he or she could do another word problem like this one:

_____Very sure I could	{ _____without help
	{ _____with help
_____Kind of sure I could	{ _____without help
	{ _____with help
_____Not very sure I could	{ _____without help

*Sequence of steps adapted from "Some Factors Influencing the Solution of Addition and Subtraction Word Problems," by E. De Corte and L. Verschaffel, 1991, in K. Durkin and B. Shire (Eds.), *Language in Mathematical Education: Research and Practice*, Buckingham, U.K.: Open University Press. Copyright 1991 by Open University Press. Adapted with permission.

References

Beathy, L., Madden, R., Gardner, E., & Karlsen, B. (1985). *Stanford Diagnostic Mathematics Test* (3rd ed.). San Antonio, TX: The Psychological Corporation.

Bezuk, N., & Cegelka, P. (1995). Effective mathematics instruction for all students. In P. Cegelka & W. Berdine (Eds.), *Effective instruction of students with learning difficulties,* (pp. 345-384). Boston: Allyn & Bacon.

Carpenter, T. (1985). Learning to add and subtract: An exercise in problem solving. In E. Silver (Ed.), *Problem solving: Multiple research perspectives.* Philadelphia: Franklin Institute Press.

Chamot, A., & O'Malley, M. (1994). *The CALLA handbook.* Reading, MA: Addison-Wesley.

Coelho, E. (1982). Language across the curriculum. *TESL Talk, 13,* 56-70.

Connolly, A. (1988). *Key Math–Revised: A Diagnostic Inventory of Essential Mathematics.* Circle Pines, MN: American Guidance Service.

Crandall, J. (1987). *ESL through content-area instruction: Mathematics, science, and social studies.* Englewood Cliffs, NJ: Prentice Hall.

Crandall, J., Dale, T., Rhodes, N., & Spanos, G. (1985). *The language of mathematics: The English barrier.* Paper presented at the Delaware Symposium of Language Studies VII, University of Delaware, Newark.

Cuevas, G. (1984). Mathematics learning in English as a second language. *Journal for Research in Mathematics Education, 15,* 134-144.

Cummins, J. (1984). *Bilingualism and special education: Issues in assessment and pedagogy.* Clevedon, Avon, England: Multilingual Matters.

De Corte, E., & Verschaffel, L. (1985). Beginning first graders' initial representation of arithmetic word problems. *Journal of Mathematical Behavior, 4,* 3-21.

De Corte, E., & Verschaffel, L. (1987). The effect of semantic structure on first graders' solution strategies of elementary addition and subtraction word problems. *Journal for Research in Mathematics Education, 18*(5), 363-81.

De Corte, E., & Verschaffel, L. (1991). Some factors influencing the solution of addition and subtraction word problems. In K. Durkin & B. Shire (Eds.), *Language in mathematical education: Research and practice*. Buckingham, U.K.: Open University Press.

Gallaudet University (1983). *Stanford Achievement Test for Hearing Impaired Students*. Washington, DC: Gallaudet University. (Available from the Center for Assessment and Demographic Studies, Gallaudet University; 800 Florida Avenue, NE; Washington, DC 20002–3695)

Garnett, K. (1989). Math learning disabilities. *LD Forum, 14*, 11-15.

Gessell, J. (1983). *Diagnostic Mathematics Inventory/Mathematics Systems*. Monterey, CA: CTB/McGraw-Hill.

Hieronymus, A., Hoover, H., & Lindquist, E. (1986). *Iowa Test of Basic Skills*. Chicago: Riverside.

Hodgkinson, J. (1979). What's right with education. *Phi Delta Kappa, 61*, 159-162.

Hudson, N. (1983). *High-interest, low-ability word problems for high school mathematics students*. Unpublished master's thesis, California State University, Chico.

Kessler, C., Quinn, M., & Hayes, C. (1985). *Processing mathematics in a second language: Problems for IEP children*. Paper presented at the Delaware Symposium of Language Studies VII, University of Delaware, Newark.

Knight, L., & Hargis, C. (1977). Math language ability: Its relationship to reading in math. *Language Arts, 54*, 423-428.

Luetke-Stahlman, B. (1998). *Language issues in deaf education*. Hillsboro, OR: Butte Publications.

Maryland State Department of Education Mathematics Framework Task Force (1987). *Mathematics: A Maryland curriculum framework*. Baltimore, MD: Maryland State Department of Education.

McCoy, K. (1995). *Teaching special learners in the general education classroom*. Denver: Love.

McLoughlin, J., & Lewis, R. (1994). *Assessing special students* (4th ed.). Upper Saddle River, NJ: Merrill.

Mercer, C., & Mercer, A. (1993). *Teaching students with learning problems*. NY: Merrill.

Montague, M., & Bos, C. (1986). The effect of cognitive strategy training on verbal math problem solving performance of learning disabled adolescents. *Journal of Learning Disabilities, 19*(1), 26-33.

National Council for Teachers of Mathematics (1989). *Curriculum and evaluation standards for school mathematics.* Reston, VA: Author.

Polloway, E., & Patton, J. (1993). *Strategies for teaching learners with special needs* (5th ed.). New York: Macmillan.

Prescott, G., Barlow, I., Hogan, T., & Farr, R. (1984). *Metropolitan Achievement Tests 6: Survey Battery.* San Antonio, TX: The Psychological Corporation.

Psychological Corporation (1989). *Stanford Achievement Test* (8th ed.). San Antonio, TX: Harcourt Brace.

Schroeder, B., & Strosnider, R. (1997). Box-and-whisker what? Deaf students learn—and write about—descriptive statistics. *Teaching Exceptional Children, 29*(3), 12-17.

Trafron, P., & Claus, A. (1994). A changing curriculum for a changing age. In C. Thornton & N. Bley (Eds.), *Windows of opportunity: Mathematics for students with special needs* (pp. 19-39). Reston, VA: National Council of Teachers of Mathematics.

Woodcock, R., & Johnson, M. (1989). *Woodcock-Johnson Psychoeducational Battery–Revised.* Chicago: Riverside.

Chapter 10

Other School Subjects and Language

School Subject Assessment

Linguistic Demands of School Subjects

Facilitating English Needed for School Subjects

Choosing Curricula

School Subject Facilitation

Using an Interpreter

Using Computers

Teaching about HIV/AIDS and Sexually
    Transmitted Disease

Resources

Appendix 10-A: Lesson Plan for Science

Appendix 10-B: Recommended Computer Programs

Appendix 10-C: Graphics Supporting the
    HIV/AIDS and STI Curriculum

When concerns arise about the academic performance of a student who is deaf or hard of hearing, team members should assess the student's ability to perform language tasks that reflect the cognitive academic demands of the school subject area. Crandall (1987) found that students who are D/HH are more motivated to use English and retain course content when team members plan mediated activities based on assessment results.

As discussed in previous chapters, given appropriate supports and services and mediated instruction, many students who are D/HH can acquire and apply the academic competencies expected at their grade level. For example, team members can use strategies to facilitate language skills while discussing content that students feel a genuine need to comprehend and express (to convey ideas, participate in discussion, write reports, and so forth). Attention to English linguistic demands and successful learning strategies used in one school subject are likely to be transferable to other subject areas as well (Crandall, 1987).

The material presented in this chapter reprises and augments discussions presented in previous chapters geared to special subject areas. It is provided here to assist team members in discussing appropriate assessment, facilitation of linguistic needs, and place-ment for *any* school subject class. Particular information is included for science, social studies, and health, including the important areas of sexually transmitted disease and HIV/AIDS.

School Subject Assessment

Guidelines for appropriate assessment discussed in previous chapters are relevant for every subject area. Assessment should be question-driven, combine formal and informal measures, and result in written goals and objectives that address any discrepancies between a particular student's abilities and those of the peer group. Assessment should be conducted by qualified personnel and under appropriate testing conditions: The room should be quiet, there should be no visual distractions, and any assistive devices should be working correctly. Curriculum-based assessment, criterion-referenced tools, analysis of written and oral work (signed and/or spoken), class tests, questionnaires, interviews, and observation are types of informal assessment that may be helpful in addressing school subject questions.

Whether school subject assessment is conducted in ASL or English depends on the purpose of the assessment. For example, if the purpose is to discern a student's ability to participate in and comprehend grade-level discussion of concepts being studied, then the student's cognitive/pragmatic skills in a given subject should be assessed in the student's dominant language (either ASL or English). (See Luetke-Stahlman, 1998, for discussions of these types of cognitive abilities and the importance of using the student's dominant language). If the purpose is to discern the student's ability to read for content and write about what has been learned, then reading and writing ability would also need to be evaluated and compared to that of hearing peers. Information on the linguistic demands of school subjects, discussed below, can be used to guide team members as they evaluate the English skills required in each subject area and in developing students' cognitive academic language proficiency (CALP; see Luetke-Stahlman, 1998, for a definition and discussion of CALP).

> **Study Guide Question**
> *What are several questions that could guide assessment of the science and social studies abilities of an elementary student who is D/HH? Write your suggestions.*

Linguistic Demands of School Subjects

Coelho (1982) provided an impressive list of language skills required of second language users across the curriculum. Her ideas have been adapted to apply to students who are D/HH and are presented with examples of the demands in specific communication areas in Figure 10–1.

Task Demands	Comprehension	Expression	Reading	Writing
Attend teacher and media presentations.	Understand formal and informal instructional language used at normal speed. Understand expository text forms (compare and contrast, sequence, and so on).	Ask questions to confirm, comprehend, define, request, obtain repetition, and obtain new information (concepts, vocabulary, spelling, pronunciation, and so on).	Read board, overheads, captioning, notes, and diagrams. Understand nonverbal representations such as figures and graphs. Read notetaker notes.	(Use a notetaker during lectures.) Take notes while reading.
Participate in discussions.	Understand conversational dialogue, idioms, informal language. Understand nonverbal language.	Demonstrate different registers and a wide variety of pragmatic skills (gain the floor, take turns, interrupt, change topics, and so on). Ask or answer questions. Express opinions, explain, defend, and so on.	Refer to text or other written material to support a point. Read notetaker notes.	Make notes about important points discussed.
Participate in labs and technical sessions.	Understand directions, procedures, warnings, and so on.	Seek advice, confer with peers. Describe parts and processes.	Understand written directions or instructions, lists and charts, and other nonverbal data.	Write lab reports and summaries. Prepare and label diagrams and charts. *cont.*

FIGURE 10–1: LANGUAGE SKILLS ACROSS THE CURRICULUM*

*From "Language Across the Curriculum," by E. Coelho, 1982, *TESL Talk, 13,* pp. 57–59. Copyright Queen's Printer for Ontario, 1982. Adapted and reproduced with permission.

FIGURE 10–1, CONT.

Task Demands	Comprehension	Expression	Reading	Writing
Use textbooks.	Understand instructions, page and paragraph references, and purposes in reading expository text.	Paraphrase, explain, discuss text, and so on.	Read to understand and retain information; read for main idea and detail; vary reading rate for specific tasks. Infer words, phrases, sentences, and paragraph meanings from context. Interpret nonverbal data, recognize bias, distinguish opinion from fact.	
Apply dictionary skills.		Choose the correct word or word form to use.	Understand pronunciation markings, short definitions, symbols used in explanations. Find information in several sources; select appropriate information. Recognize bias; distinguish opinion from fact.	Cite references and quotations. Prepare a bibliography.

cont.

388

FIGURE 10-1, CONT.

Task Demands	Comprehension	Expression	Reading	Writing
Complete assignments.	Collect information from lectures, group work, videotapes, and so on.	Conduct surveys and interviews. Give presentations that include addressing a specific audience; organizing ideas logically; designing and using visual aids; making eye contact; using language to persuade, impress, demonstrate, and so on.	Read written directions.	Select appropriate organization, vocabulary, style, and so on. Prepare an outline. Understand the functional purpose (to persuade, describe, and so on).
Take tests.		Answer questions with logic, organization, sufficient detail, and so on.		Respond to different test formats: T/F, cloze, multiple choice, matching, short answer, long answer (essay).
Interact with authority figures in academic, social, and extracurricular contexts.	Understand the sociolinguistic context (changing registers, knowing when to express oneself, and so on).	Select appropriate language and register. Request information, make appointments, ask for directions, clarify, and so on.	Understand procedures, forms, notices, announcements, school calendars, school telephone book, time tables, schedules, and so on.	Request appointments; fill in forms; respond to surveys, questionnaires, and so on. *cont.*

FIGURE 10-1, CONT.

Task Demands	Comprehension	Expression	Reading	Writing
Interact with authority figures, cont.	Understand idiomatic and nonverbal language. Understand announcements given over the public address system.			

Many of the skills listed in Figure 10–1 require higher-level thinking. Staff at the Maryland Department of Education provided a questionnaire (Figure 10–2) to assess students' capabilities for using the higher-level thinking skills demanded by school subjects. The questionnaire can also be used to facilitate cognitive academic language proficiency (CALP).

Knowledge: Identification and recall of information
Who, what, when, where, how _____?
Describe_____.

Comprehension: Organization and selection of facts and ideas
Retell _____ in your own way.
What is the main idea of _____?

Application: Use of facts, rules, principles
How is _____ related to _____?
Why is _____ significant?

Analysis: Separation of a whole into component parts
What are the parts or features of _____ ?
Classify _____ according to _____.
Outline/diagram/web _____.
How does _____ compare or contrast with _____?
What evidence can you present for _____?
cont.

FIGURE 10-2: STUDENT QUESTIONNAIRE TO ASSESS SCHOOL SUBJECT CAPABILITIES

FIGURE 10-2, CONT.

Synthesis: Combination of ideas to form a new whole
What would you predict or infer from _____ ?
What ideas can you add to _____ ?
How would you create or design a new _____ ?
What might happen if you combined _____ with _____ ?
What solutions would you suggest for _____ ?

Evaluation: Development of opinions, judgments, or decisions
Do you agree with _____ ?
What do you think about _____?

Developed and published by staff in the Division of Instruction and Staff Development, Maryland State Department of Education. Adapted with permission.

Facilitating English Needed for School Subjects

Sometimes students who are D/HH need to be taught directly to express, read, and write specific English words and phrases used to code expository information or ideas. For example, if students are expected to compare people, places, or items in a social studies class, they may first need to be taught how to formulate a statement of comparison:

> **Study Guide Question**
> *Create hypothetical evaluation data using the Maryland Student Questionnaire. What five objectives could you write for a particular student who is D/HH?*

> The population of a city *is greater than* the population of a town.

New York City and Los Angeles *are both* large cities.

Similarly, students may need to be taught words and phrases and syntactic forms required in science, health, and other subjects, including those needed for

- contrasting (*different from, either . . . or, however*)
- listing (*another, some, several, for example*)
- establishing cause and effect (*because, if, therefore, due to*)
- describing processes (*The experiment showed . . . or*, using passive voice: *The puppies are fed.*)
- time sequencing (*when, initially, first, eventually*)
- hypothesizing (*if . . . then, what if, but for*)

The CALP Threshold and the Cummins Model

Study Guide Question
Prepare a graphic organizer (such as a Venn diagram) to compare and contrast some information in a social studies or science unit. What is the specific English of comparing and contrasting required to explain or use your presentation?

If a student who is D/HH is having trouble learning and seems to lack the cognitive academic language proficiency (CALP) necessary for successful participation in a school subject class, team members might need to discuss the concept of the "threshold level of language proficiency." The threshold in this sense is the degree of linguistic ability needed to comprehend and express the cognitively demanding, context-reduced concepts taught in school subject classes (such as those presented in Figures 10–1 and 10–2). Students who have not reached this threshold will need supports and mediation to read school subject materials.

```
Appropriate CALP

THRESHOLD
_____
CALP below hearing peers
```

To facilitate CALP and thereby school subject skills, the Cummins Model of Language Proficiency (Cummins, 1980, 1984) can be used. The model can assist team members to analyze tasks, write objectives, and plan appropriate mediated activities across school subjects for students who are experiencing difficulties (Luetke-Stahlman, 1998). An example of a school subject skill that characterizes the cognitively demanding, context-reduced quadrant in the model is written in Quadrant D of Figure 10–3.

The term "mediate" used in Figure 10–3 refers to activities such as those explained in Chapter 1. The term "direct teaching" refers to the teaching of subskills in a systematic manner, always with reference to the target concept. For example, instead of using dictionary worksheets, students who cannot pronounce or discern the meaning of a word in the text they are using might be taught to look up the word in a personal, class, or standard dictionary. Then they would return to the place in the text where the word was used and apply the information obtained. The suggestions presented in Figure 10–4 can assist team members in planning for activities in Quadrants A and C (mediation) and in Quadrant B (direct teaching). Some of the mediation activities are adapted from Miller (1997).

Cognitively Demanding

Adult-**mediated** activities to accomplish the objective	Skill: *The student will understand instructional English used in the textbook.*
C	**D**

Context Embedded **A**	**B** Context Reduced
Direct teaching of subskills with **mediation**	**Direct teaching** of substeps of the objective

Cognitively Undemanding

FIGURE 10–3: THE CUMMINS MODEL APPLIED TO SCHOOL SUBJECT SKILLS

Task That Is Difficult for Student (Quadrant D)	Mediation (Quadrants A and C)	Direct Teaching (Quadrant B)
Understand instructional English used in the textbook.	■ define key words using subordinate terms and distinguishing details ■ exemplify ■ make word associations ■ list synonyms and antonyms ■ use provided or drawn pictures, newspapers, and other authentic media ■ demonstrate or model ■ link to previous knowledge ■ role play, pantomime ■ repeat and rephrase ■ write important information on an overhead transparency or on the board	■ Use a concept map to facilitate the comprehension and use of vocabulary that was not understood ■ After information is presented, paraphrase the main ideas of the instructional language, constructing a graphic organizer while doing so

FIGURE 10–4: SAMPLE MEDIATION AND DIRECTED TEACHING ACTIVITIES   *cont.*

FIGURE 10–4, CONT.

Task That Is Difficult for Student (Quadrant D)	Mediation (Quadrants A and C)	Direct Teaching (Quadrant B)
	■ use study guides and advanced organizers ■ use open-ended questioning frequently; ask students to repeat what others have said ■ compare ideas among peers ■ extend students' responses and comments ■ assist students in verbalizing their thought processes, conversing in analytical language ■ pause when oral students are taking notes, or adjust the pace of lecturing speed ■ summarize key points at the end of each session ■ provide time for questions	

School Subject Objectives

Many different objectives may be appropriate for students who are D/HH, depending on the degree to which they are expected to acquire the school curriculum competencies. The sample objectives below were written specifically to develop CALP in the context of school subject study.

The student will be able to
- write an outline of the unit material
- define 5–10 key words and concepts from the unit using a concept worksheet

Study Guide Question

Interview a teacher of science, social studies, or another subject. Which mediation activities has she or he found to be successful? Share at least two examples with your peers.

- organize information from weekly notes provided by a peer
- find three sources of information in the library and synthesize them into a paragraph or paper
- draw a graphic organizer that allows a comparison and contrast of 1–5 important points or main ideas of the material by restating or paraphrasing
- pass a unit test at 80% accuracy when questions include short answer and explanations
- orally (sign and/or speech) explain a graphic organizer or art project that emphasizes a main idea of the unit

Developing Language Skills in Context

Communication skills should be introduced within a genuine, authentic, "whole" context rather than facilitated in isolated study. A combined approach to learning can occur when audition, comprehension, speechreading, speaking, discussing, reading, and writing are facilitated simultaneously within school subject areas. Social studies, science, math, and language arts concepts can be used as the content focus as students discuss, read, and write about topics that interest them, and as they attempt to communicate ideas of personal importance to larger audiences (Chamot & O'Malley, 1994). A sample lesson plan that can be used to incorporate effective teaching practices as well as speech, audition, cognitive and linguistic objectives is provided in Appendix 10–A.

Discussions in science, social studies, and other school subject classes allow students who are D/HH opportunities for genuine language development. Many ingredients for optimal input are provided in such circumstances (relevant input; hands-on experiences; positive, small group opportunities; use of a wide range of language functions; intense vocabulary needs; literacy tasks; and so forth).

Cooperative learning groups, peer mediated learning, and small discussion groups are

> **Study Guide Question**
>
> *Observe or teach a lesson in which reading, writing, and spelling are combined and both speech and audition objectives are facilitated. What is your evaluation of the effectiveness of this lesson?*

ideal arrangements, allowing students who are D/HH to manipulate school subject concepts, vocabulary, and grammar. Other
appropriate supports and mediation strategies are presented in
Chapter 1.

Choosing Curricula

Many programs in which students who are D/HH are enrolled use
curricula designed for hearing students. For example, a nine-year-
old student who is D/HH enrolled in public school and attending a
general third grade science class might be using the general
education third grade science book. Such use is usually appropriate
if the student demonstrates the English language abilities of a typical
third grade hearing student. Even if the student who is D/HH is
able to function at grade level, however, interpreter and notetaker
services often need to be provided in a public school placement.

It may be possible for students who are D/HH to learn school
subject content and use the same textbooks that hearing peers use if
they are given appropriate supports and services. For example, a
teacher of the deaf might assist in the school subject classroom and
clarify the teacher's instructional English, ask additional comprehension questions, use question prompts (see Chapter 1), and so on.
Often additional tutoring is needed so that the material in the textbook the student is expected to read can be mediated by an adult. It
is *critical* that team members use these techniques if students who
are D/HH are to be provided access to academics and acquire age-
appropriate literacy skills.

Some teachers use materials specifically designed for students
who are D/HH, which can be appropriate when it is demonstrated
that even with supports and mediation a student cannot learn from
the general education curriculum. Team members who want to
preview and discuss adapted school subject curricula can write to
Outreach, Pre-College Programs, at Gallaudet University (see the
resources at the end of this chapter). Professionals at Gallaudet have
developed curricula for social studies, science, math, Deaf Studies,
and so forth. Team members might also consider compiling unit

notebooks of text written at a lower reading level. In addition, professionals working with hearing students who have special needs, such as cognitive impairment or learning disabilities, may be a good resource for materials and methods that can benefit students who are D/HH enrolled in a variety of school subject courses.

Students who are D/HH should participate in an established social studies program along with hearing peers unless they are enrolled in an alternative social studies program (vocational, life skills, study skills, current events, or some other adapted content). Magazines such as *Time for Kids, HIP, The World Around You, NAD Broadcaster,* or *Silent News* can be used successfully by students who need a modified program. Science and social studies magazines filled with colorful pictures and diagrams for students with low reading levels might also be appropriate. A great variety of magazines for students, as well as books like the *Eyewitness* series published by Dorling Kindersley, are available. A list of recommended science and social studies magazines is provided in the resources at the end of this chapter.

> **Study Guide Question**
>
> *Interview a teacher of the deaf about the curricula used for two different grade levels in his or her program. What are five resources this teacher recommends? Discuss these resources with a peer.*

School Subject Facilitation

Crandall (1987) and others have suggested that strategies for learning should be taught explicitly because few students generate and use strategies independently. Yet many students use strategies once they have been taught, practiced, and evaluated. McTighe (1997) suggested the following general procedure to teach learning strategies directly:

1. Introduce the strategy and explain its purpose.
2. Demonstrate and model its use.
3. Provide guided practice for students to apply the strategy; provide feedback.
4. Have students apply the strategy independently.

5. Reflect regularly on the effectiveness and appropriateness of the strategy.

In addition, many teachers cue learning strategies with tangible products such as posters, bookmarks, visual symbols, or cue cards (McTight & Lyman, 1988). Students who are D/HH may find such items helpful.

Strategies

SQ3R. Although numerous learning strategies are effective for use in school subject areas, the one that appears most frequently is SQ3R (Robinson, 1961). Using this method, students

- **Survey:** Skim the headings and graphics of the material to be read.
- **Question:** Think of questions they might be asked to answer.
- **Read:** Read the material and take notes.
- **Recite:** Repeat or answer the questions they initially formulated.
- **Review:** Reread the material and check their answers.

Concept Diagrams.* As illustrated and described in Chapter 1, Concept Diagrams and Concept Worksheets are used to facilitate student retention of content material. A Concept Worksheet that is useful for students who are D/HH when reading expository text appears in Chapter 1 (Figure 1–8). Figure 10–5 presents an example of a Concept Diagram to facilitate learning in social studies.

*Concept Diagram information and figure from "Promoting Learning in Content Classes," by B. Lenz and J. Bulgren, in *Effective Instruction of Students with Learning Difficulties*, (pp. 401–408), by P. Cegelka and W. Berdine. Copyright 1995 by Allyn & Bacon. All rights reserved. Adapted with permission. Additional information from J. Bulgren, personal communication, 1998. Adapted with the author's permission.

Key Word: Colonization

Definition: Colonization is the organized permanent settlement of an underdeveloped land by a group of people who remain under the rule of their mother country.

Characteristics present in the concept:

ALWAYS
Group of people
Rule by mother country
Organized settlement
Underdeveloped land
Plan for permanence

SOMETIMES
Rivalry for power
Economic gains
Solutions to social
   problems
Religious freedom

NEVER
Native-born people
Independent countries
Explorers who did not
   stay

EXAMPLES

(Plymouth)

(America's 13 original colonies)

(English convicts sent to Australia)

(Settlement on the moon in the 21st century)

NON-EXAMPLES

((Columbus))

((America after the War for Independence))

((Australian Aborigines))

((Armstrong and Aldrin on the moon in 1969))

Write 1–2 sentences using the target (key) word:
_____
_____
_____

Judge a definition that an adult provides as correct or incorrect.
Say the word. Fingerspell the word.
Write the key word: _____.
Discriminate (auditorially or in print) the word from two others that are similar:_____
_____

FIGURE 10-5: CONCEPT WORKSHEET

Preparing a Concept Diagram involves the following steps (J. Bulgren, personal communication, 1998):

1. Convey the concept name.
2. Offer the overall concept name.
3. Note key words.
4. Classify the always, sometimes, and never characteristics.
5. Explore examples and non-examples.
6. Practice with new items.
7. Confirm a definition.

Team members can use a Concept Diagram and teach the concept to students using the following teaching routine:

- *Cue* students' attention by naming the Concept Diagram and routine, explaining how they will help students learn, and specifying what they need to do to participate.
- *Do* the steps outlined above, working interactively with students.
- *Review* both the content information and the content analysis process.

Organizational Devices. Various organizational devices have been recommended repeatedly throughout this text, because it is essential that team members assess the need for them and use them as is appropriate. Often students who are D/HH, in order to understand subject content, need to form whole ideas of concepts and relate what they are reading or what they obtain through lectures to information from past units or life experiences. Team members can use visualizations, study or lecture guides, or oral (signed and/or spoken) cues to focus attention on the relationships among different bits of information, linking old information to new.

- *Visualizations* include time lines, continuum scales, character analysis charts, or cycles. They can be used to describe cause and effect or other structures of narrative or expository text and lectures. Examples of visualizations (graphic organizers) appear in Appendix 5–B and in *Language Issues in Deaf Education* (Luetke-Stahlman, 1998).

- *Study guides* focus attention on the information that school subject teachers feel is the most important. The most effective guides provide graphics with parts of the pictures or labels missing so that students can complete the guides (Miller, 1997). Another design provides questions on main concepts and vocabulary words from assigned passages. Advanced organizers (similar to an outline of what is to be covered) also can help students to organize input for later discussion.

- *Verbal cues* (signed or spoken) assist students who are D/HH to focus their attention on the organization of information (*"Look at this word right here, Liz"*). **Visual cues** include high lighting and pointing to help students focus. Some adults make windows (a cutout in a piece of cardboard or a 3 x 5" card) to assist students in focusing on words or phrases being read. Others use a ruler or another type of straight edge to remind students what line in a text is being read or discussed.

Understanding Devices. Providing examples which are linguistic, concrete, and/or active are understanding devices. Linguistic examples are required when concepts are defined. Concrete examples use pictures or real objects to illustrate the person, location, process, or action being discussed. Active examples demonstrate the concept (like halving an apple to show "one half").

Comparisons. Explorations of the similarities and differences between concepts being discussed typify comparisons. They are similar to examples but involve more than one concept. Verbal comparisons use single words (oral, cued, or signed) that are synonyms and antonyms, or similes, metaphors, or analogies. Active comparisons include debates and role playing. Cause-and-effect comparisons include the identification of a sequence of actions or events and a multiple-step process (Lenz & Bulgren, 1995).

Remembering Devices. Creating images, making associations, and using mnemonics are examples of remembering devices. They can be used whenever memorization of facts is required. Some of the more popular techniques are creating mental images and using familiar associations, such as an event linked to the birth of a child. An example of a rhyming device is "In 1492, Columbus sailed the ocean blue." An example of a mnemonic device is the word

HOMES, representing the first letters of the names of the Great Lakes. Lenz and Bulgren (1995) cautioned that "the research is not sufficient to determine which types of the devices . . . are most helpful in which content areas and which devices fit into common presentation formats in content-area classes. For these reasons, teachers should be cautious about the time spent instructing students in their use" (p. 408).

> **Study Guide Question**
> *How would you rate each of the facilitation strategies in terms of its usefulness for a student you know? Give reasons and examples explaining your decisions.*

Student Notetaking

A student who is D/HH often requires the services of a notetaker or access to the teacher's notes when enrolled at a public school. This is because the student cannot simultaneously speechread or watch an interpreter and also take accurate notes.

When taking notes from a written source, students who are D/HH might be asked to paraphrase important information and organize it in a useful manner. Feathers (1993) suggested that students divide a paper into two columns, labeled "Concepts" and "Details." An example is provided below.

Concepts	Details
terms	■ deaf or hard of hearing ■ not "hearing impaired"
low incidence	1 out of 1000 children

Using an Interpreter

Students who are D/HH and use an interpreter in the public school classrooms may need to discuss with the interpreter their respective responsibilities. Responsibilities like those described in Figure 10–6 can serve as a starting point for designing a successful student-interpreter contract.

Student Who is D/HH	Interpreter
1. Be on time to school and ready for classes. Ask for interpreter services before, during, and after school for all school-related activities (socializing, lunch, recess, sports, clubs, and so on). This is your right.	1. Be available to interpret for all social and academic activities that involve the student assigned to you. Facilitate socialization, team with the regular education teacher, and attend meetings as requested.
2. Use your tactile aid, hearing aid, cochlear implant, and/or FM system as needed. Always have an extra battery and cord with you.	2. Refer the student to the teacher when problems occur with an assistive listening device, unless you have been designated to help.
3. Ask for accessible seating arrangements where you can see all students, the interpreter, and the teacher well.	3. Sit or stand where the student can see you easily and where light does not shine in the student's eyes. Move with the teacher; sit beside AV monitor or screen.
4. Watch the interpreter; you are responsible for the material presented. Do not distract the interpreter or other students. Do not expect the interpreter to tell you what you missed if you have not been paying attention.	4. Interpret class instructions, lectures, and discussions as they are being presented. Become familiar with any special vocabulary. Do not change the level of the English used by the teacher unless specifically asked by the team to do so. Notify the teacher that a student appears lost if he or she does not seem to be comprehending the content.
5. Participate in class discussions. Take a role in cooperative learning activities.	5. Interpret and reverse-interpret discussions. Encourage hearing students to sign for themselves or provide them the signs they need.
6. Remember that the teacher, not the interpreter, is responsible for providing instruction, explaining lessons, answering questions, giving assignments, and being in charge of the class.	6. Refer the student's questions, concerns, and problems to the teacher. Clarify routine points for the student, but do not assume the teacher's role. Repeat the interpretation of instructions when necessary. *cont.*

FIGURE 10-6: STUDENT-INTERPRETER RELATIONSHIPS

FIGURE 10-6, CONT.

7. Read and complete all class assignments. Participate in group activities. It is your responsibility to learn the material assigned to the class.	7. Interpret assignments for the student as they are explained by the teacher. Do not do work for the student. Do not become a member of a cooperative learning group—remain in the role of interpreter.
8. Ask the teacher for clarification if you have any questions about the lesson, homework, or classwork.	8. Refer the student to the teacher for questions about classwork and assignments.
9. Keep track of all assignments, study guides, lists of key vocabulary, notes, tests, and projects assigned to the class. Ask that 2–3 peers serve as notetakers. Collect their notes at the end of class.	9. Do not remind the student about an assignment that is due. Interpret the teacher's instructions and help the student develop a habit of copying assignments from the board. Suggest that the teacher provide the student with an outline including key vocabulary. Suggest that notetakers be assigned.
10. Follow all class and school rules.	10. Follow the school's policies for educational interpreters.

Using Computers

Computers are useful tools for assisting students who are D/HH in learning school subjects. Through general reference software, subject-specific programs, the Internet, or e-mail, computers provide access to information and connections to people and resources.

Computer Software

There are many types of computer software. Interactive simulations are especially engaging because they allow students to participate in realistic science, social studies, or other experiences. Students take the role of historian, anthropologist, sociologist, biologist, chemist, pioneer on the Oregon Trail, or owner of a factory.

They address genuine, relevant issues and needs within a simulated experience (Harris & Blurton, 1989).

Various other kinds of software are available as well to assist students who are D/HH in their academic work:

- remedial and schoolwork-enhancing
- games and entertainment
- tools—word processing, desktop publishing, integrated packages, art and drawing
- reference—encyclopedias, sign language and other dictionaries, thesauruses
- telecommunications—Internet, e-mail, bulletin boards
- fingerspelling, sign system or language instruction
- speech facilitation
- auditory training

The resource list at the end of this chapter provides the names and addresses of software publishers that produce quality science, social studies, math, and writing products.

Recommended quality software programs for use in science and social studies classes are listed below. See Appendix 10–B for detailed descriptions of many of these and other software programs.

Science Software

<u>For Elementary, Middle, and High School</u>
A.D.A.M. Essentials
Eyewitness Encyclopedia of Science
How Your Body Works
Magic School Bus Series
Museum Madness
Oceans Below
San Diego Zoo Presents: Animals
Sim City 2000
Space Shuttle
Super Solvers Gizmos & Gadgets
Ultimate 3D Skeleton

Social Studies Software

<u>For Elementary School</u>
Africa Trail
Children's World Atlas
Cross Country USA
See the U.S.A.
U.S. Atlas
Where in the World Is Carmen Sandiego Series (for all ages)
World Atlas
Zip Zap Map USA

<u>For Middle and High School</u>
Amazon Trail: Rainforest Adventure
Decisions, Decisions
Maya Quest
Orange Cherry
Oregon Trail
World Atlas

Recommendations provided by Kent Luetke-Stahlman, educational computer consultant (hardware and software) and parent of two deaf daughters (see Resources)

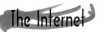

The Internet

Students who are D/HH can also learn about school subject topics by exploring the Internet. Thousands of local, national, and international Internet service providers (ISPs) offer direct access to the Internet. ISPs ranging from local telephone and cable companies to telecommunications giants are advertising that school personnel should sign up for Internet service. Many ISPs charge a flat monthly rate for unlimited access and provide good technical and customer support. These web sites provide links to major Internet service providers:

CINet ISP Comparisons
http://www.cnet.com/Content/Reviews/Compare/ISP/

ISP Finder
http://ispfinder.com

Worldwide ISPs
http://www.best.be/iap/

The ISP List
http://thelist.iworld.com

Internet Access Providers Meta-List
http://www.herbison.com/herbison/iap_meta_list.html

E-Mail

If team members want to provide e-mail for students, they can get a free account through companies such as Yahoo, Juno, or Hotmail. These companies provide e-mail service to anyone with access to a computer and a modem. Free services are paid for through selective advertising that appears within the e-mail software. If parents approve of the ad campaigns that accompany the software and are looking for an easy and cheap way to get an account, these web sites provide access for registration:

Juno
http://www.juno.com

Hotmail
http://www.hotline.com

Yahoo
http://mail.yahoo.com

Teaching about HIV/AIDS and Sexually Transmitted Disease

People who are D/HH are ten to thirty percent more likely to contract Human Immunodeficiency Virus (HIV) and Acquired Immune Deficiency Syndrome (AIDS) than are their hearing peers (AIDS Initiative for Deaf Services Task Force, 1998). This is because most of the information available on these topics requires an ability to read and understand English: messages and information about AIDS and sexually transmitted disease (STD) often are not captioned; government agencies and hearing prevention agencies often do not provide sign interpreters for meetings and workshops about HIV/AIDS and STD; and hearing and deaf sexual partners and drug users often do not communicate well about prevention.

Frustration about the lack of access to information about AIDS and STD was expressed in a *Deaf Life* "Readers' Responses" article (1995) as well as by Baker-Duncan, Dancer, Gentry, Highly, and Gibson (1997). The Baker-Duncan et al. study found deaf adolescents at greater risk for acquiring AIDS than their hearing peers because communication difficulties hinder the acquisition of accurate information. Team members must recognize their important role and responsibility in improving the education that students who are D/HH receive about STD and the deadly Human Immunodeficiency Virus (Baker-Duncan et al.; Luckner & Gonzales, 1993) and in helping to reverse this national problem (Peinkofer, 1991).

The English skills needed to understand how to practice safer sex, how to reduce the risk of contracting HIV from drug usage, how to be tested for HIV, the progression of the disease, what medications might be helpful, how or when medications are prescribed, and so forth are all potentially challenging for students who are D/HH. For example, in 1995 Van Biema reported that many students who were D/HH did not know what the English term "HIV-positive" meant. This is understandable considering the usual meaning of *positive* ("good") as compared to the negative association of being HIV-positive. Students need to be helped to understand this and other important terms. The principles of optimal language learning

(Luetke-Stahlman, 1998), effective instruction, mediated learning, and task analysis of learning as organized using the Cummins Model of Language Proficiency will all assist in facilitating effective discussions of HIV / AIDS and STD with students who are D/HH.

Available Curricula

The list of topics in Figure 10–7 is from a curriculum entitled *Serious Business about HIV/AIDS and STI (Sexual Transmitted Infections): A Kindergarten Through Twelfth Grade Prevention Curriculum for Deaf and Hard of Hearing Students.* The curriculum was developed in 1998 at the Marie H. Katzenbach School for the Deaf by Christine Gannon, Cynthia Sternfeld, and supporting authors. The curriculum includes eight appendices with materials such as listings of library resources, general resources, films and videos, references, and organizations and   contacts, as well as sign references, a sample letter to parents, and Internet contacts.   It also includes an extensive number of worksheets, guides, and other graphic materials. Some of these materials are listed in Appendix 10–C so that team members can get an idea of what is available and recognize the

> **Study Guide Questions**
> 1. *Why is the dissemination of information about STD and HIV/AIDS the responsibility of teachers of the deaf?*
>
> 2. *What is the relationship between English language abilities and STD and HIV/AIDS information when students are D/HH?*

Introduction	Kindergarten
Why do we need a curriculum	1. Healthy or Sick?
for deaf students?	2. Good Health Habits
	3. Who Can Help?
Overview	First Grade
Sequencing	4. What Do I Look Like?
Teacher Qualifications	5. Body Parts
How to Use This Curriculum	6. Body Parts II
Materials	7. Germs and How They Are Spread
Tips for Teachers	8. Treatment of Illness
Parent and School Involvement	9. Touch
Conclusion	Second Grade
	10. Everyone Is Different
	11. Name That Body Part *cont.*

FIGURE 10–7: TOPICS IN A SAMPLE STI/HIV/AIDS CURRICULUM

FIGURE 10–7, CONT.

12. Body Part Spelling Bee	44. How HIV Is Transmitted
13. Girl and Boy Body Parts	45. Dating
14. Private Parts	46. Let's Wait for Sex
15. Germs Enter the Body	
16. Communicable/Non-Communicable Illnesses	Seventh Grade
17. Illnesses Are Not All the Same	47. Anatomy Game
18. Staying Healthy	48. Teen Pregnancy
19. Some Kids Have HIV	49. Contraception
20. Some Parents Have HIV	50. Appropriate Behavior
	51. STI: What to Look for
Third Grade	52. The Immune System and HIV
21. Bodies Grow	53. How Safe Is It to Be Cool? How Cool Is It to Be Safe?
22. Drugs & the Body	
23. Serious & Not Serious Illness	
24. Treatments & Cures	Eighth Grade
25. Caring for People Who Are Sick	54. STI - Peer Education
	55. Abstinence
	56. Safer Sex & Condoms
Fourth Grade	57. HIV/AIDS - A Different STI
26. Male/Female Anatomy	58. STI & HIV/AIDS Review Game
27. Puberty	
28. The Body Protects Itself	Ninth Grade
29. Some Friends Have HIV	59. Anatomy
30. Refusal Skills	60. Puberty
31. Menstruation	61. Germs
	62. STI: What Do You Know?
Fifth Grade	63. HIV/AIDS
32. Anatomy Review #1	64. HIV Test
33. Anatomy Game	65. Wait for Sex?
34. Ways That Illnesses Are Spread	66. My Goals
35. How HIV Is *Not* Spread	67. Dating & Relationships
36. I Am Special!	
37. Friends	Tenth Grade
	68. Menstruation & Conception
Sixth Grade	69. Pathogens
38. Anatomy Review #2	70. Sexually Transmitted Infections (STI)
39. Anatomy Spelling Bee	71. STI: How Are They Transmitted?
40. Pregnancy & Conception	72. HIV/AIDS Review
41. Body Fluids	73. Immune System & HIV
42. Casual/Sexual Contact	74. The Effects of HIV on Everyone
43. High Risk Behaviors	

cont.

FIGURE 10–7, CONT.

Eleventh Grade	Twelfth Grade
75. Anatomy Reinforcement	83. Growth & Development Review
76. Contraception	84. STI and Pathogen Review
77. STI & Pathogens	85. Prevention
78. Bacterial STI	86. Perspectives on Prevention
79. Viral STI	87. Spread the News: Making an Impact
80. Fungal & Protozoa STI	88. The Media, Sex & Prevention
81. HIV/AIDS: Guided Imagery	89. What Can I Do?
82. Remembering People Who Died of AIDS: The Quilt	90. Getting Help

From *Serious Business about HIV/AIDS and STI* by C. Gannon and C. Sternfeld, 1998, Wilmington, DE: Marie H. Katzenbach School for the Deaf. Copyright 1998 by Marie H. Katzenbach School for the Deaf. Reprinted with permission.

need for such support materials. More information on this curriculum is available from the Katzenbach School or from the authors (Christine_gannon@ppfa.org; Cindi727@aol.com).

Another useful curriculum is the one developed by Warthing and Lopez (1997) for deaf people living with the HIV virus: *Me HIV+ . . . What Do? A Guide for Deaf People Living with the HIV Disease.* Because this curriculum was written by people familiar with the typical English needs of students who are D/HH, team members may find it particularly helpful. The content includes such chapters as "Now That You Know You Are HIV+," "Start Care E-A-R-L-Y," and "What HIV Does to Your Body." The graphics developed to explain difficult concepts are excellent.

> **Study Guide Question**
> *How would materials such as those listed in Appendix 10–C assist to mediate instruction when students are D/HH?*

Additional Strategies for HIV/AIDS Education ———

In addition to facilitating understanding of sexuality and STD-related concepts through discussion and use of available curricula, team members might select one or more of the following activities for working with students who are D/HH:

- Invite a deaf speaker who has been diagnosed with HIV or AIDS to share his or her experiences with students.
- Arrange for students to attend community activities (exhibits, workshops, and so on) about HIV and AIDS.

- Assist students in accessing Internet sites that focus on HIV, AIDS, and related topics.
- Make a group call (2–6 students) to the National AIDS Hotline.

Resources for HIV/AIDS Materials and Speakers

Because new information is constantly being developed, the HIV/AIDS and STD resources at the end of this chapter are not meant to be an all-inclusive list of relevant materials. The list is provided to assist team members in initiating their own collection of resources. In addition, the Captioned Films/Videos Program sponsored by the National Association of the Deaf has many films and videos that can be used as tools in discussing HIV/AIDS and STD, as well as other sexuality and health issues. A comprehensive list of their free-loan captioned films and videos can be found in their catalog. Some examples of films and videos that might assist team members in planning lessons are presented in Figure 10–8.

Abstinence: Deciding to Wait 18 minutes; Grades 9-12 (Video)	Take Charge: Sexual Health 29 minutes; Grades 9-13 (Video)
Birth Control: Your Responsibility, Your Choice 13 minutes; Grades 9-13 (Video)	Teens and AIDS: Real People, Real Stories 20 minutes; Grades 8-13 (Video)
The Body Fights Disease 13 minutes; Grades 7-12 (Film)	Teen Contraception 13 minutes; Grades 8-13(Video)
Chlamydia 9 minutes; Grades 10-13+ (Video)	What If I'm Gay? 29 minutes; Grades 9-13 (Video)
Growing Up: Body, Feelings, Behavior 12 minutes; Grades 6-13 (Video)	When Should You Tell? Abuse 14 minutes; Grades 3-6 (Video)
Sex, Drugs, and AIDS 19 minutes; Grades 8-13+ (Film/Video)	Your Body: Reproductive Systems 17 minutes; Grades 6-10 (Video)
Starting Life 15 minutes; Grades K-4 (Video)	

FIGURE 10–8: FILMS AND VIDEOS ON SEXUALITY AND HEALTH ISSUES

Films and videos by the National Association for the Deaf. Available from the Marie H. Katzenbach School for the Deaf (see Resources).

Summary

This chapter provided information useful to team members who are interested in assessing the abilities of students who are D/HH with regard to the appropriateness of placement in general classroom school subjects. Sample objectives and numerous facilitation activities for assisting students in school subjects were also presented. A student's performance in school subject content areas is unlikely to improve without team commitment to support, mediation strategies, monitoring, and problem solving as needed. Lenz and Bulgren (1995) noted that such commitment must be "consistent, systematic, and collaborative over a period of several years" (p. 414). This chapter also included a section on educating students who are D/HH about HIV/AIDS and STD. Team members assuming a role in this education can be a determining factor in preserving students' health.

Activities

1. Write several objectives for a student who is D/HH in a particular school subject area. Discuss the appropriateness of these objectives with a teacher.

2. Evaluate two magazines designed to support social studies or science curricula for use with students who are D/HH. List the strengths and weakness of each.

3. Discuss Figure 10–1 with a general education teacher. Can he or she add additional skills?

4. Teach a lesson in which you expand a student's ability to use words or phrases required in school subjects (sequencing, listing, enumeration, and so on).

5. Assess a student who is D/HH in a school subject area using the Cummins model. What type of mediation activities can you suggest?

6. Videotape yourself teaching a learning strategy to one or more students who are D/HH, and critique the videotape with a peer.

7. Videotape yourself teaching a multi-goaled lesson, and share with a peer an evaluation of three to five objectives attempted.

8. Evaluate with a peer a recommended software program for social studies or science.

9. Plan a unit for teaching about STD and HIV/AIDS to a particular student who is D/HH. Consider the English needs of the student as well as your knowledge of effective instruction.

10. Interview the school nurse in a program where students who are D/HH are enrolled. Discuss the policies regarding teaching about STD and HIV/AIDS. Summarize and share your findings with a peer.

School Subject Resources

Curricula Adapted for Students Who Are D/HH

Outreach
Pre-College Programs
Gallaudet University
800 Florida Avenue, NE
Washington, DC 20002-3695

Best Picks: Science Magazines*

Pre-K
Your Big Backyard
Ranger Rick
National Wildlife Federation
P.O. Box 777
Mount Morris, IL 61054

Grades 2–4
Super Science Level Red (1–3)
Scholastic
P.O. Box 3710
Jefferson City, MO 65102
1-800-631-1586

Grades 4–8
Science World
Level Blue (4–6)
Scholastic

Dolphin Log
The Cousteau Society
777 United Nations Plaza
New York, NY 10017

3,2,1 Contact
Children's TV Workshop
P.O. 53051
Boulder, CO 80322-0301

All grades:
Magic School Bus Magazine
Scholastic

Best Picks: Social Studies Magazines*

Grades 2–4
Kids Discover
P.O. Box 4205
Boulder, CO 80322

Grades 4–8
Cobblestone
Calliope
7 School Street
Peterborough, NH 03458-1454
603-924-7209

---

*Science and social studies magazines recommended by Joanne McDermott, Children's Librarian, Olathe Public Library, Kansas

Best Picks of Software Publishers**

Electronic Learning
Published by Scholastic Inc.
555 Broadway
New York, NY 10012
212-505-4900
http://scholastic.com/el

Grolier Electronic Publishing
95 Madison Avenue, Suite 407
New York, NY 10016

Learning & Leading with Technology
Published by ISTE (International Society for
Technology in Education)
1787 Agate Street
Eugene, OR 97403-1923
http://isteonline.uoregon.edu

Minnesota Educational Computing Consortium (MECC)
3490 Lexington Avenue N.
St. Paul, MN 55112
Micro Power & Light
12810 Hillcrest Road, Suite 120
Dallas, TX 75230

Rand McNally
P.O. Box 7600
Chicago, IL 60680

Technology & Learning
Published by Peter Li, Inc.
P.O. Box 49727
Dayton, OH 45449-0727
http://www.techlearning.com

**Software publishers recommended by Kent Luetke-Stahlman, educational computer consultant and parent of two deaf daughters [15540 So. Downing; Olathe, KS 66062]

T.H.E. Journal
Published by T.H.E. Journal L.L.C.
15021 Camino Real, Suite 112
Tustin, CA 92780-3670
http://www.thejournal.com

Tom Snyder Productions
123 Mount Auburn Street
Cambridge, MA 02138

Classroom Connect
Published by Wentworth Worldwide Media, Inc.
1866 Colonial Village Lane
Lancaster, PA 17605-0488
http://www.classroom.net
(Best information on the Internet)

HIV/AIDS and STD Resources

General Materials and Speakers

CDC National AIDS Hotline
American Social Health Association
P.O. Box 13827
Research Triangle Park, NC 27709
919-361-8454 TTY
919-361-4855 FAX
HYPERLINK mail to: chalud@ashastd.org

Holly Blake
800 Florida Avenue NE, Box 2727
Washington, DC 20002-3695
202-675-6119 TTY/Voice
HYPERLINK mail to:Bug1976@juno.com

National AIDS Hotline
1-800-AIDS-TTY or 1-800-243-7889

State of West Virginia
Dept. of Health & Human Resources
Bureau of Public Health, AIDS Program
1422 Washington Street E.
Charleston, WV 25301
800-642-8244 TTY/Voice
304-558-6335 FAX

Books and Other Written Material

AAHPERD (American Alliance for Health, Physical
Education, Recreation and Dance)
P.O. Box 385
Oxon Hill, MD 20750-0385
1-800-321-0789
301-567-9553 FAX

CDC National AIDS Clearinghouse
P.O. Box 6003
Rockville, MD 20849-6003
1-800-458-5231

ETR Associates
P.O. Box 1830
Santa Cruz, CA 95061-1830
1-800-321-4407
1-800-435-8433 FAX

Fairview Riverside Press
P.O. Box 147
Minneapolis, MN 55440-0147
1-800-544-8207

Glencoe/McGraw-Hill, Inc.
860 Taylor Station Road
Blacklick, OH 43003
1-800-334-7344

Health Impressions
A Division of WRS Group, Inc.
5045 Franklin Avenue
Waco, TX 76702
1-800-299-3366, Ext. 295
817-751-0221 FAX

J. Weston Walch
321 Valley Street (P.O. Box 658)
Portland, ME 04104-0658
1-800-341-6094
207-772-3105 FAX

Laubach Literacy/New Readers Press
1320 Jamesville Avenue
Syracuse, NY 13210
1-800-448-8878
315-422-5561 FAX

Learning Works
P.O. Box 1370
Goleta, CA 93116
1-800-235-5767

New York University Press
70 Washington Square, South
New York, NY 10012
1-800-996-6987

Planned Parenthood
Federation of America, Inc.
810 7th Avenue, 7th Floor
New York, NY 10019
1-800-669-0156
212-261-4352 FAX

SIECUS (Sexuality Information and Education Council
of the U.S.)
130 West 42nd Street, Suite 350
New York, NY 10036-7802
212-819-9770
212-819-9776 FAX

Scott Foresman/Addison Wesley School Services
1 Jacob Way
Reading, MA 01867
1-800-552-2259
1-800-333-3328 FAX

Simon & Schuster (Prentice Hall/Allyn & Bacon)
200 Old Tappan Road
Old Tappan, NJ 07675
1-800-223-2348
1-800-445-6991

Children's Books

Albert Whitman Publishers
6340 Oakton Street
Morton Grove, IL 60053
1-800-255-7675

Focus International
1160 E. Jerico Turnpike, Suite 15
Huntington, NY 11143
516-549-5320

Paperbacks for Educators
426 West Front Street
Washington, MO 63090
1-800-227-2591
1-800-514-7323 FAX

Fairview Riverside Press
P.O. Box 147
Minneapolis, MN 55440-0147
1-800-544-8207

Learning Works
P.O. Box 1370
Goleta, CA 93116
1-800-235-5767

Computer Software

The Bureau for At-Risk Youth
135 Dupont Street (P.O. Box 760)
Plainview, NY 11803-0760
1-800-99-YOUTH
516-349-5521 FAX

Diagrams, Models, and Posters

CARE, Inc.
P.O. Box 8123
Saddle Brook, NJ 07663
201-440-4324
(Contraceptive kits and pelvic models)

Ansell Public Sector
Meridian Ctr. 1 – 2 Industrial Way
Eatontown, NJ 07724
1-800-327-8659
(Condom demonstration models)

GLAD / AESD (AIDS Education / Services for the Deaf)
2222 Laverna Avenue
Los Angeles, CA 90041
213-550-4250 V / TTY
213-550-4255 FAX
(Posters)

Health Impressions
A Division of WRS Group, Inc.
5045 Franklin Avenue
Waco, TX 76702
1-800-299-3366, Ext. 295
817-751-0221 FAX
(Diagrams and Charts)

Health Connection
55 W. Oak Ridge Drive
Hagerstown, MD 21740
1-800-548-8700
301-790-9733 FAX
(Diagrams and Models)

Teach-A-Bodies
7 Dons Drive
Mission, TX 78572
210-581-9959
210-585-3089 FAX
(Anatomically correct dolls, puppets, and paper dolls)

**Materials Specifically Designed for People Who
Are Deaf or Hard of Hearing**

AIDS Education/Services for the Deaf
2222 Laverna Avenue
Los Angeles, CA 90041
213-550-4250 TDD/Voice
213-550-4255 FAX

AIDS Initiative for Deaf Services
Rich Smulley
110 Bartholomew Avenue
Hartford, CT 06106

Deaf and Hard of Hearing Services
HIV Prevention and Education Program
3951 N. Meridan Street, Suite 10
Indianapolis, IN 46208
317-920-1200 TTY/Voice
317-926-7823 FAX

GLAD/AESD (AIDS Education/Services for the Deaf
2222 Laverna Avenue
Los Angeles, CA 90041
213-550-4250 V/TTY
213-550-4255 FAX

HIV/AIDS + STD Program
Deaf Incorporated
413 Wacouta Street, Suite 300
St. Paul, MN 55101
651-297-6700 TTY/Voice
651-297-6766 FAX
HYPERLINK mail to:NancyEmery@deafinc.org
HYPERLINK http://www.deafinc.org

Minnesota Chemical Dependency Program for Deaf
and Hard of Hearing Individuals
Fairview Behavioral Services
2450 Riverside Avenue
Minneapolis, MN 55454-1400
1-800-282-DEAF V/TTY

Montrose Clinic
HIV/AIDS Services for the Deaf/Hard of Hearing
215 Westheimer
Houston, TX 77006
713-830-3077 TTY
713-830-3000 Voice

SCHI (Southwest Center for the Hearing Impaired)
6487 Whitby Road
San Antonio, TX 78240-2198
210-699-3311 V/TTY
210-696-0231 FAX

Sign Enhancers, Inc.
P.O. Box 12687
Salem, OR 97309-0687
1-800-767-4461 V/TTY
503-370-6457 FAX

Films and Videos

Films for the Humanities
P.O. Box 2053
Princeton, NJ 08543
609-275-1400
609-275-3767 FAX

Marie H. Katzenbach School for the Deaf
P.O. Box 535
Trenton, NJ 08625-0535
609-530-3136
609-530-5791 FAX

Appendix 10-A

Lesson Plan for Science*

I. Instructional Objective
Kimberly (the student) will demonstrate an ability to define ten vocabulary words by providing a subordinate term and one distinguishing detail, with 80% accuracy.

II. Materials
Ten concept sheets, science textbook, two other relevant reference resources

III. Procedure

Secure Attention
I will tell Kimberly that there is going to be a science test on Friday. I will ask her to find the unit in her book that she has been studying and to label the topic (organisms).

State Objective
I will tell Kimberly that we are going to talk about 10 vocabulary words from the unit to help her review for Friday's test.

Introduce New Material and Provide Clear Instructions
I will read a paragraph to Kimberly that contains a target word (in bold). I will ask her to spell the word and find it in the glossary at the back of the text. We will pronounce the word (speech and/or sign) and find it among three auditory-only choices.

Guide Practice
Either Kimberly or I will write a vocabulary word from the paragraph on a concept worksheet. I will give her a multiple-choice prompt to decide the subordinate term and fill it in on the worksheet. The student will then read the definition to me, and we will decide some characteristics of the term that distinguish it from others we have studied from the unit. We will discuss and record examples and non-examples on the space provided. Then the student will flip the *cont.*

*Adapted from work by Krissy Brewer, University of Kansas Deaf Education student

sheet over and say a definition in her own words.

Check Comprehension

Kimberly will decide if three definitions I provide are correct or incorrect.

Assign Independent Practice

Kimberly will continue to complete the vocabulary worksheets. When finished we will reread part of the text where the word is used. I will ask Kimberly to use the word in her own sentence. Some unfinished sheets will be sent home.

Provide Feedback

I will give Kimberly feedback as new vocabulary is introduced and practiced. When she uses the word in a sentence, I will evaluate whether the sentence is semantically correct and whether the correct technical signs or fingerspelled handshapes are being used.

IV. Questioning

I will define the vocabulary word in a sentence and ask Kimberly to judge my attempt. I will provide multiple-choice, listing, and partial answer question prompts.

V. Communication

The focus of the lesson is to define words adequately by including a subordinate term and at least one distinguishing detail. Correct syntax is not paramount if the meaning is conveyed by the student. Kimberly is asked to pronounce key vocabulary voicing the correct number of syllables. She is asked to identify key vocabulary when given a choice of three words that differ greatly in terms of phonemes included, vowel sounds, and syllable length.

VI. Evaluation

Kimberly will take the science test on Friday. Some, if not all, of the definitions of ten words will be required in fill-in-the-blank sentences.

VII. Outcome

Effectiveness of the lesson and Kimberly's success will be assessed using a general education teacher-made test.

Appendix 10-B

Recommended Computer Programs

Science Software

Body Works
Students tour every layer of many human body parts using text, movies, 3D models, and animation. Softkey.

Eyewitness Encyclopedia of Nature
Students can read about and watch videos of 250 plants, in addition to examining the effects of climate, aspects of the prehistoric world, and features of microscopic life. Dorling Kindersley.

Eyewitness Encyclopedia Series
In the science CD of this series, students can read over 1700 entries that include 20 full-motion videos, 66 animations, and other multimedia features. Material is divided into five categories: chemistry, math, physics, life science, and famous scientists. A quick access index is included. Dorling Kindersley.

How Your Body Works
Students learn about the body's processes and detailed medical information using realistic illustrations. Topics include first aid, drugs, and wellness. The program also includes a medical reference, glossary, and anatomical chart. Mindscape.

Magic School Bus
Students join Ms. Frizzle's class as it travels through three dimensions of a variety of organs. On this trip, parts of the body become animated to demonstrate their functions (for example, white blood cells become a police car to fight off germs). Students can try 12 science experiments and play 12 informative games. Microsoft. (Other *Magic School Bus* programs are available and follow a similar format.)

Oceans Below
Students explore 17 underwater destinations enhanced with 200 video clips, video narration, 125 color photos, music graphics, and text. What students cannot understand auditorially, they can read. Mindscape.

cont.

Operation Frog

Students can dissect a frog using this simulation. To do so they are required to select the proper instruments, probe and snip body parts, remove and examine body parts, and investigate body parts and systems. Students can also view a video of functioning organs. Scholastic.

San Diego Zoo Presents: The Animals 2.0

Students take an interactive walk through the zoo to see hundreds of exotic birds, mysterious mammals, and regal reptiles. This safari is made possible through 120 full-screen videos, photos, and sound. Students study the habits and habitats of the animals through narrated tours, storybook theater, and four additional programs. Hearing loss may prevent direct access to this material by some students who are D/HH. Software Toolworks.

Super Solvers Gizmos and Gadgets

Students learn the basic principles of physical science through observation and experimentation, simulations, and provided feedback. Using an interactive game approach, students can solve over 200 science puzzles that require a sequenced understanding of force, magnetism, electricity, gears, balance, energy sources, and simple machines. The Learning Company.

The Way Things Work

Students read about more than 200 inventions that are cross-linked by machine types, inventors, principles of science, and time line. There is nothing to play or solve in this program. Dorling Kindersley.

Social Studies Software

Africa Trail

Students plan and participate in a cross-country bike hike in modern-day Africa. They decide where to go and must convert currencies, manage a budget, and bargain for supplies. En route, students learn about numerous African cultures. MECC.

Amazon Trail II: Rainforest Adventure

Students find small treasures in the Amazon rainforest as they learn about the science and history of the area. MECC.

cont.

Carmen Sandiego Series

Students travel as detectives throughout a particular location as they try to find Carmen Sandiego and her gang. To solve cases, students must research the answers to geography clues. Broderbund.

Children's World Atlas

Students learn about world using a format similar to that in the *World Atlas and Almanac* (see below). Six educational games are provided.
Rand McNally.

Cross Country USA

Students are truck drivers who locate and deliver commodities to 180 American cities. To succeed, they must learn the geography of the country, read maps, estimate expenses, and plan cost-effective routes from coast to coast. Didatech.

Decisions, Decisions

Students engage in discussions about the environment, building a nation, ancient empires, feudalism, colonization, immigration, revolutions and wars, foreign policy, balancing the national budget, and so on. Tom Snyder.

Maya Quest

Students are detectives and explore back in the time of the Mayan people of South America. They use high-tech tools to solve mysteries, navigate wild bike paths, and save priceless artifacts from being stolen. *Maya Quest* combines archeology, history, culture, and geography with adventure and mystery. MECC.

Museum Madness

Students must put together a museum that comes to life after hours. In doing so, historical facts, scientific information, logic, and creativity are used to work with artifacts and objects from American, world, and natural history; technology; and air and space exploration. MECC.

Oregon Trail

Students travel west during the 1800s by choosing one of three trails. They confront challenges and make decisions about how to proceed when they face inclement weather, health complications, and other hazards. During their adventure, students see rendered towns and forts, talk to historical characters, and hunt to survive. MECC.

cont.

See the USA
Students take fact-finding trips across the United States and learn about states, capitals, famous people, and places. Compton's.

Time Traveler
Students are able to explore 6,000 years of history, including important events, inventions, and cultures. Articles read are enhanced by audio and visual clips. Orange Cherry.

U.S. Atlas and Almanac
Students explore the United States using a format similar to that in the *World Atlas and Almanac*. Mindscape.

World Atlas and Almanac
Students are able to view more than 150 video clips and satellite photography, listen to audiotaped national anthems, and explore an extensive almanac to learn about world landmarks. Mindscape.

Zip Zap Map USA
Students can play one of three games that entertain while they teach. Students earn points as they move geographic features onto their correct location on the map. Arcade sound effects alert students as they zap geographic features into place. National Geographic.

Appendix 10-C

Graphics Supporting the HIV/AIDS and STI Curriculum:
Serious Business about HIV/AIDS and STI *

Kindergarten
Here is a picture of me when I am
sick . . .
Treatment Approaches

First Grade
Body Parts (words)
List of Body Parts
Body Outline
Treatment Approaches
Touch
Touch II
My Circles of Touch
"My Choice"

Second Grade
Body Outline
Body Parts (pictures)
Girl and Boy Body Parts
Private Parts
Germs Enter the Body
Illnesses and Their Symptoms

Third Grade
Bodies Grow I & II
Serious and Not Serious
   Illnesses I & II
Treatment Approaches
Ailment Cards

Fourth Grade
Male Reproductive Organs
Female Reproductive Organs
Male Reproductive Organs
Worksheets
Female Reproductive Organs
Worksheets
Body Outline
"Alex, the Kid with AIDS"
"Alex, the Kid with AIDS" Concept
   Map
If I Knew Someone with HIV
"I Can Say No" Cartoons

Fifth Grade
"Male, Female, Both" Signs
Male Reproductive Organs
Female Reproductive Organs
Reproductive Organs & Their
   Function
Body Parts I, II, & III
Menstrual Cycle Guide
Menstrual Cycle
How HIV Is *Not* Transmitted
Body Outline

Sixth Grade
"Male, Female, Both" Signs
Male Reproductive Organs
Female Reproductive Organs
Reproductive Cycle

cont.

*From *Serious Business about HIV/AIDS and STI* by C. Gannon and C. Sternfeld, 1998, Wilmington, DE: Marie H. Katzenbach School for the Deaf. Copyright 1998 by Marie H. Katzenbach School for the Deaf. Reprinted with permission.

Conception
Body Fluids/Body Parts Match-up
Risk Behavior Signs

Seventh Grade
Male Reproductive Organs
Female Reproductive Organs
Male Reproductive Organs
   Worksheets
Female Reproductive Organs
   Worksheets
Teen Pregnancy I & II
Choices of Appropriate Behavior
STI Chart
STI: What to Look for
HIV & the Body I–V
T-cells and HIV Infection
HIV & the Body Worksheet

Eighth Grade
Chlamydia Outline
Gonorrhea Outline
Genital Warts Outline
Herpes Outline
Syphilis Outline
Vaginitis Outline
Hepatitis B Outline
HIV/AIDS Outline
Condom Guide

Ninth Grade
Male Reproductive Organs
Female Reproductive Organs
Male Anatomy Match-up
Female Anatomy Match-up
Puberty
Modes of Germ Transmission

Germ Transmission
Fluids That Transmit HIV
Risk Signs
Behavior Guide
Behavior Signs

Tenth Grade
Menstrual Cycle
Reproductive Cycle
Conception
Menstrual Cycle Worksheet
Pathogen Guide
Characteristics of Pathogens
Casual/Sexual Contact
Body Parts and Body Fluids
STI: How Do They Spread?
STI: How Do They Spread?
   Worksheet
HIV & the Body I–V
HIV & the Body Worksheet
T-cells and HIV Infection

Eleventh Grade
Male Reproductive Organs
Female Reproductive Organs
Contraception
Barrier Contraception Graph
Non-Barrier Contraception Graph
Pathogen Guide
STI Pathogens
STI Pathogens Worksheet
Bacterial STI Guide
STI Vocabulary List
Bacterial STI
Chlamydia Outline
Gonorrhea Outline
Syphilis Outline
Vaginosis Outline

cont.

Bacterial STI–Compare/Contrast
Viral STI Guide
Viral STI
HIV/AIDS Outline
Herpes Outline
Genital Warts Outline
Hepatitis B Outline
Viral STI–Compare/Contrast
Fungi and Protozoa STI Guide
Fungus and Protozoa STI
Candidiasis Outline
Pediculosis Outline
Scabies Outline
Trichomoniasis Outline
Fungus and Protozoa STI–
    Compare/Contrast
Sample Calculation

Twelfth Grade
Pathogens I–III
Role Play Scenarios
The Influences in My Life
Spread the News
What Can I DO?
"Getting Help" Scenarios

References

AIDS Initiative for Deaf Services Task Force (1998). Unpublished data; 110 Bartholomew Avenue, Hartford, CT 06106 (806-951-4791 V/TTY).

Baker-Duncan, N., Dancer, J., Gentry, B., Highly, P., & Gibson, B. (1997). Deaf adolescents' knowledge of AIDS: Grade and gender effects. *American Annals of the Deaf, 142*(5), 368-372.

Cegelka, P., & Berdine, W. (1995). *Effective instruction of students with learning difficulties.* Boston: Allyn & Bacon.

Chamot, A., & O'Malley, M. (1994). *The CALLA handbook.* Boston: Addison-Wesley.

Coelho, E..(1982). Language across the curriculum. *TESL Talk, 13,* 56-70.

Crandall, J. (1987). *ESL through content-area instruction: Mathematics, science, and social studies.* Englewood Cliffs, NJ: Prentice Hall.

Cummins, J. (1980). The construction of language proficiency in bilingual education. In J. Alatis (Ed.), *Current issues in bilingual education.* Washington, DC: Georgetown University Press.

Cummins, J. (1984). *Bilingualism and special education: Issues in assessment and pedagogy.* Clevedon, Avon, England: Multilingual Matters.

Do you feel that there's enough HIV/AIDS education for Deaf people? (December, 1995). *Deaf Life,* 30.

Feathers, K. (1993). *Infotext: Reading and learning.* Scarborough, Ontario; Canada: Pippin.

Gannon, C. & Sternfeld, C. (1998). *Serious business about HIV/AIDS and STI.* Trenton, NJ: Marie H. Katzenbach School for the Deaf.

Harris, S., & Blurton, C. (1989). Promote positive cognitive and affective outcomes for students with special needs: Integrate computers in the social studies curriculum. *Reading, Writing, and Learning Disabilities, 5,* 85-102.

Lenz, B., & Bulgren, J. (1995). Promoting learning in content classes. In P. Cegelka & W. Berdine, (Eds.) *Effective instruction of students with learning difficulties* (pp. 385-417). Boston: Allyn & Bacon.

Luckner, J., & Gonzales, R. (1993). What deaf and hard of hearing adolescents know and think about AIDS. *American Annals of the Deaf, 138*(4), 338-342.

Luetke-Stahlman, B. (1998). *Language issues in deaf education.* Hillsboro, OR: Butte Publications.

Maryland State Department of Education. *Student questionnaire to assess school subject capabilities.*

McTighe, T. (1997). What happens between assessments? *Educational Leadership, 54*(4), 6-13. Effingham, IL: World Color.

McTight, J., & Lyman, F. (1988). Cueing thinking in the classroom: The promise of theory-embedded tools. *Educational Leadership, 45*(7), 18-24.

Miller, W. (1997). *Reading and writing remediation kit.* West Nyack, NY: Center for Applied Research.

Peinkofer, J. (1991). HIV education for the deaf, a vulnerable minority. *Public Health Reports*, 390-396.

Robinson, F. (1961). *Effective study.* New York: Harper & Row.

Van Biema, D. (1995). AIDS. *Deaf Life*, 29.

Warthing, D., & Lopez, S. (1997). *Me HIV + . . . what do? A guide for deaf people living with the HIV disease.* Austin, TX: AIDS Services (512-458-AIDS).

Index

Note: Page numbers in this index identify the first page of the section in which the subject is discussed.

A

academic subjects — see school subjects

academic supports and services, 2

activating learning, 21

activities, adaptation (in general classroom), 11

AIDS education, 407, 429

analytical conversation, 19

assessment
    of audition, 62
    of math, 358
    of reading, 191
    of school subjects, 384
    of social interaction, 155
    of speech, 112
    of speechreading, 106
    of spelling, 330
    of writing, 296

assignment completion (in general classroom), 12

audition, 59
    assessment, 62
    Cummins model and, 86
    facilitation, 80
        auditory training curricula, 79
        cognitive challenge, 87
            games for, 87

B

books
children's, about deafness, 182
choosing appropriately, 197
for reluctant readers, 288
holding while signing, 198
multimedia books, 200

C

checklist, social interaction, 158

Circle of Friends, 165

cognition, and math, 360

cognitive academic language proficiency (CALP), 384, 385, 391, 393

cognitive challenge, games for, 87

collaboration, team members and administration, 33

communication services, 3

comprehension checking (in general classroom), 11

computers
for school subject facilitation, 403
for writing facilitation, 316
software, 403, 425

concepts, academic
Concept Worksheets and Diagrams, 22, 397
facilitating retention of, 22

conversation, analytical, 19

cooperative learning, 27

Cummins model
        audition facilitation and, 86
        math facilitation and, 360
        mediation and, 18
        school subjects facilitation and, 391
        speech facilitation and, 125
        speechreading facilitation and, 108
        spelling facilitation and, 334

curricula
        auditory, 79
        HIV/AIDS and sexually transmitted disease, 407, 429
        school subjects, 395
        social interaction, 160

D
decoding skills and strategies, 209, 255

E
e-mail, 406

F
facilitation
        Cummins model and — see Cummins model
        of audition, 80
        of HIV/AIDS education, 407
        of math, 370
        of reading, 193, 199, 251
        of school subjects, 390
        of social interaction, 162
                curricula, 160
                strategies, 162
        of speech, 118
                when auditory feedback not possible, 129
        of speechreading, 110
        of spelling, 334
        of writing, 301, 303

family sign classes — see signing

G

GASP

> subtest 1, 68
> subtest 2, 72
> subtest 3, 77

general education, general classroom, 2
> activities, adaptation in, 11
> assignment completion in, 12
> comprehension checking in, 11
> instructional format in, 7
> lesson format in, 10
> materials for, 11
> monitoring learning in, 12
> placement in, 13
> rapport and affect in, 6
> supports and services for, 2, 35

grading and tests, 5

graphic organizers, 29, 234, 255, 399

H

HIV / AIDS education, 407, 429

I

independence, facilitation of, 32

instruction
> direct, of social skills, 167
> format of (in general classroom), 7
> mediated — see mediated instruction
> principles of effective, 22
> > incorporating into lessons, 52

instructional language, 9

instructional level (level + 1), 197, 253

Internet, 405

interpreting, 2, 401

L

language
>math and, 357, 361, 363
>reading and, 189, 213, 217, 255
>school subjects and, 384, 385, 390
>social interaction and, 153

learning strategies, 31

lesson format (in general classroom), 10

level + 1 — see instructional level

linguistic supports and services, 4

listening
>environment for, 4
>to speech, motivation for, 61

M

materials, general classroom, 11

math, 357
>assessment, 358
>cognition and, 360
>Cummins model and, 360
>facilitation, 370
>language and, 361, 363, 365
>time and money, 364
>word problems, 365, 378

mediated instruction/mediation, 13
>Cummins model and, 18
>elaboration strategies, 28
>reciprocity, 25
>spelling and, 334
>strategies, 19

monitoring learning (in general classroom), 12

N

name signs — see signing

new and old information, linkages, 21

notetaking, 401

objectives
for auditory comprehension, 78
for auditory discrimination, 74
for school subjects, 393
for social interaction, 160

organizational structure, as a support service, 6

organizational support, 33

P

peer signing — see signing
peer teaching, 27

phonetic speech evaluation, 114

phonological awareness, 209
decoding strategies, 209, 255
phonics and spelling monitoring form, 348
students who are D/HH and, 333

phonological speech evaluation, 117

physical environment, 5

placement in general classroom, 13

print, concepts of, 206, 253

problem solving, active, 28

process writing — see writing

program and curricular modifications, 1
        checklist, 35
        examples using, 43

Q

question prompts, 25

questionnaires, for social interaction, 158

R

rapport and affect (in general classroom), 6

reading
        adults reading to students, 187
                adult skills quiz, 230
        assessment, 191
        at home, 285
        choosing appropriate text, 197
        concepts of print, 206, 253
        essential practices, 199
                examples, 222
        extending, at home or school, 265, 285
        facilitation, 193, 199, 251
        getting ready to read, 197
        graphic organizers for, 234
        holding the book while signing, 198
        independent reading, 269
        instructional level reading, 197, 253
        level, choosing appropriate, 197, 269
        reluctant readers, encouraging, 288
        rereading, 253
        sight vocabulary list, 346
        students reading to adults, 251, 280
                adult skills quiz, 274

S

school subjects, 383
    assessment, 384
    Cummins model and, 391
    curricula, choosing, 395
    facilitation, 1, 390, 396
    language and, 383
    linguistic demands of, 385

science, 383, 423

sexually transmitted disease education, 407

signing
    family classes, 174
    holding books while, 198
    in schools, 173
        signed story time, 176
    name signs, 175
    peer signing, 173
    sign print and words, 175

Six Sound Hearing Test, 66

Six Trait rubrics for writing, 314, 320

social interaction, 153
    adult's role in, 168
    assessment, 155
    cooperative play and work, 170
    evaluation, 171
    facilitation, 162
    goals and objectives, 160
    modeling, 169
    questionnaires for, 158

social skills, direct instruction of, 167

social studies, 383

speech, 105
      assessment, 112
      Cummins model and, 125
      developing precursory, 129
      facilitation, 118
      intelligibility, 117
      suprasegmentals, speech facilitation and, 120
      tracking speech targets, 138

speechreading, 105
      assessment, 106
      Cummins model and, 107
      facilitation, 110

spelling, 329
      assessment, 330
      Cummins model and, 334
      facilitation, 331, 334
      mediation, 334
      monitoring, 348
      phonological awareness and, 333

strategies
      for auditory training, 80
      for HIV/AIDS education, 407
      for math, 373
      for reading, 199, 255, 284
      for school subjects, 397
      for social integration, 162
      for speech, 118
      for speechreading, 110
      for spelling, 331, 334
      learning, 31
      mediation, 19

supports and services, 2

T

tests
- auditory detection assessment, closed- and open-set, 70
- auditory identification assessment, 75
- GASP — see GASP
- Meaningful Auditory Integration Scale, 70, 94
- Meaningful Use of Speech Scale, 117, 142
- reading, 191
- Six Sound Hearing Test, 66
- social interaction, 179

tests and grading, 5

text structure, 207, 236

W

word recognition, 209, 255

word work, 258

writing, 258, 295
- assessment, 296
- beginning writers, 301
- computers and, 316
- dialogue journals, 315
- facilitation, 301, 303
- process writing, 303
- reading about, 315
- Six Trait rubrics for, 314, 320

OTHER TITLES AVAILABLE BY BARBARA LUETKE-STAHLMAN

LANGUAGE ISSUES IN DEAF EDUCATION

An issues text designed for teachers and related service providers. Includes explanations of relevant linguistic theories and issues: assessment and facilitation of use, meaning, and form skills; definitions of languages and systems; ASL nomative data, bi-bi models, language tips for general educators, and more. Also includes practical ideas, diagrams and examples, study questions, resources and suggestions for applied activities. A must have for teachers in training.

Butte Publications, Inc. P.O. Box 1328, Hillsboro, OR 97123.

HANNIE

Fourth and fifth graders will enjoy reading this novel about a year in the life of a hearing girl who has two sisters who are deaf and attends public school with both hearing and deaf peers. A good reader for students who are experiencing cultural diversity and are educated with children who have special needs. Issues involving Quakerism and adoption also highlighted. Provides valuable insights in an entertaining and easy-to-read format. Includes maps and pictures in almost every chapter.

Butte Publications, Inc., P.O. Box 1328, Hillsboro, OR 97123.

ONE MOTHER'S STORY

The story of raising her daughters is told by a professor in Deaf Education who became a parent of first one deaf toddler and then a deaf preschooler. Barbara is married to Kent Luetke-Stahlman and also has two older hearing daughters. All members of the family strive to provide an environment in which audition, speech, language and socialization skills are developed and ASL respected. Parents of children who are deaf or hard of hearing, as well as teachers and interpreters, will find this book packed with ideas for living and growing with toddlers, preschoolers, and young school-aged children. Barbara tells of her struggles and joys in a way that will encourage us all to work together to improve deaf education in the years to come. Modern Signs Press, Los Alamitos, CA 90720.

THE SIGNING FAMILY
What Every Parent Should Know about Sign Communication
by David A. Stewart and Barbara Luetke-Stahlman

Parents of deaf children will welcome the straightforward, reader-friendly information presented in a style both positive and pragmatic. The authors employ common-sense reasoning to establish the importance of teaching deaf children language fundamentals as early as possible.

Gallaudet University Press, Washington, DC 20002.